COGNITIVE AGING

Progress in Understanding and Opportunities for Action

Committee on the Public Health Dimensions
of Cognitive Aging

Board on Health Sciences Policy

Dan G. Blazer, Kristine Yaffe, and Catharyn T. Liverman, *Editors*

INSTITUTE OF MEDICINE
OF THE NATIONAL ACADEMIES

THE NATIONAL ACADEMIES PRESS
Washington, D.C.
www.nap.edu

THE NATIONAL ACADEMIES PRESS • 500 Fifth Street, NW • Washington, DC 20001

NOTICE: The project that is the subject of this report was approved by the Governing Board of the National Research Council, whose members are drawn from the councils of the National Academy of Sciences, the National Academy of Engineering, and the Institute of Medicine.

This project was supported by the McKnight Brain Research Foundation; by Contract No. HHSN26300034 between the National Academy of Sciences and the National Institutes of Health (National Institute of Neurological Disorders and Stroke, National Institute on Aging); by Contract No. 200-2011-38807 between the National Academy of Sciences and the Centers for Disease Control and Prevention; by The Retirement Research Foundation; and by AARP. The views presented in this publication are those of the editors and attributing authors and do not necessarily reflect the view of the organizations or agencies that provided support for this project.

Library of Congress Cataloging-in-Publication Data

Institute of Medicine (U.S.). Committee on the Public Health Dimensions of Cognitive Aging, author.
 Cognitive aging : progress in understanding and opportunities for action / Committee on the Public Health Dimensions of Cognitive Aging, Board on Health Sciences Policy, Institute of Medicine of the National Academies ; Dan G. Blazer, Kristine Yaffe, and Catharyn T. Liverman, editors.
 p. ; cm.
 Includes bibliographical references.
 ISBN 978-0-309-36862-9 (hardcover) — ISBN 978-0-309-36863-6 (pdf)
 I. Blazer, Dan G., II (Dan German), 1944- , editor. II. Yaffe, Kristine, editor. III. Liverman, Catharyn T., editor. IV. Title.
 [DNLM: 1. Aging—physiology. 2. Cognition—physiology. 3. Cognition Disorders—prevention & control. 4. Health Policy. 5. Policy Making. 6. Risk Factors. WT 145]
 QP356
 612.8'233—dc23
                    2015020490

Additional copies of this report available for sale from the National Academies Press, 500 Fifth Street, NW, Keck 360, Washington, DC 20001; (800) 624-6242 or (202) 334-3313; http://www.nap.edu.

For more information about the Institute of Medicine, visit the IOM home page at: www.iom.edu.

Copyright 2015 by the National Academy of Sciences. All rights reserved.

Printed in the United States of America

The serpent has been a symbol of long life, healing, and knowledge among almost all cultures and religions since the beginning of recorded history. The serpent adopted as a logotype by the Institute of Medicine is a relief carving from ancient Greece, now held by the Staatliche Museen in Berlin.

Suggested citation: IOM (Institute of Medicine). 2015. *Cognitive aging: Progress in understanding and opportunities for action*. Washington, DC: The National Academies Press.

*"Knowing is not enough; we must apply.
Willing is not enough; we must do."*
—Goethe

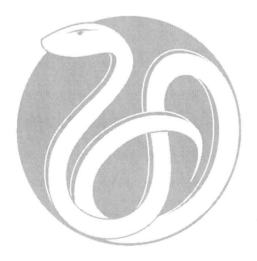

INSTITUTE OF MEDICINE
OF THE NATIONAL ACADEMIES

Advising the Nation. Improving Health.

THE NATIONAL ACADEMIES
Advisers to the Nation on Science, Engineering, and Medicine

The **National Academy of Sciences** is a private, nonprofit, self-perpetuating society of distinguished scholars engaged in scientific and engineering research, dedicated to the furtherance of science and technology and to their use for the general welfare. Upon the authority of the charter granted to it by the Congress in 1863, the Academy has a mandate that requires it to advise the federal government on scientific and technical matters. Dr. Ralph J. Cicerone is president of the National Academy of Sciences.

The **National Academy of Engineering** was established in 1964, under the charter of the National Academy of Sciences, as a parallel organization of outstanding engineers. It is autonomous in its administration and in the selection of its members, sharing with the National Academy of Sciences the responsibility for advising the federal government. The National Academy of Engineering also sponsors engineering programs aimed at meeting national needs, encourages education and research, and recognizes the superior achievements of engineers. Dr. C. D. Mote, Jr., is president of the National Academy of Engineering.

The **Institute of Medicine** was established in 1970 by the National Academy of Sciences to secure the services of eminent members of appropriate professions in the examination of policy matters pertaining to the health of the public. The Institute acts under the responsibility given to the National Academy of Sciences by its congressional charter to be an adviser to the federal government and, upon its own initiative, to identify issues of medical care, research, and education. Dr. Victor J. Dzau is president of the Institute of Medicine.

The **National Research Council** was organized by the National Academy of Sciences in 1916 to associate the broad community of science and technology with the Academy's purposes of furthering knowledge and advising the federal government. Functioning in accordance with general policies determined by the Academy, the Council has become the principal operating agency of both the National Academy of Sciences and the National Academy of Engineering in providing services to the government, the public, and the scientific and engineering communities. The Council is administered jointly by both Academies and the Institute of Medicine. Dr. Ralph J. Cicerone and Dr. C. D. Mote, Jr., are chair and vice chair, respectively, of the National Research Council.

www.national-academies.org

COMMITTEE ON THE PUBLIC HEALTH DIMENSIONS OF COGNITIVE AGING

DAN G. BLAZER (*Chair*), J. P. Gibbons Professor of Psychiatry Emeritus, Duke University Medical Center
KRISTINE YAFFE (*Vice Chair*), Scola Endowed Chair, Professor of Psychiatry, Neurology and Epidemiology, University of California, San Francisco
MARILYN ALBERT, Professor of Neurology, Director of the Division of Cognitive Neuroscience, Johns Hopkins University School of Medicine
SARA J. CZAJA, Leonard M. Miller Professor of Psychiatry and Behavioral Sciences, Scientific Director, Center on Aging, University of Miami Miller School of Medicine
DONNA FICK, Distinguished Professor of Nursing, Co-Director, Hartford Center of Geriatric Nursing Excellence, Pennsylvania State University
LISA P. GWYTHER, Director, Family Support Program, Center for Aging, Duke University
FELICIA HILL-BRIGGS, Professor of Medicine, Departments of Physical Medicine and Rehabilitation, and Health Behavior and Society, Johns Hopkins University
SHARON K. INOUYE, Professor of Medicine, Harvard Medical School; Milton and Shirley F. Levy Family Chair; and Director, Aging Brain Center, Institute for Aging Research, Hebrew SeniorLife
JASON KARLAWISH, Professor of Medicine, Medical Ethics and Health Policy, University of Pennsylvania
ARTHUR F. KRAMER, Professor and Director, Beckman Institute for Advanced Science & Technology, University of Illinois at Urbana-Champaign
ANDREA Z. LaCROIX, Professor and Chief of Epidemiology and Director, Women's Health Center of Excellence, University of California, San Diego
JOHN H. MORRISON, Dean of Basic Sciences and the Graduate School of Biomedical Sciences, Icahn School of Medicine at Mount Sinai
TIA POWELL, Director, Montefiore Einstein Center for Bioethics, Professor of Clinical Epidemiology and Clinical Psychiatry, Albert Einstein College of Medicine
DAVID REUBEN, Director, Multicampus Program in Geriatric Medicine and Gerontology, Chief, Division of Geriatrics, University of California, Los Angeles

LESLIE SNYDER, Professor, Department of Communication Sciences, University of Connecticut
ROBERT B. WALLACE, Irene Ensminger Stecher Professor of Epidemiogy and Internal Medicine, Center on Aging, University of Iowa College of Public Health

IOM Staff

CATHY LIVERMAN, Study Director
SARAH DOMNITZ, Program Officer
CLAIRE GIAMMARIA, Research Associate
JUDY ESTEP, Program Associate
JEANETTE GAIDA, Senior Program Assistant
ANDREW M. POPE, Director, Board on Health Sciences Policy

IOM Scholar-in-Residence

KATIE MASLOW

Reviewers

This report has been reviewed in draft form by individuals chosen for their diverse perspectives and technical expertise, in accordance with procedures approved by the National Research Council's Report Review Committee. The purpose of this independent review is to provide candid and critical comments that will assist the institution in making its published report as sound as possible and to ensure that the report meets institutional standards for objectivity, evidence, and responsiveness to the study charge. The review comments and draft manuscript remain confidential to protect the integrity of the deliberative process. We wish to thank the following individuals for their review of this report:

Julie Bynum, The Geisel School of Medicine at Dartmouth
Laura Carstensen, Stanford University
Mark E. Frisse, Vanderbilt University
Fred Gage, The Salk Institute for Biological Studies
Adam Gazzaley, University of California, San Francisco
Charlene Harrington, University of California, San Francisco
Dilip V. Jeste, University of California, San Diego
K. Ranga Krishnan, Duke-National University of Singapore Graduate Medical School
Nancy E. Lane, University of California, Davis, Health System
Kenneth M. Langa, University of Michigan, Ann Arbor
Eric B. Larson, Group Health Research Institute
Sally C. Morton, University of Pittsburgh
Ruth M. Parker, Emory University

Ronald C. Petersen, Mayo Clinic
Brenda Plassman, Duke University School of Medicine
Thomas R. Prohaska, George Mason University
George Rebok, Johns Hopkins University

Although the reviewers listed above have provided many constructive comments and suggestions, they did not see the final draft of the report before its release. The review of this report was overseen by **Nancy Fugate Woods,** Dean Emeritus, University of Washington School of Nursing, and **Bradford H. Gray,** Editor Emeritus, The Urban Institute. Appointed by the Institute of Medicine, they were responsible for making certain that an independent examination of this report was carried out in accordance with institutional procedures and that all review comments were carefully considered. Responsibility for the final content of this report rests entirely with the authoring committee and the institution.

Preface

Of the abilities people hope will remain intact as they get older, perhaps the most treasured is to "stay sharp"—to think clearly, remember accurately, and make decisions with careful thought. Yet the brain ages. Cognitive functioning in older adults can improve in some areas, such as those related to wisdom and experience, and can decline in others, such as memory, attention, and speed of processing. Individuals vary widely in the specific cognitive changes that occur with age, in the nature and extent of cognitive aging, as well as in the ways these changes affect daily life.

This Institute of Medicine (IOM) study focused on the public health dimensions of cognitive aging as separate from neurodegenerative diseases, such as Alzheimer's disease and other dementias. To accomplish its task, the IOM committee looked at cognitive aging through a broad lens and explored its implications for individuals, for their families, and for society. Its report comes at a time ripe for change in how society responds to cognitive aging. The population of older Americans is rapidly growing, and this frontier of science and health is achieving a marked increase in understanding of the brain, cognition, and aging.

The report greatly benefited from the efforts of many individuals and organizations. We thank the study sponsors for their support and for their work in bringing the topic of cognitive aging to the forefront of discussion: the McKnight Brain Research Foundation, the National Institute of Neurological Disorders and Stroke, the National Institute on Aging, the Centers for Disease Control and Prevention, The Retirement Research Foundation, and AARP. Further, we thank each of the workshop speakers for their presentations and for the time and expertise that they and others shared with the committee. We are grateful to the reviewers whose insights strengthened this report.

The committee is especially indebted to the IOM staff who worked with us tirelessly and most competently. Cathy Liverman led the effort with her usual quiet and effective guidance. She was assisted by Sarah Domnitz, Claire Giammaria, Judy Estep, and Jeanette Gaida. Katie Maslow, IOM Scholar-in-Residence, provided a wealth of insights into this complex topic. As is usually the case, staff were full colleagues in the process of producing this report while retaining their specific duties in support of the committee. We also thank Andrew Pope, Director of the Board on Health Sciences Policy, who shepherded the report from its inception to completion.

The report's findings and recommendations result from the deliberations of a dedicated and hardworking committee. It was our pleasure and privilege to have the opportunity to work with these colleagues—each of whom brought energy, commitment, and intellectual curiosity and rigor to this endeavor. This committee was intrigued and engaged by this most challenging of public health issues encountered by older adults, and such engagement was crucial in our deliberations.

We and our colleagues on the committee hope this report focuses attention and action on cognitive aging. Much can be done by older adults and their families and a wide range of stakeholders—at every level of society, from the local community to national policy and research priorities—to address the opportunities and challenges of cognitive aging and to ensure that older adults live the full and independent lives they desire.

Dan G. Blazer, *Chair*
Kristine Yaffe, *Vice-Chair*
Committee on the Public Health Dimensions of Cognitive Aging

Contents

SUMMARY		1
1	INTRODUCTION	17
2	CHARACTERIZING AND ASSESSING COGNITIVE AGING	31
3	POPULATION-BASED INFORMATION ABOUT COGNITIVE AGING	75
4A	RISK AND PROTECTIVE FACTORS AND INTERVENTIONS: LIFESTYLE AND PHYSICAL ENVIRONMENT	109
4B	RISK AND PROTECTIVE FACTORS AND INTERVENTIONS: HEALTH AND MEDICAL FACTORS	149
4C	RISK AND PROTECTIVE FACTORS AND INTERVENTIONS: GENERAL COGNITIVE AGING INTERVENTIONS AND NEXT STEPS	187
5	HEALTH CARE RESPONSE TO COGNITIVE AGING	209

6	COMMUNITY ACTION: HEALTH, FINANCIAL MANAGEMENT, DRIVING, TECHNOLOGY, AND CONSUMER DECISIONS	227
7	PUBLIC EDUCATION AND KEY MESSAGES	257
8	OPPORTUNITIES FOR ACTION	295

APPENDIXES

A	Meeting Agendas	299
B	U.S. Surveys and Studies That Include One or More Items to Measure Cognition	307
C	Committee Biographies	311

Summary

People forget things—a name, where they put their keys, a phone number—and yet what is dismissed as a minor inconvenience at 25 years of age can evolve into a momentary anxiety at 35, and a major source of personal worry at age 55 or 60. Forgetfulness at older ages is often equated with a decline in cognition—a public health issue that goes beyond memory lapses and one that can have significant impacts on independent living and healthy aging. The term "cognition" covers many mental abilities and processes, including decision making, memory, attention, and problem solving. Collectively, these different domains of cognition are critical for successfully engaging in the various activities involved in daily functioning such as paying household bills, following a recipe to cook a meal, and driving to a doctor's appointment. As human life expectancy increases, maintaining one's cognitive abilities is key to assuring the quality of those added years.

Cognitive aging is a public health concern from many perspectives. Individuals are deeply concerned about declines in memory and decision-making abilities as they age and may also be worried about whether these declines are early signs of a neurodegenerative disease, particularly Alzheimer's disease. They may fear that cognitive decline will lead to a loss of independence and a reduced quality of life and health. In a 2012 survey of its members, AARP found that "staying mentally sharp" was a top concern of 87 percent of respondents. Cognitive decline affects not only the individual but also his or her family and community, and an array of health, public health, social, and other services may be required to provide necessary assistance and support. Lost independence may stem from impaired decision making, which can reduce an individual's ability to drive or increase the individual's vulnerability to financial abuse or exploitation. Cognitive impairment also affects society and the public's quality of life.

At this point in time, when the older population is rapidly growing in the United States and across the globe, it is important to carefully examine what is known about cognitive aging, to identify the positive steps that can be taken to maintain and improve cognitive health, and then to take action to implement those changes by informing and activating the public, the health sector, nonprofit and professional associations, the private sector, and government agencies. In the past several decades rapid gains have been made in understanding the non-disease changes in cognitive function that may occur with aging and in elucidating the range of cognitive changes, from those that are normal with aging to those that are the result of disease; much remains to be learned yet the science is readily advancing.

This Institute of Medicine (IOM) study examines cognitive aging, a natural process associated with advancing years. The IOM committee was charged with assessing the public health dimensions of cognitive aging with an emphasis on definitions and terminology, epidemiology and surveillance, prevention and intervention, education of health professionals, and public awareness and education.

WHAT IS COGNITIVE AGING?

This report focuses on one aspect of health in older adults—cognitive health. Cognition refers to the mental functions involved in attention, thinking, understanding, learning, remembering, solving problems, and making decisions. It is a fundamental aspect of an individual's ability to engage in activities, accomplish goals, and successfully negotiate the world. Although cognition is sometimes equated with memory, cognition is multidimensional because it involves a number of interrelated abilities that depend on brain anatomy and physiology. Distinguishing among these component abilities is important since they play different roles in the processing of information and behavior and are differentially impacted by aging.

The committee provides a conceptual definition of cognitive aging as a process of gradual, ongoing, yet highly variable changes in cognitive functions that occur as people get older. Cognitive aging is a lifelong process. It is not a disease or a quantifiable level of function. However, for the purposes of this report the focus is primarily on later life. In the context of aging, cognitive health is exemplified by an individual who maintains his or her optimal cognitive function with age.

Box S-1 provides the committee's characterization of cognitive aging. Cognitive aging is too complex and nuanced to define succinctly, and therefore it is appropriately characterized through this longer description. Efforts

**BOX S-1
Characterizing Cognitive Aging**

- **Key Features:**
  - Inherent in humans and animals as they age.
  - Occurs across the spectrum of individuals as they age regardless of initial cognitive function.
  - Highly dynamic process with variability within and between individuals.
  - Includes some cognitive domains that may not change, may decline, or may actually improve with aging, and there is the potential for older adults to strengthen some cognitive abilities.
  - Only now beginning to be understood biologically, yet clearly involves structural and functional brain changes.
  - Not a clinically defined neurological or psychiatric disease such as Alzheimer's disease and does not inevitably lead to neuronal death and neurodegenerative dementia (such as Alzheimer's disease).

- **Risk and Protective Factors:**
  - Health and environmental factors over the life span influence cognitive aging.
  - Modifiable and non-modifiable factors include genetics, culture, education, medical comorbidities, acute illness, physical activity, and other health behaviors.
  - Cognitive aging can be influenced by development beginning in utero, infancy, and childhood.

- **Assessment:**
  - Cognitive aging is not easily defined by clear thresholds on cognitive tests since many factors—including culture, occupation, education, environmental context, and health variables (e.g., medications, delirium)—influence test performance and norms.
  - For an individual, cognitive performance is best assessed at several points in time.

- **Impact on Daily Life:**
  - Day-to-day functions, such as driving, making financial and health care decisions, and understanding instructions given by health care professionals, may be affected.
  - Experience, expertise, and environmental support aids (e.g., lists) can help compensate for declines in cognition.
  - The challenges of cognitive aging may be more apparent in environments that require individuals to engage in highly technical and fast-paced or timed tasks, in situations that involve new learning, and in stressful situations (i.e., emotional, physical, or health-related), and may be less apparent in highly familiar situations.

are needed to develop operational definitions of cognitive aging in order to allow comparisons across studies.

CHARACTERIZING AND ASSESSING COGNITIVE AGING

Age-related changes in cognition are highly variable from one individual to the next. This variability is explained in part by differences in life experience, health status, lifestyles, education, attitudinal and emotional factors, socioeconomic status, and genetics. The trajectory of cognitive change also varies for different cognitive functions—memory, decision making, learning, speed of processing, and so on. Further, older age is not associated only with decline; some aspects of cognition, such as wisdom, remain stable in the older decades and aspects of intelligence, such as knowledge, may actually increase with age until the very later decades.

A wide variety of tools and measures are available to test for cognitive change; however, not all may be relevant to real-world activities. Studies use different methods, measures, and definitions that make comparison difficult, and the cognitive aging literature has some significant gaps. Studies of brain tissue in both humans and in animal models have sought to examine the underlying neural mechanisms that may be responsible for the age-related changes in cognition. These include studies of neuronal number, synaptic integrity, and neurotransmitter changes. Overall, they show that neuronal number remains relatively stable, although changes do occur in neuronal structure and neurotransmitter receptors. (The stability in the number of neurons—that is, the lack of neuron death in areas supporting cognition—seen with aging is in contrast to the extensive neuron loss that occurs in Alzheimer's disease.)

> **Recommendation 1:** *Increase Research and Tools for Assessing Cognitive Aging and Cognitive Trajectories*
> The National Institutes of Health, the Centers for Disease Control and Prevention, research foundations, academic research institutions, and private-sector companies should expand research on the trajectories of cognitive aging and improve the tools used to assess cognitive changes and their effects on daily function.
> Specific needs include
> - Studies using a range of assessments (e.g., neuronal injury biomarkers, neuroimaging, postmortem assessments of neuronal integrity) to explore the physiological and structural basis of cognitive aging;
> - Non-human animal studies that examine the mechanisms and clinical correlates of cognitive aging and that are designed to inform human cognitive aging;

- Studies to examine the mechanisms underlying interventions that affect the cognitive trajectory;
- Studies to identify and validate novel tools and measures of function that capture the complexities of real-world tasks and are sensitive to early changes in cognition and function; and
- An update of the norms for cognitive function in older adults (including those in the most advanced age groups) to include the consideration of disease, literacy, language, racial and ethnic diversity, culture, and socioeconomic factors.

UNDERSTANDING THE POPULATION IMPACT

While a great deal of research has examined the occurrence, causes, natural history, pathogenesis, and clinical management of dementia, including Alzheimer's disease, less attention has been paid to cognitive aging per se, particularly from a public health perspective. Population-based information about the nature and extent of cognitive aging provides a basis for building public awareness and understanding and can be used to engage individuals and their families in maintaining cognitive health; to inform health care professionals, financial professionals, and others as they educate and advise their older patients and clients; and to guide program development and implementation.

Recommendation 2: *Collect and Disseminate Population-Based Data on Cognitive Aging*
The Centers for Disease Control and Prevention (CDC), state health agencies, and other relevant government agencies, as well as nonprofit organizations, research foundations, and academic research institutions, should strengthen efforts to collect and disseminate population-based data on cognitive aging. These efforts should identify the nature and extent of cognitive aging throughout the population, including high-risk and underserved populations, with the goal of informing the general public and improving relevant policies, programs, and services.

Specifically, expanded cognitive aging data collection and dissemination efforts should include
- A focus on the cognitive health of older adults as separate from dementia or other clinical neurodegenerative diseases.
- The development of operational definitions of cognitive aging for use in research and public health surveillance and also the development of a process for periodic reexamination. Analyses of existing longitudinal datasets of older persons should be used to inform these efforts.

- Expanded data collection efforts and further analyses of representative surveys involving geographically diverse and high-risk populations. These efforts should include cognitive testing when standardized, feasible, and clinically credible and also self-reports of perceptions or concerns regarding cognitive aging, personal and social adaptations, and self-care and other management practices.
- Longitudinal assessments of changes in cognitive performance and risk behaviors in diverse populations.
- Inclusion of cognition-related questions in the core instrument of the Behavioral Risk Factor Surveillance System, rather than an optional module.
- Exploration of other available relevant data on cognitive health such as health insurance claims data, sales and marketing data for cognition-related products and treatments, data on financial and banking transactions as well as on financial fraud and scams, and data on automobile insurance claims.
- Active dissemination of data on cognitive aging in the population. An annual or biennial report to the U.S. public should be issued by the CDC or other federal agency on the nature and extent of cognitive aging in the U.S. population.

REDUCING RISKS AND DEVELOPING INTERVENTIONS

The brain is subject to a lifetime of demands and exposures, both beneficial and deleterious. Given the importance to the public's health of preventing individuals' cognitive impairment and promoting their cognitive health, it is important to develop an in-depth understanding of these various beneficial and deleterious factors to guide prevention and remediation efforts. However, much remains to be learned about the relationship between lifestyle and risk factors and the maintenance of cognitive health throughout the adult life span. While many studies have examined dementia-based outcomes, few have examined non-dementia-related cognitive changes. Most of the interventions developed to date focus on prevention, although researchers are exploring some remediation strategies. For products that claim to enhance cognitive function or to maintain current levels of function (including cognitive training products, nutriceuticals, supplements, or medications), a review of policies and regulatory guidance is needed. Although there is wide variability in cognitive function among individuals, a number of specific actions can be taken to maintain cognitive health and reduce the effects of cognitive aging.

Recommendation 3: *Take Actions to Reduce Risks of Cognitive Decline with Aging*
Individuals of all ages and their families should take actions to maintain and sustain their cognitive health, realizing that there is wide variability in cognitive health among individuals.
Specifically, individuals should:
- Be physically active.
- Reduce and manage cardiovascular disease risk factors (including hypertension, diabetes, smoking).
- Regularly discuss and review health conditions and medications that might influence cognitive health with a health care professional.
- Take additional actions that may promote cognitive health, including
  - Be socially and intellectually engaged, and engage in lifelong learning;
  - Get adequate sleep and receive treatment for sleep disorders if needed;
  - Take steps to avoid the risk of cognitive changes due to delirium if hospitalized; and
  - Carefully evaluate products advertised to consumers to improve cognitive health, such as medications, nutritionals, and cognitive training.

Recommendation 4: *Increase Research on Risk and Protective Factors and Interventions to Promote Cognitive Health and Prevent or Reduce Cognitive Decline*
The National Institutes of Health, the Centers for Disease Control and Prevention, other relevant government agencies, nonprofit organizations, and research foundations should expand research on risk and protective factors for cognitive aging and on interventions aimed at preventing or reducing cognitive decline and maintaining cognitive health.
Research efforts should:
- Develop collaborative approaches between ongoing longitudinal studies across the life span that focus on cognitive aging outcomes in order to maximize the amount and comparability of data available on risk and protective factors.
- Examine risk factors and interventions in under-studied and vulnerable populations, including people 85 years and older and those with childhood or youth trauma or developmental delay, mental illness, learning disabilities, or genetic intellectual disabilities, and spanning ethnic/cultural and socioeconomic groups.

- Conduct single- and multicomponent clinical trials of promising interventions to promote cognitive health and prevent cognitive decline, testing for both cognitive status and functional outcomes.
- Assess cognitive outcomes in clinical trials that target the reduction of cardiovascular and other risk factors likely related to cognitive health.
- Explore older adults' preferences and values regarding cognitive health and aging and regarding specific cognitive interventions and training modalities.
- Identify effective approaches to sustaining behavior changes that promote healthy cognition across the life span.

Recommendation 5: *Ensure Appropriate Review, Policies, and Guidelines for Products That Affect Cognitive Function or Assert Claims Regarding Cognitive Health*
The Food and Drug Administration and the Federal Trade Commission, in conjunction with other relevant federal agencies and consumer organizations, should determine the appropriate regulatory review, policies, and guidelines for

- over-the-counter medications (such as antihistamines, sedatives, and other medications that have strong anticholinergic activity) that may affect cognitive function, and
- interventions (such as cognitive training, nutriceuticals, supplements, or medications) that do not target a disease but may assert claims about cognitive enhancement or maintaining cognitive abilities such as memory or attention.

IMPROVE HEALTH CARE PROFESSIONAL EDUCATION AND USE OF WELLNESS VISITS

As a result of the aging of the population, older adults constitute an increasingly larger portion of the patients seen by health care professionals both in acute and ambulatory care settings. Moreover, with increased public awareness of and concern about cognitive impairment and dementia in older age, individuals and families are turning to health care professionals for information and advice about brain health. Health care professionals are trusted sources of information on cognitive aging and need to be fully informed and ready to respond to patient queries. Further efforts are needed by health professional schools, continuing education organizations, and professional associations to establish and reinforce the core competencies needed to respond to patient and family concerns about cognitive aging as well to proactively recommend effective steps to maximize cognitive health.

Furthermore, attention needs to be paid to certain medications that may cause cognitive impairment as well as to delirium and associated cognitive decline that may occur in older adults during hospitalization and post-surgery recovery.

Recommendation 6: *Develop and Implement Core Competencies and Curricula in Cognitive Aging for Health Professionals*
The Department of Health and Human Services, the Department of Veterans Affairs, and educational, professional, and interdisciplinary associations and organizations involved in the health care of older adults (including, but not limited to, the Association of American Medical Colleges, the American Association of Colleges of Nursing, the National Association of Social Workers, the American Psychological Association, and the American Public Health Association) should develop and disseminate core competencies, curricula, and continuing education opportunities, including for primary care providers, that focus on cognitive aging as distinct from clinical cognitive syndromes and diseases, such as dementia.

Recommendation 7: *Promote Cognitive Health in Wellness and Medical Visits*
Public health agencies (including the Centers for Disease Control and Prevention and state health departments), health care systems (including the Veterans Health Administration), the Centers for Medicare & Medicaid Services (CMS), health insurance companies, health care professional schools and organizations, health care professionals, and individuals and their families should promote cognitive health in regular medical and wellness visits among people of all ages. Attention should also be given to cognitive outcomes during hospital stays and post-surgery.

Specifically, health care professionals should use patient visits to:
- identify risk factors for cognitive decline and recommend measures to minimize risk; and review patient medications, paying attention to medications known to have an impact on cognition;
- provide patients and families with information on cognitive aging (as distinct from dementia) and actions that they can take to maintain cognitive health and prevent cognitive decline; and
- encourage individuals and family members to discuss their concerns and questions regarding cognitive health.

In addition, other components of the health care system have a cognitive health promotion role:
- CMS should develop and implement demonstration projects to identify best practices for clinicians in assessing cognitive change and functional impairment and in providing appropriate counseling and prevention messages during, for example, the Medicare Annual Wellness Visit or other health care visits.
- Health care systems and private and public health insurance companies should develop evidence-based programs and materials on cognitive health across the life span.
- During and after hospital stays and post-surgery, health care providers, patients, and families should be alert to potential cognitive changes and delirium.

COMMUNITY ACTIONS: HEALTH, FINANCES, DRIVING, TECHNOLOGY, AND CONSUMER DECISIONS

Cognitive aging can affect everyday life for older adults and their families. These effects can manifest themselves as decreased judgment in determining when to make a left turn while in a busy intersection, uncertainty about whether a new financial investment is a wise choice or a financial scam, or determining the best way to take care of one's overall health. Furthermore, cognitive aging has significant impacts on society. In addition to significant financial losses (that older adults lose an estimated $2.9 billion per year, directly and indirectly, to financial fraud), an array of health, public health, social, and other services may be required to provide necessary assistance and support. Improving the quality of life for older adults is a societal value that for cognitive aging has widespread consequences and requires action in many sectors.

Communities across the country have been working to improve independence, health, and quality of life for older adults. Efforts are under way in many areas, but challenges remain in knowing how best to help older adults identify and address the potential impacts of cognitive aging.

Recommendation 8: *Develop Consumer Product Evaluation Criteria and an Independent Information Gateway*
The Centers for Disease Control and Prevention, National Institutes of Health, and the Administration for Community Living, in conjunction with other health and consumer protection agencies, nonprofit organizations, and professional associations, should develop, test, and implement cognitive aging information resources and tools that can

help individuals and families make more informed decisions regarding cognitive health.

Specifically,
- A central, user-friendly, easily navigated website should be available to provide independent, evidence-based information and links relevant to cognitive aging, including information on the promotion of protective behaviors and links to effective programs and services. The information should be presented in a way that takes health literacy into account.
- Consumer-relevant criteria should be developed and widely disseminated to provide individuals and families with guidance on evaluating cognition-related products (e.g., cognitive training products, nutriceuticals, and medications).

Recommendation 9: *Expand Services to Better Meet the Needs of Older Adults and Their Families with Respect to Cognitive Health*
Relevant federal and state agencies (including the Administration for Community Living [ACL], the Centers for Disease Control and Prevention [CDC], the National Highway Traffic Safety Administration [NHTSA], and the Consumer Financial Protection Bureau), nonprofit organizations (such as the Financial Industry Regulatory Authority), professional associations, and relevant private-sector companies and consumer organizations should develop, expand, implement, and evaluate programs and services used by older adults relevant to cognitive aging with the goal of helping older adults avoid exploitation, optimize their independence, improve their function in daily life, and aid their decision making.

Specifically,
- Financial decision making:
  - The banking and financial services industries and state and federal banking and financial regulators should develop and disseminate banking and financial policies, services, and information materials that assist older adults and their families in making decisions that meet their financial means and objectives, that reduce the opportunities for unsuitable decisions, and that mitigate the harms of such decisions.
  - Surrogacy mechanisms, such as powers of attorney or multiparty accounts should have appropriate safeguards to protect the interests of the older adult.
  - The financial services industries and relevant state and federal agencies should develop, strengthen, and implement systems approaches, best practices, training, and

laws and regulations to help verify that financial transactions are not fraudulent or the result of diminished capacity or undue influence.
- Systems should be strengthened for reporting or taking other protective actions against potential financial fraud, exploitation, or abuse to relevant enforcement and investigative officials. Laws and regulations should be revised to mitigate civil liability and professional harms resulting from such protective actions.

- Driving and transportation:
  - NHTSA, states' departments of motor vehicles, and relevant professional and consumer organizations such as the American Automobile Association should expand, validate, and disseminate tools and informational materials to assist older adults in maintaining and assessing their driving skills and to assist older adults and their families in making decisions about safe driving.
  - The automobile industry should expand and evaluate technologies that enhance decision making and safety for older drivers.
  - State and local transportation authorities, local planning commissions, private developers, and community groups should expand efforts to develop and implement alternative transportation options to accommodate changes that occur with cognitive aging, including efforts to ensure safe and walkable communities.

- Technology:
  - Technology industries should develop and adapt hardware, software, and emerging technologies to accommodate the needs of older adults that are related to cognitive aging.
  - The CDC, ACL, and other relevant agencies, organizations, and private-sector companies should support evidence-based programs that educate older adults in the use of emerging technologies.

- Health information:
  - Health information providers, including private-sector companies and government agencies, should ensure that their websites (including patient health portals), packaging (including medication packaging), and other consumer health information relevant to cognitive aging meet health literacy standards.

EXPAND PUBLIC EDUCATION AND ENGAGEMENT

Meeting the public health goal of maintaining cognitive health requires clear and effective communication featuring accurate, up-to-date, and consistent messages that resonate with individuals and their communities and encourage behavior that promotes cognitive health. Attention needs to be paid to whether different segments of the population are exposed to relevant information, persuaded to act accordingly, and have the environmental supports in place to change and maintain behaviors that are supportive of cognitive health. Since new research findings are constantly becoming available, stakeholders also need a reliable means of keeping up with this rapidly changing field.

As noted throughout this report, cognitive aging is not synonymous with Alzheimer's disease. Major challenges for public information campaigns about cognitive aging are to differentiate the messages from those about Alzheimer's disease and other dementias and to promote actions to enhance or maintain cognitive health and to prevent or reduce cognitive decline.

> **Recommendation 10:** *Expand Public Communications Efforts and Promote Key Messages and Actions*
> The Centers for Disease Control and Prevention, the Administration for Community Living, the National Institutes of Health, other relevant federal agencies, state and local government agencies, relevant nonprofit and advocacy organizations and foundations, professional societies, and private-sector companies should develop, evaluate, and communicate key evidence-based messages about cognitive aging through social marketing and media campaigns; work to ensure accurate news and storylines about cognitive aging through media relations; and promote effective services related to cognitive health in order to increase public understanding about cognitive aging and support actions that people can do to maintain their cognitive health.
>
> Public communications efforts should:
> - Reach the diverse U.S. population with campaigns and programs targeted to all relevant groups;
> - Be sensitive to existing differences in knowledge, literacy, health literacy, perceived risk, cognitive aging–related behavior, communication practices, cultures and beliefs, speech and hearing declines, and skills and self-efficacy among target groups;
> - Include evaluation components to assess outreach efficacy in the short and long term, and research the optimal com-

munication strategies for the key messages among the target groups;
- Be updated as new evidence is gained on cognitive aging;
- Emphasize a lifelong approach to cognitive health;
- Promote succinct and actionable key messages that are understandable, memorable, and relevant to the target groups;

BOX S-2
Opportunities for Action

Many of the following actions require multiple efforts involving a number of agencies, organizations, and sectors as well as individuals and families. These efforts will be greatly strengthened by joint and collaborative efforts.

Individuals and families:
- Be physically active and intellectually and socially engaged, monitor medications, and engage in healthy lifestyles and behavior;
- Talk with health care professionals about cognitive aging concerns;
- Be aware of the potential for financial fraud and abuse, impaired driving skills, and poor consumer decision making;
- Make health, finance, and consumer decisions based on reliable evidence from trusted sources.

Communities, community organizations, senior centers, residential facilities, housing and transportation planners, local governments:
- Provide opportunities for physical activity, social and intellectual engagement, lifelong learning, and education on cognitive aging; expand relevant programs and facilities;
- Improve walkability and public transportation options in neighborhoods, communities, and cities.

Health care professionals and professional associations and health care systems:
- Learn about cognitive aging and engage patients and families in discussions;
- Pay attention to cognition during wellness visits, prescribing and reviews of medications, and during hospital stays and post-surgery;
- Identify useful and evidence-based community and patient resources and make sure patients and families know about them;
- Develop core professional competencies in cognitive aging as distinct from dementia and other neurodegenerative diseases in treatment and in counseling patients and families;
- Address factors that lead to delirium in hospitalized patients.

- Focus on sustaining changes in behaviors that promote cognitive health; and
- Promote effective evidence-based tools for maintenance of cognitive health and cognitive change assessment, as well as the information gateway on cognitive aging (see Recommendation 8).

Public health agencies at the federal, state, and local levels; aging organizations; media; professional associations; and consumer groups:
- Strengthen efforts to collect and disseminate population-based data on cognitive aging as separate from dementia and other neurodegenerative diseases;
- Develop and widely disseminate independent authoritative information resources on cognitive aging and criteria for consumer evaluation of products and medications that claim to enhance cognition;
- Develop, test, and disseminate key messages regarding cognitive aging through social marketing campaigns, media awareness efforts, and other approaches to increase public understanding about cognitive aging; and promote activities that help maintain cognitive health.

Research funders and researchers:
- Explore cognitive aging as separate from dementia and other neurodegenerative diseases in basic, applied, and clinical research;
- Expand research on the trajectories of cognitive aging and improve assessments of cognitive changes and impacts on daily function;
- Focus research on risk and protective factors for cognitive aging and on developing and improving the implementation of interventions aimed at preventing or reducing cognitive decline and maintaining cognitive health.

Policy makers, regulators, and consumer advocacy and support organizations:
- Support the resources needed to understand and address cognitive aging;
- Determine (or provide input into the appropriate regulatory review) policies and guidelines for products, medications, and other interventions that claim to enhance cognitive function or that have a negative impact on cognition;
- Develop, validate, and disseminate policies, products, services, and informational materials focused on cognitive aging and addressing potential financial, health, and safety impacts, harms, and vulnerabilities.

Private-sector businesses, including the financial, transportation, and technology industries:
- Develop, validate, and disseminate policies, products, services, and informational materials focused on cognitive aging and addressing potential financial, health, and safety impacts, harms, and vulnerabilities.

OPPORTUNITIES FOR ACTION

Aging is inevitable, but individuals, families, communities, and society can take actions that may help prevent or ameliorate the impact of aging on cognition, create greater understanding about its impact, and help older adults live fuller and more independent lives. One of the major concerns of older adults is "Will I stay sharp?" Although changes in cognitive function vary widely among individuals, there are a number of actions that would make a difference and promote cognitive health; these are summarized in Box S-2 and detailed throughout the discussion and recommendations in this report. Cognitive aging is not just an individual or family or health care system challenge—it is an issue that affects the fabric of society and requires actions by many and varied stakeholders. How society responds to these challenges will reflect the value it places on older adults and how it views their continued involvement and contribution to their families, social networks, and communities.

The committee heard throughout its work on this study that cognitive aging is a concern to many people across all cultural groups and income levels. In recent years a vigorous public health, research, and community response has focused on Alzheimer's disease and other neurodegenerative dementias. These efforts should continue to be strengthened. At the same time, similar efforts should be made in the field of cognitive aging. Attention needs to be paid to the cognitive vulnerabilities of the vast majority of older adults who may experience cognitive decline that is not caused by a neurodegenerative disease. They, too, want to maintain their cognitive health to the fullest extent possible. The committee hopes that a commitment to addressing cognitive aging by many sectors of society will bring about further effective interventions, greater understanding of risk and protective factors, and a society that values and sustains cognitive health.

1

Introduction

People forget things—a name, where they put their keys, a phone number—and yet what is dismissed as a minor inconvenience at 25 years of age can evolve into a momentary anxiety at 35, and a major source of personal worry at age 55 or 60. Forgetfulness at older ages is often equated with a decline in cognition—a public health issue that goes beyond memory lapses and one that can have significant impacts on independent living and healthy aging. The term "cognition" covers many mental abilities and processes, including decision making, memory, attention, and problem solving. Collectively, these different domains of cognition are critical for successfully engaging in the various activities involved in daily functioning such as paying household bills, following a recipe to cook a meal, and driving to a doctor's appointment. As human life expectancy increases, maintaining one's cognitive abilities is key to assuring the quality of those added years.

Cognitive aging is a public health concern from many perspectives. Individuals are deeply concerned about declines in memory and decision-making abilities as they age and may also be worried about whether these declines are early signs of a neurodegenerative disease, particularly Alzheimer's disease. They may fear that cognitive decline will lead to a loss of independence and a reduced quality of life and health. Cognitive decline affects not only the individual but also his or her family and community, and an array of health, public health, social, and other services may be required to provide necessary assistance and support. Lost independence may stem from impaired decision making, which can reduce an individual's ability to drive a car or increase the individual's vulnerability to financial abuse or exploitation. Cognitive impairment also affects society and the public's quality of health and life.

At this point in time, when the older population is rapidly growing in the United States and across the globe, it is important to carefully examine what is known about cognitive aging, to identify the positive steps that can be taken to maintain and improve cognitive health, and then to take action to implement those changes by informing and activating the public, the health sector, nonprofit and professional associations, the private sector, and government agencies. In the past several decades rapid gains have been made in understanding the non-disease changes in cognitive function that may occur with aging and in elucidating the range of cognitive changes, from those that are normal with aging to those that are the result of disease; much remains to be learned yet the science is readily advancing.

This Institute of Medicine (IOM) study examines the public health dimensions of cognitive aging with an emphasis on definitions and terminology, epidemiology and surveillance, prevention and intervention, education of health professionals, and public awareness and education (see Box 1-1).

To complete this task the IOM appointed the 16-member Committee on the Public Health Dimensions of Cognitive Aging whose members have expertise in cognitive neuroscience, geriatric medicine and nursing, gerontology, neurology, psychology, psychiatry, behavioral sciences, communication, public health, epidemiology, social work, and ethics. The study was sponsored by the McKnight Brain Research Foundation, the National Institute of Neurological Disorders and Stroke, the National Institute on Aging, the Centers for Disease Control and Prevention, The Retirement Research Foundation, and AARP.

The committee held five meetings during the course of its work, two of which included public workshops during which a number of speakers provided their expertise on the study topics (see Appendix A). The committee also heard from various speakers at its first meeting in February 2014 and in public conference call meetings in August and September 2014. In addition to the input received through these workshops and meetings, the committee examined the scientific literature and other available evidence. The committee focused on providing a report for a broad audience, including the general public; health care and human services providers; local, state, and national policy makers; researchers; and foundations and nonprofit organizations.

WHAT IS COGNITION?

This report focuses on one aspect of health in older adults—cognitive health. Cognition refers to the mental functions involved in attention, thinking, understanding, learning, remembering, solving problems, and making decisions. It is a fundamental aspect of an individual's ability to engage in

> **BOX 1-1**
> **Statement of Task**
>
> The Institute of Medicine will conduct a study to examine cognitive health and aging, as distinct from Alzheimer's disease. The committee will make recommendations focused on the public health aspects of cognitive aging with an emphasis on the following:
>
> - Definitions and terminology—The study will explore relevant definitions and terminology with consideration given to preventing unintended consequences of terminology.
> - Epidemiology and surveillance—The focus of the study will be on identifying efforts needed to better understand the public health implications of cognitive aging and its risk and preventive factors, as well as the development of relevant surveillance or monitoring tools and methodologies.
> - Prevention and intervention opportunities—The study will examine opportunities for prevention and intervention taking into account the multiple aspects of enhancing cognitive capacity, prevention of impairment, amelioration of cognitive decline, and promoting cognitive resilience. This will include relevant research on human behavior change and the evidence-based approaches needed to ensure the retention of healthy practices to maintain cognitive health and remediate cognitive decline.
> - Education of health professionals—This study will explore the education of health professionals related to cognitive health and decline and will identify examples of best practices for educating health professions to ensure high quality care and education for older adults and their families about cognitive aging and its possible consequences.
> - Public awareness and education—The study will consider new approaches for enhancing awareness and disseminating information (with cultural, ethical, and health literacy considerations) to the public and to older adults and their families and caregivers.
>
> The committee will hold information-gathering workshops open to the public during the course of its work. The report will not focus on setting an agenda for basic and biomedical science research as this has been the topic of recent reports and forums. Biomedical research will, however, inform the committee's deliberations and will serve as the foundation for the evidence base of the report.

activities, accomplish goals, and successfully negotiate the world. Although cognition is sometimes equated with memory, cognition is multidimensional because it involves a number of interrelated abilities that depend on brain anatomy and physiology. Distinguishing among these component abilities is important since they play different roles in the processing of information and behavior and are differentially affected by aging.

While cognitive abilities do not neatly map to single discrete regions of the brain, generalizations can be drawn between brain regions and key cognitive abilities that individuals need for their day-to-day function, well-being, and flourishing. For example, decision making, organizing, and planning, and other related processes, are collectively referred to as "executive function." The prefrontal cortex is the region of the brain that is active in executive functions, such as the planning and multitasking required for cooking a meal. In contrast, memory, such as is involved in remembering the list of food items needed at the supermarket, is largely controlled by the hippocampus. Other brain areas play key roles in other functions. Clinicians use different tests to measure and evaluate various cognitive dimensions depending on the type of cognition or brain region (see Chapter 2).

THE INTERSECTION OF COGNITION AND AGING

What Is Cognitive Aging?

The committee provides a conceptual definition of cognitive aging as a process of gradual, ongoing, yet highly variable changes in cognitive functions that occur as people get older. Cognitive aging is a lifelong process. It is not a disease or a quantifiable level of function. However, for the purposes of this report the focus is primarily on later life. In the context of aging, cognitive health is exemplified by an individual who maintains his or her optimal cognitive function with age.

Box 1-2 provides the committee's characterization of cognitive aging. Cognitive aging is too complex and nuanced to define succinctly, and therefore it is appropriately characterized through this longer description. Efforts are needed to develop operational definitions of cognitive aging in order to allow comparisons across studies (see Chapter 3).

Prior Terminology and Definitions

The literature on cognitive aging includes a wide array of terms to describe the various aspects of cognitive aging. For instance, Rowe and Kahn (1987) differentiated "usual aging" from "successful aging." "Usual cognitive aging" referred to such commonly found changes as reductions in processing speed and working memory, and also common pathological changes, such as those associated with cardiovascular disease. In contrast, the phrase "successful aging" was used to refer to the amelioration or prevention of changes that have a substantial and negative impact, often by adopting a healthy lifestyle. Rowe and Kahn argued that scientists, physicians, and the general public were all too ready to accept that significant and deleterious changes associated with age were inevitable. This complacency, in their view, ignored both the great variation in changes with age as well as the variation over time within an individual, and it undermined

BOX 1-2
Characterizing Cognitive Aging

- **Key Features:**
  - Inherent in humans and animals as they age.
  - Occurs across the spectrum of individuals as they age regardless of initial cognitive function.
  - Highly dynamic process with variability within and between individuals.
  - Includes some cognitive domains that may not change, may decline, or may actually improve with aging, and there is the potential for older adults to strengthen some cognitive abilities.
  - Only now beginning to be understood biologically, yet clearly involves structural and functional brain changes.
  - Not a clinically defined neurological or psychiatric disease such as Alzheimer's disease and does not inevitably lead to neuronal death and neurodegenerative dementia (such as Alzheimer's disease).

- **Risk and Protective Factors:**
  - Health and environmental factors over the life span influence cognitive aging.
  - Modifiable and non-modifiable factors include genetics, culture, education, medical comorbidities, acute illness, physical activity, and other health behaviors.
  - Cognitive aging can be influenced by development beginning in utero, infancy, and childhood.

- **Assessment:**
  - Cognitive aging is not easily defined by clear thresholds on cognitive tests since many factors—including culture, occupation, education, environmental context, and health variables (e.g., medications, delirium)—influence test performance and norms.
  - For an individual, cognitive performance is best assessed at several points in time.

- **Impact on Daily Life:**
  - Day-to-day functions, such as driving, making financial and health care decisions, and understanding instructions given by health care professionals, may be affected.
  - Experience, expertise, and environmental support aids (e.g., lists) can help compensate for declines in cognition.
  - The challenges of cognitive aging may be more apparent in environments that require individuals to engage in highly technical and fast-paced or timed tasks, in situations that involve new learning, and in stressful situations (i.e., emotional, physical, or health-related), and may be less apparent in highly familiar situations.

the search for reversible causes of such changes. The committee appreciates the important distinctions made by Rowe and Kahn, but it decided not to adopt the term "successful aging" because it may suggest a value judgment regarding those with greater or lesser preservation of cognitive capacity.

Similarly, the committee did not adopt the term "normal aging" because it is confusing. Some authors use this term to refer to standard or common aspects of cognitive aging (Aine et al., 2011), while others suggest that "normal" aging is the optimal state and refers to those aspects of aging change that remain when all disease-related changes have been ruled out (Jagust, 2013). (A detailed discussion of the development of norms in aging research is provided in Chapter 2.) Despite variability in the terminology across investigators and clinicians, there is wide agreement that preserving cognitive function is a key component of desirable aging (Warsch and Wright, 2010).

The committee uses the term "cognitive aging" to emphasize that the human brain changes with age, both in its physical structures and in its ability to carry out various functions. Indeed, it would be surprising if the brain did not age, given that all other organs and body structures age. Kidneys and muscles, for example, show a range of age-related changes in structure and function (Cohen et al., 2014; Keller and Engelhardt, 2013). And it is not only humans whose brains age. A considerable body of literature demonstrates that there is remarkable consistency across mammalian species in age-related neural and cognitive changes (Samson and Barnes, 2013; also see Chapter 2).

The brain is the locus for a vast array of functions, including reasoning, emotion, memory, judgment, sensory processing, learning, and motor skills. These many brain functions and the neural structures and networks that support them change at different rates and in different ways over time, with the particular changes based on a large number of interacting factors, including genetic makeup, education, environment, lifestyle, and trauma. A clear body of evidence indicates that as individuals age a decline occurs in specific brain functions that cannot be attributed to disease processes in the brain, such as neurodegeneration from Alzheimer's disease or stroke. For instance, most older adults process information less quickly than they did when they were younger (Birren, 1970). Researchers face a daunting task in distinguishing between changes that are the consequences of aging and those that are attributable to specific neurological diseases and conditions, which may or may not have potentially reversible attributes.

What Are the Potential Impacts of Cognitive Aging?

Age-related changes in cognition can affect not only memory but also decision making, judgment, processing speed, and learning. (For more details on the many elements of cognition, see Chapter 2.) These changes can in turn affect an older person's capacity to live independently, to preserve a sense of identity grounded in autonomy, and to pursue treasured activities. The more that a society values an ethic of independence and a respect for autonomy, the more cognitive aging will be perceived as a social, cultural, and individual challenge. In fact, some people have reported that they are reluctant to tell their physicians or family members about their difficulties with cognition out of fear that they will lose their independence or their driving privileges (Ralston et al., 2001).

In a 2012 survey of its members, AARP found that "staying mentally sharp" was a top concern of 87 percent of respondents (AARP, 2013). Changes in cognition also have the potential to affect health directly by impairing a patient's ability to take the proper medication dose on the correct schedule or to understand risks and benefits when choosing a treatment option or health insurance plan (IOM, 2014).

However, identity is shaped by a person's capacity for interdependence as much as it is for a capacity for independence. Each person is defined by his or her relationships with family, colleagues, co-worshipers, and communities. The ability to help others, to collaborate, and to, at times, receive help are crucial human qualities. Ironically, the ability to appropriately seek and accept help when needed can be a critical factor in maintaining independence. One key message for this report is that although the brain will change with age, numerous opportunities exist to prevent, ameliorate, or adapt to cognitive changes. These opportunities can allow older adults to continue to function both independently and interdependently.

Family members of older adults also worry about how their loved one's changes in cognition could affect their daily functioning. A 2010 survey found that 40 percent of children with parents age 65 years or older were concerned that their parents would have difficulty handling their personal finances (Investor Protection Trust, 2015).

Although most of the focus on cognitive aging is on its negative implications, noteworthy positive changes also can occur as the brain ages. For example, wisdom and knowledge increase with age (Grossmann et al., 2010), and happiness follows a U-shaped curve relative to age, with people reporting they are happiest in youth, less happy in midlife, and happiest again much later in life (Stone et al., 2010). Furthermore, levels of stress, worry, and anger all decline with increasing age (Stone et al., 2010).

Various groups and industries have taken note of the public health and societal impacts of cognitive changes in later life and are attempting to minimize the negative effects of cognitive aging, to make more resources available to more people, and to raise public knowledge. Examples of this heightened attention can be seen in actions by government at the federal, state, and local levels; by nonprofit organizations focused on older adults; and by companies in the relevant industries, including the financial services industries and the physical activity, transportation, food, and insurance industries (see Chapter 6). Given the demographics and the aging of society (see section below), the market for cognitive-related sales is significant, and older adults and their families will need to make evidence-based decisions.

CHANGING DEMOGRAPHICS

The population of the United States, like that of many other countries, is getting older. Thus, cognitive aging will affect an ever-increasing number and proportion of Americans. Life expectancy in the United States has increased dramatically over the past century. In 1900, the average life expectancy at birth was 46.3 years for men and 48.3 years for women; by 2010 it had increased to 76.2 years for men and 81.0 years for women (NCHS, 2014). While the mortality rate among children and young adults has decreased, thanks to a variety of advances, age-adjusted mortality rates have also declined in the population over age 65 years (Hoyert, 2012). Decreases in mortality are attributable to, among other factors, reductions in smoking, better control of chronic diseases (e.g., especially heart disease), and improved education (Cutler et al., 2007).

Increased life expectancy, changes in birth and mortality rates, and other factors are leading to major changes in the demographic composition of the U.S. and global population. In 1900, 4.1 percent of the U.S. population was 65 years or older (just over 3 million people); by 2012 that age group accounted for 13.7 percent of the population (more than 40 million people) (AoA, 2013; West et al., 2014). By 2050 people 65 years and older are expected to make up 21 percent of the U.S. population (see Figure 1-1; U.S. Census Bureau, 2012b). The "oldest old" demographic—people age 85 years and older—is expected to increase from 6.3 million (1.96 percent of the population) in 2015 to just over 18 million (4.5 percent) in 2050 (Suzman and Riley 1985; U.S. Census Bureau, 2012a,b). In the past three decades the percentage of the population that is age 90 years and older has tripled, and in the next four decades it is expected to more than quadruple (He and Muenchrath, 2011).

Similar aging trends are occurring in developed countries around the globe. Japan's 65-years-and-older population is almost one-fourth of its total population, with similar percentages seen in Germany and Italy (both more than 20 percent) (Jacobsen et al., 2011). Even though the public health implications of cognitive aging may be unique for each country due to their distinct social, cultural, and economic conditions, the challenges and opportunities that these countries face are all related.

Diversity

In addition to increasing in total number, the U.S. population 65 years and older is expected to diversify racially and ethnically by 2050. In 2010,

INTRODUCTION

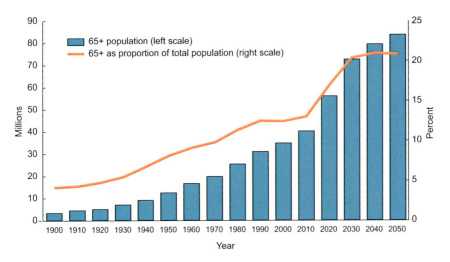

FIGURE 1-1 Population age 65 years and older, 1900 to 2050.
SOURCE: West et al., 2014.

the non-Hispanic white demographic made up 80 percent of this group, but this share is projected to decrease to 58 percent by 2050. While the Hispanic population accounted for 7 percent of the 65-years-and-older population in 2010, it is projected to grow to 20 percent in 2050 (increasing from 3 million individuals in 2010 to 17.5 million in 2050); the black population will account for 12 percent of the 65-years-and-older population in 2050, up from 9 percent in 2010 (from 3.4 million to 10.5 million people); and the Asian population will increase from 6 percent to 9 percent of the 65-years-and-older population (from 1.3 million in 2010 to 7.5 million in 2050) (FIFARS, 2012). This increasing diversity of the population calls for a focus on improving cognitive measurement techniques and the development of appropriate metrics and interventions for diverse ethnic, cultural, and racial groups as part of the broad effort to improve cognitive health in the aging population.

Health Status

The health status of older Americans has improved over the past several decades (West et al., 2014). In 2010 roughly three-fourths of adults age 65 years and older reported their health status to be "excellent," "very good," or "good" (Schiller et al., 2012). However, the percentage of adults reporting excellent or very good health decreases with age.

Despite good self-rated health, a large majority of older adults have at least one chronic disease (e.g., hypertension, arthritis) that requires ongo-

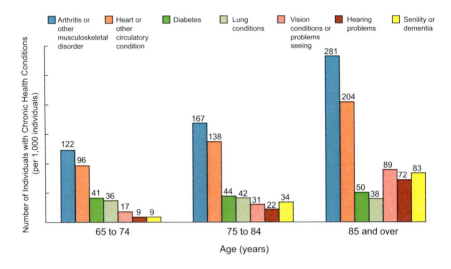

FIGURE 1-2 Limitations of activity caused by chronic health conditions by age, 2006–2007 (per 1,000 individuals).
NOTE: Data are from the 2006–2007 National Health Interview Surveys, which cover the civilian noninstitutionalized population.
SOURCE: West et al., 2014.

ing care. In addition, many older adults experience one or more clinical conditions that do not fit into discrete disease categories (e.g., incontinence, frailty) (see Figure 1-2; West et al., 2014). The care needed for these syndromes and diseases—both acute and chronic—presents older adults with decisions that will lead to ethical and economic outcomes that can substantially affect their well-being and quality of life. Cognitive aging can add to the challenges that older adults face when making these decisions.

CROSS-CUTTING THEMES

Cognitive aging is a broad topic with sweeping implications and challenges. This report focuses on the public health dimensions of cognitive aging and touches only briefly on the numerous basic science questions and neuropsychological assessment challenges related to cognitive aging. In addressing the public health challenges of cognitive aging, the committee identified several cross-cutting themes and key messages (see Chapter 7):

- **Cognitive health should be promoted across the life span. Actions can be taken by individuals to help maintain cognitive health.**

Healthy cognition facilitates an individual's capacity to function. It allows people to learn, to make appropriate choices, and to express current and future preferences. Cognitive abilities enable people to accomplish the tasks of daily living, to understand information and apply it to personal situations through appreciation and reasoning, and to effectively assess emotions such as trust. It enables people to maintain the essence of self. Actions to maintain cognitive health are discussed throughout the report.

- **Cognition is memory plus much more; there are multiple dimensions of cognition.** Cognitive abilities range from the capacities for decision making and processing time to memory, attention, and more (see Chapter 2).
- **Cognitive functioning levels vary among individuals and throughout the life span.** From infancy through young adulthood and old age, the brain continues to change. Within the predictable level of change at each stage of life, there is also great variability among individuals.
- **Cognitive function is affected by multiple factors. Neuroplasticity persists throughout the life span so that there is potential for older adults to strengthen cognitive abilities.** Due to the complexity of the human brain, numerous risk and protective factors may affect cognitive abilities (including genetics, physical activity, traumatic brain injury, sleep quality, comorbidities, acute illness, delirium, and medications) (see Chapters 4A, 4B, 4C).
- **Cognitive changes are not necessarily signs of neurodegenerative disease (such as Alzheimer's disease) or other neurological diseases.** There are many potential causes of cognitive decline, some of which may be at least partly preventable or treatable (e.g., recent changes in medications associated with short-term delirium).
- **Cognitive aging can affect daily activities and independent living.** The significance of cognitive aging can be seen especially in its potential effects on daily tasks and decision making. Cognitive decline caused by cognitive aging may occur gradually and with few overt symptoms or signs. As a result, individuals or their close friends or family may not notice deterioration in driving, financial decisions, food choices, and other everyday activities until it becomes severe.
- **Age affects all organ systems. The brain, as with all organs, is affected by aging.** Over the span of life, connectivity is lost between some neuronal synapses and other changes occur.
- **Aging can have positive effects on cognition.** The experiences and knowledge gained over a lifetime can provide individuals with positive cognitive benefits (e.g., wisdom learned from experience).

OVERVIEW OF THE REPORT

This report explores the multiple issues involved in considering cognitive aging from a public health perspective. Chapter 2 explores the challenges of characterizing and measuring changes in cognition, highlights the impact of cognitive aging on daily function, and discusses the variability among individuals particularly as related to setting norms. Chapter 3 focuses on collecting and understanding population-based data on cognitive aging. Chapters 4A, 4B, and 4C provide an overview of the epidemiologic research on risk and protective factors for cognitive aging and discuss the research on a range of prevention and treatment interventions. Chapter 5 focuses on health care's response to cognitive aging, with discussions on increasing the abilities of health professionals to assess cognitive aging and to use wellness visits to discuss these issues with their patients. The community's response to cognitive aging is discussed in Chapter 6, which describes the wide variety of resources that are currently available and that need to be developed for older adults and their families facing decisions on personal finances, driving, technology, and cognitive-related products. Chapter 7 offers key messages on cognitive aging and highlights efforts that are needed to raise awareness of these issues among members of the general public. The report concludes in Chapter 8 with a call to action for individuals, government agencies, private-sector corporations, and nonprofit and professional organizations.

REFERENCES

AARP. 2013. *2012 member opinion survey issue spotlight: Interests and concerns.* http://www.aarp.org/politics-society/advocacy/info-01-2013/interests-concerns-member-opinion-survey-issue-spotlight.html (accessed December 4, 2014).

Aine, C. J., L. Sanfratello, J. C. Adair, J. E. Knoefel, A. Caprihan, and J. M. Stephen. 2011. Development and decline of memory functions in normal, pathological and healthy successful aging. *Brain Topography* 24(3-4):323-339.

AoA (Administration on Aging). 2013. *A profile of older Americans: 2013.* http://www.aoa.gov/Aging_Statistics/Profile/Index.aspx (accessed December 5, 2014).

Birren, J. E. 1970. Toward an experimental psychology of aging. *American Psychologist* 25(2):124-135.

Cohen, E., Y. Nardi, I. Krause, E. Goldberg, G. Milo, M. Garty, and I. Krause. 2014. A longitudinal assessment of the natural rate of decline in renal function with age. *Journal of Nephrology* 27(6):635-641.

Cutler, D. M., E. L. Glaeser, and A. B. Rosen. 2007. Is the U.S. population behaving healthier? *National Bureau of Economic Research Working Paper 13013.* http://www.nber.org/papers/w13013 (accessed December 5, 2014).

FIFARS (Federal Interagency Forum on Aging-Related Statistics). 2012. *Older Americans 2012: Key indicators of well-being.* http://www.agingstats.gov/agingstatsdotnet/Main_Site/Data/2012_Documents/docs/EntireChartbook.pdf (accessed December 5, 2014).

INTRODUCTION

Grossmann, I., J. Na, M. E. Varnum, D. C. Park, S. Kitayama, and R. E. Nisbett. 2010. Reasoning about social conflicts improves into old age. *Proceedings of the National Academy of Sciences of the United States of America* 107(16):7246-7250.

He, W., and M. N. Muenchrath. 2011. 90+ in the United States: 2006-2008. *U.S. Census Bureau American Community Survey Reports.* http://www.census.gov/prod/2011pubs/acs-17.pdf (accessed December 5, 2014).

Hoyert, D. L. 2012. 75 years of mortality in the United States, 1935-2010. *NCHS Data Brief*, No. 88. http://www.cdc.gov/nchs/data/databriefs/db88.pdf (accessed December 5, 2014).

Investor Protection Trust. 2015. *IPT activities: 06.15.2010—IPT Elder Investor Fraud Survey: 1 out of 5 older Americans are financial swindle victims.* http://www.investorprotection.org/ipt-activities/?fa=research (accessed February 19, 2015).

IOM (Institute of Medicine). 2014. *Health literacy and numeracy: Workshop summary.* Washington, DC: The National Academies Press.

Jacobsen, L. A., M. Kent, M. Lee, and M. Mather. 2011. America's aging population. *Population Bulletin* 66(1). http://www.prb.org/pdf11/aging-in-america.pdf (accessed December 5, 2014).

Jagust, W. 2013. Vulnerable neural systems and the borderland of brain aging and neurodegeneration. *Neuron* 77(2):219-234.

Keller, K., and M. Engelhardt. 2013. Strength and muscle mass loss with aging process. Age and strength loss. *Muscles, Ligaments, and Tendons Journal* 3(4):346-350.

NCHS (National Center for Health Statistics). 2014. *Health, United States, 2013: With special feature on prescription drugs. 2013.* http://www.cdcgov/nchs/data/hus/hus13.pdf (accessed December 5, 2014).

Ralston, L. S., S. L. Bell, J. K. Mote, T. B. Rainey, S. Brayman, and M. Shotwell. 2001. Giving up the car keys. *Physical & Occupational Therapy in Geriatrics* 19(4):59-70.

Rowe, J. W., and R. L. Kahn. 1987. Human aging: Usual and successful. *Science* 237(4811):143-149.

Samson, R. D., and C. A. Barnes. 2013. Impact of aging brain circuits on cognition. *European Journal of Neuroscience* 37(12):1903-1915.

Schiller, J. S., J. W. Lucas, B. W. Ward, and J. A. Peregoy. 2012. *Summary health statistics for U.S. adults: National Health Interview Survey, 2010.* http://www.cdc.gov/nchs/data/series/sr_10/sr10_252.pdf (accessed January 8, 2015).

Stone, A. A., J. E. Schwartz, J. E. Broderick, and A. Deaton. 2010. A snapshot of the age distribution of psychological well-being in the United States. *Proceedings of the National Academy of Sciences of the United States of America* 107(22):9985-9990.

Suzman, R., and M. W. Riley. 1985. Introducing the "oldest old." *The Milbank Memorial Fund Quarterly: Health and Society* 63(2):177-186.

U.S. Census Bureau. 2012a. *Table 2. Projections of the population by selected age groups and sex for the United States: 2015 to 2060.* https://www.census.gov/population/projections/data/national/2012/summarytables.html (accessed December 5, 2014).

———. 2012b. *Table 3. Percent distribution of the projected population by selected age groups and sex for the United States: 2015-2060.* https://www.census.gov/population/projections/data/national/2012/summarytables.html (accessed December 5, 2014).

Warsch, J. R., and C. B. Wright. 2010. The aging mind: Vascular health in normal cognitive aging. *Journal of the American Geriatrics Society* 58(Suppl 2):S319-S324.

West, L. A., S. Cole, D. Goodkind, and W. He. 2014. *65+ in the United States: 2010. U.S. Census Bureau Special Studies.* http://www.census.gov/content/dam/Census/library/publications/2014/demo/p23-212.pdf (accessed January 8, 2015).

2

Characterizing and Assessing Cognitive Aging

Many people are concerned about the effects that changes related to cognitive aging may have on their capacity for living independently and making autonomous choices. This chapter will clarify the concept of cognitive aging and explain how it differs from disease. The chapter will review the many different elements of cognition, how they are measured, what is known about the patterns of age-related changes in cognition in both humans and animals, the implications of these changes for everyday functioning, and important concepts such as adaptability and plasticity. The chapter then details the age-related changes observed in human cognition and discusses how research findings from non-human animal models may explain the biological basis for these changes. Next is a summary of the evidence concerning the neural mechanisms that contribute to age-related changes in cognition and the implications of these changes. The background offered in this chapter provides a framework to understand how cognition is assessed, with particular attention to the challenges of creating norms and applying them in cognitive tests, especially given that such tests are often used by non-experts outside of carefully monitored research settings.

Numerous age-related changes in cognitive abilities are highly relevant to everyday activities and have substantial importance to the public. For example, declines in cognitive abilities increase the risk that older adults will make errors in financial decisions, select options that have less than optimal financial rewards, and suffer financial fraud and abuse (Agarwal et al., 2009; Denburg et al., 2007; Samanez-Larkin et al., 2012). Older adults generally have limited opportunities for employment for a variety of reasons, and they also tend to have less time to recover any financial losses. Age-related changes in cognition can impair driving performance, which has safety and public health implications (e.g., Ball et al., 1998; Clay et al., 2005; and see Chapter 6 for further discussion of these topics). Current research indicates that age-related changes in cognitive processes affect performance on technology-based tasks such as searching the Internet for health information (e.g., Czaja et al., 2013; Sharit et al., 2008) and using health care providers' patient portals (Taha et al., 2013). Given the ubiquitous use of computers and the Internet for many routine interactions with businesses, public services, and social events, this has substantial implications for older adults' ability to participate in many domains of life.

AGE-RELATED CHANGES IN HUMAN COGNITION

There is tremendous inter-individual and intra-individual variability in age-related changes in cognitive abilities. This vast heterogeneity among older adults increases the challenges associated with understanding cognitive aging. The trajectory is not the same for everyone, and an individual's performance on measures of ability may change across evaluation occasions (see Figure 2-1). Differences in the degree to which individuals' cognitive function changes with age are due in part to a lifetime of differences in experiences, health status, lifestyles, education, attitudinal and emotional factors, socioeconomic status, and genetics. The trajectory also varies for different cognitive functions. Some aspects of cognition decline with age while others show improvement or remain stable until the much later decades of life. In addition, performance on laboratory tasks is not always representative of performance in everyday functioning. While age-related declines on many standardized tests of cognitive abilities are well documented, older adults may still maintain high levels of competence on most everyday activities because they are often able to compensate for declines in cognitive abilities with expertise and experience or environmental cues or support. The age-related changes seen in several domains of cognition have implications for behavior and function. This section provides descriptions of the primary domains of cognition (also known as neurocognition) along with summaries of what is known about the age-related changes in each. Box 2-1 offers examples of how each domain of cognition can be evaluated.

Speed of Information Processing

Speed of information processing reflects the efficiency of cognitive operations. One of the hallmarks of cognitive aging is a generalized slowing of processing speed, which is reflected in both perceptual and cognitive operations (e.g., Birren, 1970). Generally, it takes longer for older people to process information and give a response. These age-related changes have

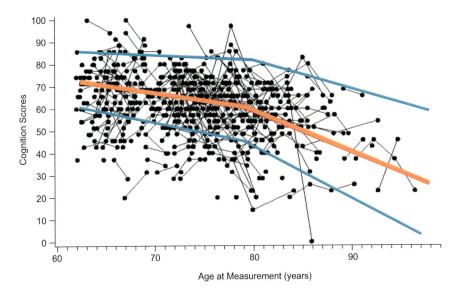

FIGURE 2-1 Intra-individual changes in cognition scores over time for a random sample of approximately 500 adults who were enrolled in the Health and Retirement Study.
NOTE: Lines connect dots that represent the scores of the same individual at different ages. The orange line represents the average score for all individuals, and the two blue lines represent 1 standard deviation above and below the average. Scores for some individuals increased over time even though, as indicated by the orange line representing the average score at each age, there was a general decline over time.
SOURCE: McArdle, 2011. Reprinted with permission.

an influence on the efficiency of other cognitive operations, such as working memory, attention, and speech processing, and have tremendous implications for behavior and interactions with others. For example, making the appropriate responses in driving, such as determining when to turn or when to stop at a red traffic light are heavily dependent on processing speed.

Declines in processing speed can also affect a person's ability to remember spoken instructions, attend to important information, or perform tasks that have pacing demands. As will be discussed in more detail later in this chapter, age-related declines in processing speed can be offset to some extent by experience. For example, a study of skilled typists ranging in age from 19 to 72 years old found that although the older typists were slower on standard measures of reaction time and key tapping, they were not slower in typing speed (Salthouse, 1984). This was due to the older typists' experience, which helped them anticipate the next characters that would have to be typed.

BOX 2-1
Examples of Cognitive Assessments

Numerous cognitive tests have been developed and validated. A few commonly used measures for key cognitive domains are

Speed of processing: The Pattern Comparison Processing Speed Test asks a person to determine whether a set of two pictures placed side by side are the same. The participant is given 90 seconds to evaluate as many sets of pictures as possible. The Digit Symbol Substitution Test, another timed measure of speed of processing, consists of nine digit–symbol pairs. The participant is given a list of digits and asked to write the corresponding symbol for each.

Sustained attention: The Connors Continuous Performance Test presents individuals with a repetitive task and asks them to maintain their focus for a period of time in order to respond to targets. For example, they will see or hear the number "1" or "2" and are told to respond when presented with a visual or auditory "1" but not when presented with "2."

Selective attention: In visual search tasks, an individual is asked to search a visual display for a target, such as a letter, that is surrounded by other, non-target letters. The task can be made more difficult by making the target and non-target letters more similar or by increasing the density of the display. In the Stroop Test, another measure of attention, a person is asked to name the color of ink in which another color word is printed (e.g., the word "red" printed in the color green).

Episodic memory: The Picture Sequence Memory Test entails recalling increasingly long series of 6 to 18 illustrated objects and activities presented in a certain order on a computer screen. Participants are asked to recall the sequence of pictures presented over two learning trials.

Working memory: There are multiple common tests of working memory that include giving participants a list of items (letters, numbers, words) and asking them to repeat the items back in order. Performance on these tests is usually measured in terms of the longest sequence of letters, numbers, or words that are remembered correctly. For example, in the List Sorting Test, participants are shown pictures of different foods and animals along with the written text and audio recording that correspond to the item displayed. Then the participant is asked to recite the items back in order of size from smallest to largest, first within a single category (e.g., animals) and then in two categories (e.g., foods, then animals).

Semantic memory: In the Category Fluency Test, individuals are given a category, such as animals, and asked to name all of the items they can that belong to that category in 1 minute. In the Boston Naming Test, an individual is shown a series of pictures and asked to name each picture within 20 seconds (Kaplan et al., 1983).

Executive function: The Wisconsin Card Sorting Test is a measure of cognitive flexibility in which an individual is asked to match two sets of cards according to some characteristic—the color, shape, or number of items on the cards—but the participant is not told which characteristic is to be used. Feedback is provided after each match so that the participant can figure out the correct system of classification. After a fixed number of correct matches, the classification is changed without notice, and the participant must learn the new rule of classification. In the Trail Making Test (Reitan, 1955)—a test of attention and set-shifting—the individual has to connect 25 consecutive items on paper or a computer screen. In the first part of the test, the participant is asked to connect numbers in sequential order (1, 2, 3, etc.), and in the second part of the test, the participant is asked to alternate between numbers and letters.

Reasoning: The Letter Sets Test consists of five sets of four letters. The participant has to decide which one of the five sets is dissimilar in the sense that it does not follow a rule used to generate the other four sets. Tests of inference are used to measure the ability to reason and draw conclusions from information presented in statements.

Language: There are a variety of tests that can be used to measure language skills depending on the particular aspect of language being assessed. For example, studies have used a word-by-word reading paradigm to assess comprehension of sentences (e.g., Kemtes and Kemper, 1997). Other studies use word-by-word reading time (e.g., Stine, 1990) or recall of text (Stine-Morrow et al., 1996). Another frequently used measure of language comprehension is the Token Test. A common test of word retrieval skills is the Boston Naming Test. The Category Fluency Test measures the ability to retrieve words rapidly from a semantic lexicon. The Boston Diagnostic Aphasia Examination is an example of a test of repetition of phrases and written communication skills. Finally, measures of prosody examine inflection and rhythm.

Spatial ability: In the Paper Folding Test, participants are shown a series of folds in a piece of paper through which a set of holes is then punched. The participants are asked to choose which of a set of unfolded papers with holes matches the original. In the Mental Rotations Test, participants are asked to compare several three-dimensional objects, often rotated on some axis, and state whether they are the same image or mirror images. A complex three-dimensional task is the Block Design subtest of the Wechsler Adult Intelligence Scale (WAIS). The participant is presented with a two-dimensional drawing in red and white of a target design and a set of three-dimensional blocks (some sides of the blocks are red, some sides are white, and some are half red and half white). The participant is asked to arrange the blocks within a specified time limit so that they mimic the drawing.

Intelligence: A common measure of intelligence used with older adults is the WAIS, 4th version. It consists of 10 core subtests and 5 supplemental subtests. The core subtests provide the intelligence quotient, which is derived from four index scores: Verbal Comprehension Index, Perceptual Reasoning Index, Working Memory Index, and Processing Speed Index. Sometimes a distinction is made between crystallized and fluid intelligence. The vocabulary and verbal subscale of the WAIS is often used as a measure of crystallized intelligence, whereas the other subtests are often used to assess fluid intelligence.

Additional measures: These measures provide an assessment of an individual's mental status and include the Montreal Cognitive Assessment Battery, the Mini-Mental State Examination, and the Telephone Interview for Cognitive Status.

Attention

Attention is the capacity for processing information. Humans have limits in the amount of information they can process at any given time. Performing tasks at levels near full capacity for long periods of time can be tiring, especially for older adults (Kramer and Madden, 2008; Zanto and Gazzaley, 2014). When capacity limits are exceeded, performance tends to decline and be prone to error (Zanto and Gazzaley, 2014). There are several types of attention.

Selective attention refers to the ability to filter information and focus on select items despite the presence of other information. Examples include searching a visual display for a specific letter that is surrounded by other letters, identifying a road sign on a highway cluttered with billboards and advertisements, or finding relevant information on a highly cluttered website. This becomes more difficult with increasing amounts of clutter and irrelevant information, especially for older adults. In general, older adults have more trouble discriminating between relevant and irrelevant stimuli and locating relevant information in the presence of distracting background information (McDowd and Shaw, 2000).

Divided attention is the ability to split one's focus between competing activities or multiple sources of information—also known as multitasking—and can involve the processing of multiple pieces of information or the performance of multiple tasks simultaneously. Reading an instruction manual while listening to music is one example of divided attention. A dangerous example is driving while typing a text message on a cell phone. Generally, older adults have more difficulty with multitasking than do younger adults (McDowd and Shaw, 2000; Tsang and Shaner, 1998; Verhaeghen and Cerella, 2002).

Sustained attention refers to the ability to maintain concentration on a task for a long period of time. It is required when a person must continuously monitor a situation in which important, but usually infrequent and unpredictable, events may occur. These types of tasks are typically referred to as vigilance tasks and are common in the work of air traffic controllers, inspection and quality control personnel, and others engaged in monitoring and surveillance. The literature suggests that sustained attention generally does not show age-related decrements (Berardi et al., 2001; Carriere et al., 2010).

Memory

Declines in **memory** are one of the most common complaints among older adults and can cause psychological distress and worry. Survey data from 21 states indicated that approximately 13 percent of Americans age 60 years and older reported confusion and memory loss (CDC, 2013).

As discussed below, there are many forms of memory. Some elements of memory are fairly stable in older adulthood, while others decline, and, as emphasized throughout this chapter, considerable variability exists among individuals. The aspects of memory discussed here were chosen because they are important to everyday functioning and have been thoroughly examined in the literature.

Working memory refers to the ability to temporarily hold information in one's mind while it is processed or used. It encompasses the active manipulation of information or the maintenance of some information while dealing concurrently with further incoming information. For example, people listening to instructions on how to take a particular medication rely on working memory to hold the instructions in memory while they process the information for use at a later time. Working memory plays a central role in many activities, such as adherence to a medication schedule (e.g., Insel et al., 2006), and it is a fundamental element of other cognitive abilities such as processing language, solving problems, and making decisions. Working memory is also important to new learning. The rich literature available on the effects of aging on working memory indicates that working memory generally declines with age, especially for complex tasks (e.g., Salthouse, 1994; Zacks et al., 2000).

Long-term memory is the system for relatively permanent memory storage and is the repository of a person's knowledge. There are multiple types of long-term memory.

Semantic long-term memory stores factual information acquired over a lifetime and is often not associated with a particular time or place. Semantic memory is used when a person provides answers to factual questions, such as naming the current president of the United States or a state capital. Older adults typically perform as well as young adults on tasks testing this type of memory (Craik and Jennings, 1992; Nilsson, 2003; Spaniol et al., 2006). In fact, an individual's accumulated semantic knowledge and memory increase into the sixth and seventh decades of life and only a slight decline may be seen subsequently (Brickman and Stern, 2009). People may have some difficulty with retrieving semantic information if it has not been accessed for some time, but generally the information can be retrieved with the appropriate cues.

Episodic memory is the memory of autobiographical events, including times, places, associated emotions, and other contextual information. Episodic memory is relevant to events of both the recent and the distant past. This type of memory tends to decline with age, and the declines are greater when the task demands are more complex or when there are few environmental supports or cues available (e.g., writing a note to oneself about where the car was parked this morning) (Craik and McDowd, 1987; Mitchell, 1989).

Prospective memory is another type of long-term memory. It is the ability to remember to do something in the future, such as take a medication or pick up the dry cleaning, and it can be time-based or event-based. Time-based prospective memory is remembering to do something at a later time, such as to go to a doctor's appointment next Tuesday at 2 p.m. Event-based prospective memory is remembering to do something after an event, such as meeting a friend after the appointment. Age-related declines occur in both types of prospective memory, but the declines are usually greater for time-based prospective memory (Henry et al., 2004; Maylor et al., 2002). The declines appear more pronounced for event-based tasks that require higher levels of controlled processing (e.g., effortful processing, which requires attentional capacity) than for those supported by relatively more automatic processes (e.g., very well-learned tasks, which require little attentional capacity). In addition, the effects of age on prospective memory appear to be greater when tested in laboratory tasks than when tested using more naturalistic tasks (Henry et al., 2004).

Procedural memory, also known as skill learning, refers to learning and remembering how to perform an activity such as driving a car, riding a bicycle, cooking a favorite recipe, or using a software program. Generally, this type of memory is built up gradually over time as a function of practice. Well-learned procedures such as driving or typing become automatic and can be performed without high levels of conscious processing or attentional resources. Older adults do not usually have trouble doing procedures that are automatic or well learned, and they can learn to do new procedures with practice (Backman et al., 2001). Distinguishing between performance time, learning, and memory for a task is important. For example, older adults may perform tasks more slowly when procedural memory is required, and they may learn procedural sequences at a slower rate than younger adults, but they can still maintain the procedural aspects of the task (e.g., how to type) and can learn new procedures (Brickman and Stern, 2009).

Finally, there is **source memory,** which relates to the context or details surrounding an event, particular fact, or piece of information. This is different from remembering the content of the information. For example, people might remember a news story but forget when they first received the information or whether they read it in a newspaper or heard it on television. Similarly, they might remember that a friend is retiring but forget who told them the information. Research findings indicate that source memory can decline with age and that aging has a greater effect on source memory than it does on the memory of content (Glisky et al., 2001; Spencer and Raz, 1995; Trott et al., 1997).

Executive Function

Executive function refers to the cognitive skills used to regulate behavior and modify responses based on environmental cues. This includes the ability to plan actions (e.g., paying bills or creating schedules), to organize information, to think abstractly, to allocate mental resources (cognitive flexibility), to reason, to solve novel problems, to adapt to new situations, and to act appropriately during social interactions. Generally, executive function declines with age (Zelazo et al., 2004).

Tests evaluating set-shifting (i.e., the ability to move back and forth between tasks) show significant changes with age. For example, performance on the Visual-Verbal Test (in which participants are asked to look at a series of cards and indicate how three of the four objects on each card are alike in one way and then indicate how three of the objects are alike in another way) declines substantially with age. These changes appear to be related to the difficulty that older participants have with switching from one abstract answer to another (e.g., they tend to get the first item correct but the second item wrong) (Albert et al., 1990).

Series completion tests also show substantial declines with age. These tests generally require the participant to examine a series of letters or numbers and to determine the rule that governs the sequencing of the items in the series. Cross-sectional and longitudinal data both demonstrate age-related declines on tasks of this sort (e.g., Lachman and Jelalian, 1984; Schaie, 1983).

Proverb interpretation tests, which require the participant to provide the general meaning of a proverb (e.g., "Barking dogs seldom bite."), also demonstrate age-related declines (Albert et al., 1990). This is true whether participants are asked to provide the meaning of the proverb or are given alternative choices of interpretation.

Declines in executive functioning can affect a person's ability to make decisions, to inhibit responses, and to simultaneously process relevant and irrelevant information. These declines have been linked to declines in ability to perform instrumental activities of daily living, such as medication management (Bell-McGinty et al., 2002).

Reasoning Abilities

Reasoning ability, which is sometimes considered an aspect of executive function, also declines with age. It reflects logical thinking, or the process of drawing conclusions from information to inform problem solving or make decisions, such as medical or financial decisions. (The societal implications of declines in reasoning ability are discussed in detail in Chapter 6.) There is a distinction between deductive and inductive reasoning. Deductive reasoning allows a person to draw conclusions about specific events or situations based on premises or general theories assumed to be true, whereas inductive reasoning allows a person to draw general conclusions based on specific observations. Overall, the literature from laboratory tests of reasoning indicates that both of these abilities decline with age in a fairly linear way, beginning in middle adulthood (e.g., Salthouse, 2004).

Language

Language function consists of an array of abilities, including understanding and producing speech, reading, writing, and naming. It is a fundamental component of human behavior and a primary mechanism for communication. Language processing is a critical element of cognitive tasks (e.g., the ability to understand written and spoken instructions) and social interactions. For example, older adults whose hearing loss impedes their understanding of spoken language may withdraw from social interaction (Mick et al., 2014). This is noteworthy not only because social interaction is important to quality of life for many people but also because limited social interaction may contribute to cognitive decline (see Chapter 4B).

Age-related effects on language abilities vary as a function of the ability being investigated: Some aspects of language function decline, while others do not. Although vocabulary does not decline until very old age (Burke and Shafto, 2008; Schaie, 1994, 2005), language production skills do decline with age. These are word-finding failures and language disfluencies, such as the phenomenon of "having a word on tip of the tongue" or pausing for longer intervals while speaking (Burke and Shafto, 2008; Kemper and Herman, 2006). The syntactic complexity of spoken language also tends to decline with age (Kemper and Sumner, 2001), and older adults generally produce sentences with lower idea density than younger adults (for a review, see Burke and Shafto, 2008). Older adults may also experience more difficulty spelling familiar words (Abrams and Stanley, 2004). However, the comprehension of the meaning of words is typically well-preserved in older age. With respect to speech comprehension, older adults generally have difficulty understanding spoken language that is distorted or too rapid (Wingfield and Grossman, 2006; Wingfield et al., 1999). Thus, it may be difficult for them to comprehend loudspeaker messages such as gate announcements in airports, or synthetic speech messages such as those used in interactive telephone messaging systems.

Spatial Ability

Spatial ability—the maintenance and manipulation of visual images—also generally declines with age (Techentin et al., 2014; Willis and Schaie,

1986). More specifically, spatial ability includes the abilities to produce figures, to recognize familiar faces, to form relationships among spatial locations, and to copy and match objects and pictures. Older adults do not perform as well as younger adults on spatial tasks requiring mental rotation, visualization abilities, or remembering the location of objects (e.g., Dobson et al., 1995; Hertzog and Rypma, 1991; Light and Zelinski, 1983). These abilities are important for tasks such as learning environmental layouts and routes, wayfinding, map reading, and translating directions. They also influence performance on computer tasks, such as editing text and using a spreadsheet, and searching map- and computer-based information (Pak et al., 2006b), and navigating telephone menu systems (Pak et al., 2006a).

Furthermore, compared to younger individuals, older people are less able to depict and perceive the three-dimensionality of drawings. In one study in which young and old adults (mean ages 21 and 67 years, respectively) were asked to draw a cube, the drawings by the older adults were rated as less accurate than those of the younger adults (Plude et al., 1986). The older participants were also less accurate in determining the adequacy of drawings of cubes that were distorted to varying degrees. They were, however, equally capable of copying an image of a cube when they were given cues about the size of the lines.

Intelligence

In the course of day-to-day activity, individuals combine many of these previously described cognitive domains in order to function. **Intelligence** is a multifaceted construct that refers to the ability to solve problems, plan, think abstractly, and adapt to and learn from everyday experiences. Cognitive abilities are the underlying processes or mechanisms of intelligence.

Intelligence is most commonly measured on one or more standardized tests that produce an intelligence quotient (IQ) score, which indicates how far an individual deviates from the average for that person's age group. Different types of intelligence are discussed in the literature, including emotional intelligence (the ability to monitor one's own and other people's emotions, discriminate among different types of emotions, and use emotional information to guide behavior) and practical intelligence, or everyday competence.

Differentiating between crystallized intelligence and fluid intelligence can be useful when discussing aging and cognition. **Crystallized intelligence,** or **crystallized abilities,** reflects a person's knowledge, such as language skills or knowledge about a particular topic, while **fluid intelligence,** or **fluid abilities,** is involved in processing current or new information, such as learning to play chess. Fluid abilities reflect a person's capacity to think logically and solve problems in novel situations, and they aid in skill acquisition and learning. Data from both cross-sectional (comparisons among different age groups at a single point in time) and longitudinal (examination of a change in a cohort over time) studies indicate that crystallized abilities tend to remain stable, with only modest age-related decline until the very latter decades, whereas declines in fluid abilities begin earlier and are more gradual across the life span (Schaie, 1996).

Wisdom

Like intelligence, **wisdom**, a construct that has a relatively short history of independent investigation within the realm of cognitive aging, is multidimensional and has been viewed from a number of theoretical perspectives and defined in a variety of ways. The definition most germane to this report considers wisdom to be an expert knowledge system and emphasizes the amount and use of knowledge that someone has accumulated in life and how that person is able to use and apply this knowledge (Baltes and Smith, 1990; Kunzmann and Baltes, 2003). Wisdom encompasses expertise and mastery of life matters that require insight, judgment, management of life circumstances and events, life planning, and personal conduct.

Wisdom goes beyond descriptive knowledge and entails a deeper interpretive understanding of knowledge (Ardelt and Hunhui, 2010). Overall, wisdom includes cognitive, reflective, and affective elements (Ardelt, 2004). For example, wisdom-related expertise is important in providing advice on relationship conflicts or in planning for retirement. With respect to aging, wisdom needs to be examined from a life span perspective in the sense that it begins developing in adolescence and early adulthood. Wisdom-related knowledge often remains stable in older adulthood (e.g., Baltes and Smith, 1990; Staudinger, 1999). However, studies comparing age differences in wisdom are relatively few and, just as there are differences in definitions of wisdom, the manner in which wisdom is measured also varies (for a review, see Jeste and Oswald, 2014).

Assessment of Cognitive Abilities

Examples of standard measures used to evaluate each domain of cognition are in Box 2-1. A wide variety of such measures is available for research and clinical use, and there is some controversy about which measures are optimal for each domain and population of interest. For example, people from racial or ethnic minority backgrounds might not do as well on certain tests as the rest of the population even though their cognitive ability being tested may be perfectly intact. The National Institutes of Health (NIH) has developed the NIH Toolbox for the Assessment of Neurological and Behavioral Function® to harmonize the measurement of functioning across diverse study designs and settings. The NIH Toolbox® includes a set of brief measures (validated for use in individuals who are ages 3 to 85 years old) that can be used to assess cognitive, emotional, motor, and sensory function (Weintraub et al., 2013). The specific cognitive functions measured are executive function, episodic memory, language, processing speed, working memory, and attention.

At one time it was thought that specific cognitive functions were located within certain regions of the brain. For example, poor performance on the Wisconsin Card Sorting Test, a measure of executive function, was thought to be indicative of damage to the dorsolateral frontal lobes, but performance on this test is now known to be affected by damage to a number of different structures and neuronal pathways that serve this aspect of executive function. In fact, the vast majority of cognitive processes, such as memory, executive function, visuospatial abilities, and processing speed, are known to be related to highly sophisticated networks containing tens of millions of neurons. This emphasizes the need for continued development of sophisticated neurocognitive batteries as well as neuroimaging modalities that allow for structural analysis of brain connectivity. As will be discussed below, additional information can be derived from studying the associations between functional capabilities and performance on neuropsychological tests.

VARIABILITY IN COGNITIVE CHANGES

A few important caveats need to be noted concerning the above discussion. Life expectancy has increased due to changes in lifestyle and advances in medical care, and increasing numbers of people are living into their 80s, 90s, and beyond (see Chapter 1). People at 60 or 70 years of age are typically very different from people in their 80s, who are different from those 90 years or older. The prevalence of various diseases that affect cognition, such as cardiovascular diseases, diabetes, and dementia, increases greatly with advancing age, and sensory declines also may be magnified. Careful consideration needs to be given to what defines cognitive aging for younger older adults as compared to the oldest older adults. Even though there is limited research examining cognition in very old age, the available evidence shows deterioration in cognitive functioning in this population. A 6-year study examining changes in cognitive abilities in a sample of twin pairs age 80 years and older who did not have dementia found that all aspects of cognition that were assessed (memory, reasoning, processing speed, and verbal ability) declined in a linear fashion during that period (Johansson et al., 2004). The decline was evident even for those aspects of cognition that are less vulnerable to age-related effects, such as verbal abilities. Similarly, 6-year longitudinal data from a sample of adults age 70 years and older who were enrolled in the Berlin Aging Study demonstrated that perceptual speed, memory, and fluency declined with age, while knowledge remained stable up to about 90 years of age and then declined thereafter (Singer et al., 2003).

Another key caveat, stated previously, is that the aging population is extremely heterogeneous, with older adults varying in their abilities and in the longitudinal course of their cognitive aging because of differences in genetics and experiences over the life span. Studies examining aging and cognition or aging and learning often differentiate between two types of variability: Inter-individual variability refers to the differences among people or groups of people, and intra-individual variability refers to the changes that occur within one person over time.

One type of inter-individual variability is the variability observed in comparisons of people in different age groups. When comparing younger and older adults on a variety of performance measures (e.g., processing speed or working memory), researchers often find that older adults, as a group, do not perform as well as younger people (e.g., Schaie, 1996). However, there is such tremendous variability in performance that some older people might perform as well as or better than some younger adults. For example, a study examining Internet search abilities among older and younger people indicated that, on average, the younger adults performed better on the search problems. However, some older participants performed at the same level as or better than the younger participants (e.g., Sharit et al., 2008). Also, sometimes differences found in these types of studies may not be entirely due to the effects of aging but may also be a function of cohort or generational differences. For example, skill using a computer or the Internet demonstrates a cohort difference between today's younger and older adults; unlike younger adults, today's older adults did not grow up using computers and therefore would not be expected to be as fluent with computer and Internet use.

Inter-individual variability also occurs among individuals within the same age group. Older adults vary widely in educational background, health status, literacy, culture, ethnicity, skills, abilities, and life experiences. These differences contribute to vast inter-individual variability among people of the same age and can make predicting performance based solely on age less precise as people increase in age and their differences in experience add up. Intra-individual variability, by contrast, is examined in studies that measure performance across two or more sessions. In longitudinal studies, these sessions are typically spread over a period of years, with the performance of the same people measured every 5 or 10 years. Intra-individual variability can also be seen over shorter periods of time, even days, due to such factors as fatigue, acute illness, distractions, or attention lapses.

A third caveat is that the cognitive trajectory over time is not necessarily smooth or linear but rather may be a dynamic process with ups and downs due, for example, to environmental stressors, medications, or illnesses. Many of these factors are reversible, and there is much that can be done to prevent declines (see Chapters 4A, 4B, and 4C).

A fourth caveat is that aging is not just a picture of decline. As will be discussed later in this chapter, neural plasticity is retained as people age, so older adults can learn new skills and their performance can improve. For example, results from the ACTIVE trial, which examined the benefits of cognitive training on various aspects of cognitive ability, showed that training in speed of processing and reasoning resulted in cognitive improvements in a sample of older adults (e.g., Ball et al., 2002). Older adults also can and do successfully employ compensatory strategies to offset cognitive declines, and they have a wealth of knowledge, skills, and experience that younger adults may not have.

BOUNDARY CONDITIONS

As noted in Chapter 1, this report focuses on cognitive aging as opposed to the cognitive changes associated with age-related diseases of the brain, such as neurodegenerative dementias, including Alzheimer's disease. The committee recognizes that much remains to be done to fully understand the boundary between cognitive aging and the initial phase of a neurodegenerative disorder, but it has concluded that a sufficient body of knowledge concerning cognitive aging exists to support distinguishing it from neurodegeneration and therefore to draw meaningful conclusions about cognitive aging and to make substantive recommendations for future directions.

The challenge of identifying boundaries between conditions is not unique. In the field of neurocognitive disorders, for example, the syndrome of mild cognitive impairment (MCI)[1] is considered an interim clinical diagnostic phase between the time when an individual's cognitive function falls within the normal range and the time when that person meets criteria for dementia. International studies have focused on participants with MCI (Petersen, 2004; Winblad et al., 2004), and consensus criteria have been established that are in wide use (Albert et al., 2011; Dubois et al., 2014). Nevertheless, it remains challenging to determine the boundary between cognitive aging and MCI. These diagnostic challenges remain for several reasons: (1) The clinical diagnosis of MCI is usually based not only on whether a person's performance falls within the "normal range" on cognitive testing but also on how well that individual is functioning on a daily

---

[1] The *Diagnostic and Statistical Manual of Mental Disorders, 5th Edition*, refers to MCI as "mild neurocognitive disorder" (APA, 2013).

basis, and information about this usually depends on inherently subjective self-reports or the reports of an informant who knows the individual well. (2) Medical illnesses or life stressors can have a temporary effect on cognition such that when the conditions are alleviated, a person previously thought to be on a downward trajectory may recover cognitive functions. (3) A range of disorders can cause progressive cognitive decline, and the symptoms of these disorders are quite varied, which means that the group of individuals that meets the criteria for MCI can be heterogeneous in terms of cognition and function. MCI is a syndromic label, capturing a variety of causes which include neurodegenerative diseases and cognitive aging. Differentiating between these causes can be challenging because the symptoms and signs are mild. It requires a clinical assessment and sometimes a series of assessments. Cognitive testing and imaging can help to distinguish among individuals with neurodegeneration or cognitive aging. For all of the foregoing reasons, not all individuals with MCI progress to dementia, and some may even improve over time. These diagnostic challenges are particularly problematic in epidemiological settings, where it may be difficult to obtain reliable information from an informant who knows the individual well. For similar reasons, it is often difficult to determine whether an individual is in the late phase of MCI or the early phase of dementia, as this distinction typically depends on the person's degree of functional impairment in daily life, and functional impairment is often difficult to quantify because it depends on the subjective report of another person who knows the individual well. These diagnostic challenges can result in mislabeling an individual as irreversibly impaired.

Substantial efforts are under way to improve the accuracy of cognition-related diagnoses by using biological measures of underlying pathology, often referred to as "biomarkers." For example, the revised diagnostic criteria for MCI and dementia due to Alzheimer's disease now include the use of biomarkers to facilitate the determination of whether the underlying neurodegenerative process of Alzheimer's disease is the cause of the observed cognitive decline. The use of biomarkers as criteria for diagnosis is an active and evolving area of research (Albert et al., 2011; McKhann et al., 2011; Sperling et al., 2011).

Similar challenges exist in the study of depression with, for example, the difficulty of distinguishing the boundaries between sadness, grief, and depression. Nevertheless, despite the difficulty in determining definitive boundaries between mental states, objective studies using operational criteria have permitted the study of depression in populations and led to improved treatments.

An emerging challenge to defining the boundaries between cognitive aging and disease is the more recent recognition of preclinical stages of neurodegenerative diseases such as Alzheimer's and Parkinson's diseases

(Sperling et al., 2011; Wu et al., 2011). The term describes a novel but not yet validated stage for which identification does not rely on a patient's signs and symptoms, such as disabling impairments in cognition or movement, but instead measures pathobiology, such as the presence of amyloid as measured by imaging or the presence of autosomal dominant genes. If diagnosis at this stage of disease becomes part of clinical practice, then investigators of cognitive aging will need to decide whether to include otherwise healthy persons who have preclinical disease in future studies of cognitive aging. This issue is further examined later in this chapter in the section on norms.

AGE-RELATED CHANGES IN COGNITION—
INSIGHTS FROM ANIMAL MODELS

The central premise of studying animal models is that if age-related changes in cognition found in humans are also found in other species, it increases the likelihood that the cognitive changes are related to aging and not to early signs of neurodegenerative disorders common in humans, such as Alzheimer's disease. Studies in animals, like those in humans, have focused on subjects that are healthy, with the added advantage that animal models do not develop human neurodegenerative disorders. As a result, research in animal models has been particularly important in demonstrating that the cognitive changes seen with advancing age are related to aging, as opposed to disease.

The two areas of cognition that have been most widely studied across species are memory, as mediated by the hippocampus and other areas of the medial temporal lobe, and executive function, which is highly dependent on the prefrontal cortex. Given the extensive involvement of these two brain regions in the cognitive functions vulnerable to aging, most studies aimed at revealing the biological basis of cognitive aging have targeted these regions.

The following sections of the chapter review how animal models inform the neuropsychological and biological basis of age-related cognitive changes and the mechanisms that may explain these changes. While some cognitive functions, such as language, do not correlate well between humans and animals, others do allow comparable measures. This report focuses on three that do: attention, memory, and executive function.

Attention

Functions related to attention, including vigilance, orienting of attention, and cognitive flexibility, have a vulnerability to aging that can be observed in animal models. Aged rats show impairments in choice reaction time tasks that are thought to reflect vigilance (Jones et al., 1995; Moore et al., 1992; Muir et al., 1999), and these impairments are similar to age-related declines in vigilance in humans (Parasuraman et al., 1989). The ability to focus attention on a designated spatial location in the environment appears to be largely spared in older monkeys (Baxter and Voytko, 1996), mirroring the relative preservation of this function in older adult humans without dementia (Greenwood et al., 1993). Cognitive flexibility and the capacity to shift attention to different sensory inputs in the course of problem-solving is impaired in aged rodents (Barense et al., 2002) as it is in older humans (Robbins et al., 1998). In short, a substantial correspondence in multiple domains of attention has been observed in both animal models and humans. (For a review, see Bizon et al., 2012.)

Memory

Episodic memory performance has been studied extensively in healthy monkeys and rodents across their life spans. The Delayed NonMatching to Sample task (DNMS) is used to assess recognition memory in the nonhuman primate. In this task, the monkey is required to indicate which of two objects was most recently presented. Monkeys may show either a deficit on learning the task, which likely involves the prefrontal cortex, or a deficit in memory as the delay gets longer, which is more likely to reflect hippocampal function. Studies using the DNMS have demonstrated that aged monkeys are impaired at learning the nonmatching principle but are only mildly impaired by increasing the delay (Arnsten and Goldman-Rakic, 1990; Bachevalier et al., 1991; Moss et al., 1988; Presty et al., 1987; Rapp and Amaral, 1989). Thus, as is the case for humans, as monkeys age they take longer to learn something new but retain the information reasonably well. Age-related changes can be seen on a very difficult memory task, such as the Delayed Recognition Span Test (DRST). This test requires a monkey to identify a new stimulus from an increasingly large selection of items with which the monkey is familiar. The goal is to keep track of as many stimuli as possible without making a mistake. Middle-aged monkeys are impaired on the spatial version of the DRST but not on the color version (Herndon et al., 1997). Older monkeys are impaired on both versions of the task (Moss et al., 1997). Thus, the performance of monkeys on the spatial version of the test may be functionally equivalent to the performance of humans on difficult delayed recall tests. As with aging humans, performance varies considerably in aging monkeys. Among the oldest animals, some perform as well as younger animals, but the performance average of the group declines substantially with age.

Rodents also display age-related declines in memory tasks. For example, older rats show less exploration than younger rats in a task similar to the visual paired comparison task (Cavoy and Delacour, 1993). Older rats are also impaired, relative to young and middle-aged rats, on the Morris water maze task, in which animals are required to find a platform that is under water (Rapp et al., 1987). Rodents' performance on this task has been shown to be highly dependent on the hippocampus (Morris et al., 1982). These deficits are highly stable over time when a specific combination of learning trials and probe trials are used. Moreover, as with humans and monkeys, there is considerable variability in performance among older rodents: A substantial subgroup shows age-related declines in performance, but some older rodents perform on par with young animals (Rapp et al., 1987).

Executive Function

Changes in executive function in non-human primates have been examined primarily by using reversal learning paradigms (Bartus et al., 1979; Rapp, 1990) or a form of delayed response (Bachevalier, 1993). Reversal learning entails responding to a change in reinforcement rules by first unlearning, or breaking, the initial stimulus–reinforcement bond that had been learned, and then shifting to a new one. In this way, reversal learning can be a measure of executive function and, by extension, a reflection of the integrity of the prefrontal cortex. Data show that when compared to young monkeys, older monkeys have trouble unlearning established stimulus–reward contingencies, particularly when they are based on spatial location, thus demonstrating impaired spatial reversal learning (Lai et al., 1995). Moreover, in tests of both spatial and object reversal learning, older adult monkeys tend to continue making the same response even though it is not rewarded.

Comparable findings have been reported on a task called the Conceptual Set Shifting Task, which was developed for non-human primates as an equivalent to the Wisconsin Card Sorting Test in humans (Moore et al., 2003). In the version for non-human primates, a pattern of responding is developed on the basis of rewards for responses to a specific visual pattern. The animal maintains this response pattern for a while, and then the reward contingency changes. One can therefore examine the number of errors prior to attainment of the initial abstraction rule as well as the number of perseverative responses after the rule changes. Older adult monkeys are impaired relative to young monkeys on both the concept formation and the set-shifting aspects of the task (Moore et al., 2003).

Executive function is dependent on working memory, which is also mediated by the prefrontal cortex. Working memory can be tested in monkeys by using a delayed response task, which requires the monkey to remember an initial visual stimulus over extended delays and to choose it in preference to a new stimulus when the two are presented simultaneously (Rapp and

Amaral, 1989). Monkeys show age-related declines in this task, particularly as the delays lengthen (Rapp and Amaral, 1989; Wang et al., 2011).

NEURAL MECHANISMS THAT CONTRIBUTE TO AGE-RELATED CHANGE IN COGNITIVE FUNCTION

Studies of brain tissue both in humans and in animal models have sought to examine the underlying neural mechanisms that may be responsible for the age-related changes in cognition described above. This research includes studies of neuronal number, synaptic integrity, and neurotransmitter changes. Overall, the studies show that while the number of neurons remains relatively stable, changes occur in their structure and in their neurotransmitter receptors—changes that likely explain the cognitive declines discussed above. The stability in the number of neurons number—that is, the lack of neuron death in areas supporting cognition—seen with aging in these studies is in contrast to the extensive neuron loss that occurs in Alzheimer's disease.

Neuronal Number in Aging

A wealth of human anatomical data indicates that in the cortex neuronal loss with advancing age is either not significant or not as extensive as reports had suggested prior to 1984 (Anderson et al., 1983; Brody, 1955, 1970; Colon, 1972; Henderson et al., 1980; Shefer, 1973). Although large neurons appear to shrink, few are lost (Terry et al., 1987).

Interestingly, research in monkeys has produced comparable findings. The absence of neuron loss with increasing age in monkeys has been shown in multiple cortical areas, including the prefrontal cortex (O'Donnell et al., 1999; Peters et al., 1994; Vincent et al., 1989). These conclusions are based both on a comparison of the number of neurons in young and old monkeys and on an examination of the cortical tissue by electron microscopy (Peters et al., 1998). Studies in rodents have reported comparable findings (Rapp et al., 2002).

Post-mortem data from humans and monkeys show that age-related neuronal loss does not occur in the hippocampus (Amaral, 1993; Gomez-Isla et al., 1996; Rosene, 1993; West, 1993) or in the entorhinal cortex (Gazzaley et al., 1997), which is tightly linked to the hippocampus both structurally and functionally. Equivalent data have been reported in rodents: Even in the subset of animals with declines on a memory task that depends on the hippocampus, there was no decrease in the number of neurons in the various regions of the hippocampus (Rapp and Gallagher, 1996). Thus, while there are clear age-related declines in cognitive functions mediated by the hippocampus and prefrontal cortex, they are not due to a loss of neurons.

These findings are in striking contrast to the extensive neuronal loss seen in Alzheimer's disease, and they support the conclusion that age-related cognitive decline does not result simply from a milder form of neuron loss; rather, it is more likely to involve changes in neurons that are still living yet functionally compromised. (For a more detailed review of these issues, see Morrison and Hof, 1997.)

Synaptic Integrity

Even though there does not appear to be enough neuronal loss to account for age-related cognitive change, other changes in neuronal function—specifically, the number and function of synapses—may contribute to age-related cognitive changes. Studies in non-human primates have shown that with advancing age, specific subclasses of dendritic spines are selectively lost in the dorsolateral prefrontal cortex, and the density of these spines correlates with working memory performance (Dumitriu et al., 2010). The specific loss of the spines is important because they are known to be the most plastic spines, suggesting that it is not just a loss of synapses with aging that drives cognitive decline but, more specifically, it is the loss of synaptic plasticity that is key (Morrison and Baxter, 2012).

In contrast, in the hippocampus it is the largest, most stable, and most complex synapses that are selectively lost with age, and their number correlates with memory performance (Hara et al., 2012; Morrison and Baxter, 2012). Studies in rodents show comparable changes. For example, older rodents with spatial learning deficits display substantial decreases in the number of synapses (Smith et al., 2000) and alterations in synapse function, suggesting that a loss of synaptic plasticity with aging leads to memory deficits (Norris et al., 1996; Rosenzweig and Barnes, 2003).

Neurotransmitter Changes

The age-related synaptic alterations described above have been linked with neurotransmitter changes, particularly in the functioning of the AMPA receptor (α-amino-3-hydroxy-5-methyl-4-isoxazolepropionic acid receptor). AMPA receptors have been linked to learning, memory, and synaptic plasticity. For example, within some synapses in the hippocampus of monkeys there is an age-related decrease in the number of AMPA receptors, and the extent of the decrease is predictive of declines in performance on a memory task (Hara et al., 2012). Additionally, alterations in certain regions that project to the cortex in humans and animals (e.g., the basal forebrain and the locus coeruleus) are likely responsible for decreases in the production of neurotransmitters, such as norepinephrine, which is important for cognitive function (Robbins and Arnsten, 2009).

White Matter Changes

Studies have found age-related alterations in the brain's white matter—the myelin sheath surrounding neuronal axons (Nielsen and Peters, 2000; Peters, 1996; Peters et al., 1994). Evidence from non-human primates suggests that the oligodendrocytes, which are responsible for forming white matter, may be less efficient with age. For example, a comparison of the oligodendrocytes of young and old monkeys showed that the myelin sheaths in the old monkeys were abnormal and appeared to be degenerating (Peters, 1996). However, when investigators compared the number of axons in old and young monkeys, the axon number was largely unchanged, and relatively few degenerating axons were found in the old monkeys (Nielsen and Peters, 2000). Because the myelin sheath enhances signal conduction down the axon, these age-related alterations may explain some of the age-related changes seen in neural processing speed.

Neuronal Proliferation in the Adult Brain

The adult brain has the capacity for neuronal replacement. Ample evidence indicates that new neurons are generated in the hippocampus and olfactory system in both monkeys (Gould et al., 1999; Kornack and Rakic, 1999) and humans (Eriksson et al., 1998). The proliferation of new neurons decreases with age. In rodents, there appears to be a gradual increase in total numbers of neurons; in primates, such an accumulation is less certain. It has been suggested that the number of neurons in the primate hippocampus is constant, with a balance maintained between the generation of new neurons and the rate of neuron death and cell removal (Kornack and Rakic, 1999).

Summary of Findings from Animal Models

When the findings in animal models are juxtaposed with observations from humans, together they suggest that the variability seen in cognitive changes with advancing age among healthy individuals is related to variations in synaptic integrity and synaptic plasticity in specific brain circuits that are tightly linked to cognitive functions, such as memory and executive function (see Morrison and Baxter, 2014, for a more detailed discussion). The fact that comparable changes are found among both healthy non-human primates and healthy rodents increases the likelihood that such changes in humans are not the result of a neurodegenerative disorder such as Alzheimer's disease.

These age-associated alterations have a clear effect on daily function, which will be discussed later in this chapter. Importantly, synapse loss is potentially reversible, whereas neuron death is not, which suggests a natural therapeutic target for sustaining synaptic and cognitive health. Synapse loss has been described in humans very early in the transition from normal cognitive function to cognitive decline that may represent the earliest stages of Alzheimer's disease (Scheff et al., 2006). Synaptic alterations in humans may leave certain neurons vulnerable to the degeneration that occurs in Alzheimer's disease, which suggests that early intervention at the synaptic level may be key to preventing the transition to Alzheimer's disease.

While it appears that the loss of synapses without significant neuron loss contributes to cognitive decline, the cause of synapse loss is unknown, as is the extent to which such loss is linked to other age-related brain changes (e.g., vascular changes). In fact, pathologic alterations (e.g., tau and beta-amyloid accumulation) that have been linked to Alzheimer's disease have also been seen in older adults with unimpaired cognition, although the changes in these cases are less clearly linked to neuron death than they are in Alzheimer's disease dementia cases, and the degree to which this more moderate pathology promotes synapse loss is not known. In addition, pathology can differ by brain region, with virtually all adults approximately 70 years of age or older having some tau deposits in the entorhinal cortex (Bouras et al., 1994), but it is not clear how such restricted pathology affects cognitive function. It is also important to acknowledge that there are many protective factors that influence cognitive aging, as noted elsewhere in this report. Taken together, these findings suggest that cognitive aging represents a balance of lifelong risk and protective factors that include both neuropathologies and other factors that preserve or impair the organization and maintenance of brain structures and circuits. While the pathologic conditions associated with Alzheimer's disease have been linked to neuron loss and dementia, the middle ground, where events lead to cognitive aging in the absence of neurodegeneration, remains poorly understood and requires further investigation both in humans and in animal models.

COGNITIVE RESERVE AND PLASTICITY

Though all brains age, they do not all age at the same rate or in the same way. For example, multiple studies have demonstrated that a person may function well and yet have the pathology characteristic of Alzheimer's disease at autopsy (Crystal et al., 1988; Katzman et al., 1988; Morris et al., 1996; Price and Morris, 1999).

Why do some people have good cognitive function despite a level of brain injury that impairs function in others? The concept of cognitive reserve has been proposed as an explanation for why some people are able to tolerate the brain alterations associated with dementia (and other illnesses) without exhibiting the associated symptoms (Scarmeas and Stern, 2004). Factors that may contribute to cognitive reserve include education, occupational attainment, physical activity, and engagement in intellectual and social activities (Tucker and Stern, 2011). Though some factors that increase risk for cognitive decline and dementia, such as genes, are not readily modified, a number of factors that contribute to cognitive reserve can be enhanced, even later in life. Various studies have shown a positive effect in older adults from maintaining an active social network (Graham et al., 2014; Magnezi et al., 2014) and keeping physically fit, although the quality of evidence in some studies is not strong (Anderson et al., 2014; Carvalho et al., 2014; also see Chapter 4A).

The proposed mechanism by which cognitive reserve operates is through enhancement of neural plasticity. Animal studies indicate that certain factors inhibit or promote the brain's capacity to generate new neurons, even in adulthood. Negative factors include inflammation, damage from free radical forms of oxygen, and vascular changes associated with age, while positive factors include exercise and mental stimulation (Lee et al., 2012). People with greater cognitive reserve also appear more readily able to access alternate neural networks when their primary networks are damaged (Tucker and Stern, 2011).

In sum, cognitive function in an older person is not solely determined by the amount of pathology associated with brain-related diseases such as Alzheimer's disease. Rather, the level of cognitive function may represent a balance between the extent of changes in the brain and the brain's ability to compensate through cognitive reserve.

CHALLENGES AND OPPORTUNITIES IN DEFINING AND ASSESSING COGNITIVE AGING

Relationship Between Cognitive Aging and Functioning in Daily Life

Age-associated changes in cognitive abilities can challenge older people's ability to perform everyday tasks such as managing medications or finances, negotiating complex environments, or learning something new. This is especially salient in a technology-driven world where people regularly need to learn and interact with new systems and new ways of performing routine tasks. Technology is integral to many aspects of life and is changing how people work, communicate, manage finances and health care, shop, and perform other routine activities. The rapid pace of technological innovation will require that people continue to learn and adapt to new ways of doing things. Being able to successfully manage these adaptations and to learn new systems and tasks requires cognitive skills and abilities. In essence, cognitive function depends on one's ability to meet the sensory and cognitive demands imposed by the system, tasks (requirements implicit in the use of the system), and the environment. A thorough understanding of these demands and how cognitive aging affects an older person's ability to meet them is needed for the development of strategies to successfully negotiate the environment, perform routine tasks, learn new things, and live independently. This in turn requires outcome and performance measures that capture the relevant and critical elements of real-world tasks and environments while maintaining sound psychometric properties.

A broad array of neuropsychological measures can be used to assess and characterize age-related changes in cognition, as detailed earlier in this chapter (see Box 2-1). These measures provide information that is essential to understanding cognitive aging. Furthermore, strong relationships exist between performance on these measures and functional performance, such that individuals who demonstrate higher performance on measures of component cognitive abilities also generally demonstrate higher performance on functional tasks. For example, performance on measures that use working memory and reasoning is indicative of performance on computer-based tasks such as searching the Internet (e.g., Czaja et al., 2010) and the ability to manage medications (Insel et al., 2006; Stilley et al., 2010). Similarly, processing speed and attention are predictors of driving performance (Ball and Owsley, 2003; Ball et al., 1998; Edwards et al., 2008).

However, standard neuropsychological measures do not capture the complexity of real-world activities or a person's knowledge of everyday tasks. Everyday activities involve a combination of component cognitive abilities and knowledge, and they occur within a context that shapes the demands of a task (Hertzog et al., 2009). For example, an older person using an automated teller machine (ATM) for a banking transaction uses such abilities as working memory and executive function to perform this task. However, using an ATM occurs within a certain context and requires some knowledge of how to use the machine. Performance on this task is likely to be less efficient if the person has limited familiarity with the use of ATMs, if the ATM is located in a sunny area where the display is difficult to read, or if there is a line of people waiting to use the machine, which can create social pressure and anxiety. More generally, performance in any situation is shaped by a number of factors, including the environmental and social contexts, knowledge and prior experience, health status, the demands of the activity, and available support.

Older adults with cognitive impairment are more likely to fall than those with no impairment. Specifically, attentional capacity, as measured by dual-task or time-sharing paradigms, is linked to gait impairment and the risk of falls. Impairments in executive function may also increase risk of falling (for a review, see Segev-Jacubovski et al., 2011). With regard to spatial abilities, one study found a correlation between impaired spatial cognition and a history of falling, although the sample size was small (Newell et al., 2011). Multimodal interventions that focus on both mobility and cognition may be effective in reducing risk of falling (e.g., Segev-Jacubovski et al., 2011).

Numerous examples in the literature demonstrate that, despite age-related declines on measures of component cognitive abilities, performance on well-learned tasks often shows little decline. For example, although working memory—which typically declines with age—is important to chess performance, it is well-maintained in older adults who actively engage in chess playing (Roring and Charness, 2007). Additionally, studies have shown a relationship between measures of cognitive ability and job performance (e.g., Schmidt and Hunter, 1998, 2004), yet several meta-analyses of age and work performance have found little evidence that older workers are any less productive than younger workers (McEvoy and Cascio, 1989; Waldman and Avolio, 1986). Important factors in the relationship between age and work performance include the demands of the task (e.g., physical demands), worker experience, and the type of performance measures (e.g., supervisory ratings versus some objective measure of performance). Standardized measures of cognition do not capture the complexity of work situations, and for many work tasks older workers are able to use their knowledge, experience, and contextual support mechanisms to compensate for their age-related changes in cognitive ability. In most day-to-day tasks, people are rarely pressed to perform at their maximum level, in contrast to the standards for neuropsychological tests, where the typical expectation is to perform at one's maximum potential.

Another approach to understanding functional competence is to gather information for a given individual from multiple sources. Individuals may overestimate their performance abilities or have inaccurate judgments regarding the presence of cognitive impairment. An informant, such as a spouse, can be another source of information about functional competence. One study showed that informants could reliably assess cognitive change in individuals with MCI, and their ratings correlated with ratings from objective measures of performance (Tsang et al., 2012). Additional sources of information may be especially important for obtaining reliable data because informant ratings may indicate a greater loss of everyday functional ability and cognitive competency than patient ratings. Informant ratings may also have a greater association with objective measures of cognitive performance than patient ratings (Schinka, 2010). Importantly, informant and self-ratings of performance may not always provide information as to sources of performance difficulties, as they tend to focus on global aspects of performance.

Understanding everyday cognition may require a more ecological approach and the identification of measures that have external and ecological validity. Ecological validity is the ability to generalize results to natural or real-world situations, and it depends on capturing the key elements of environments, tasks, and behaviors. In this case, ecological validity is the extent to which outcome measures capture the relevant features of real-world tasks and environments for activities such as driving, health care, financial management, and so on. There is an ongoing focus on developing and validating these types of measures. For example, the Everyday Cognition Battery (Allaire and Marsiske, 1999) is a set of paper-and-pencil tests that include assessment stimuli related to four everyday activities: medication use, financial planning, food preparation, and nutrition. The Everyday Problems Test is another paper-and-pencil measure designed to assess performance on instrumental activities of daily living (Willis and Marsiske, 1993), including problems with telephone use, shopping, meal preparation, housekeeping, transportation, medication use, and finance. The measure assesses a person's ability to solve cognitively challenging everyday tasks related to these domains but does not assess the person's actual ability to perform these tasks in a natural setting. The Revised Observed Tasks of Daily Living (OTDL-R) is a performance measure of everyday problem solving. It includes nine tasks involving medication use, telephone use, and financial management (Diehl et al., 2005). Performance on the OTDL-R has been found to be significantly associated with age, education, self-rated health, paper-and-pencil measures of everyday problem solving, and measures of basic cognitive functioning. However, while competence in basic cognitive abilities is necessary for successfully solving everyday problems, it is not sufficient.

Other investigators have developed ecologically valid simulations of common technology-based work tasks (e.g., Czaja et al., 2001; Sharit and Czaja, 1999) and have also shown that while cognitive abilities are important for performing tasks, other factors such as prior technology experience and the amount of task practice are also important predictors of performance. Researchers have developed a battery of computer-based simulations of common everyday activities, such as the use of an ATM, refilling a prescription, using a ticket kiosk, and medication management (Czaja et al., 2014). Preliminary data indicate that use of the battery is feasible with diverse populations of older adults: It is sensitive to individual differences in abilities, and performance on the battery correlates with performance on standard measures of cognition. And, because real-time performance measures are captured, use of the battery also permits the identification of sources of difficulties in task performance. Such data are critical to the development of strategies that can be used to improve performance. However, these measures need to be validated and normed with larger populations.

Norms and Norming for Cognitive Tests

The cognitive changes seen in aging humans have been documented through cognitive testing in research settings. In the coming years, as a result of public health and health care policy initiatives designed to preserve cognitive health and prevent cognitive losses, cognitive testing will likely become more common outside of these carefully supervised settings, especially among people age 65 years and older. The Centers for Disease Control and Prevention's Healthy Brain Initiative includes action items to improve surveillance, monitoring, and public awareness of cognitive health and impairment (Alzheimer's Association and CDC, 2013). *Healthy People 2020*, the nation's roadmap for health, has among its goals improving the "health, function, and quality of life of older adults" (HHS, 2014).

Medicare beneficiaries have access to cognitive assessment through the Annual Wellness Exam that includes the detection of "any cognitive impairment" (CMS, 2013). Activities and health insurance benefits such as these will increase the likelihood that older adults will undergo cognitive testing, and the dissemination of computer-based, self-administered technologies will likely facilitate testing in settings where the expertise of a neuropsychologist is not available. Automated technologies to test cognition are increasingly common, such as computer-based, Internet-accessed cognitive testing and "brain exercises." Typically, these technologies include feedback to participants about whether their performance is "normal." Although not all of these tests are equally reliable, they may be used by consumers to assess whether they have had cognitive changes that require medical evaluation.

As cognitive testing becomes an increasing part of adults' lives and of how they conceive of their health, society has a collective interest in ensuring that testing is performed responsibly and accurately. The failure to do so may result in people receiving inappropriate labels concerning their cognitive abilities—labels that can lead to stigma, demoralization, and discrimination, or, on the other hand, false reassurance. It may also thwart the ability of policy makers and public health officials to monitor cognitive health and to estimate the prevalence and severity of cognitive impairment and, therefore, the size and urgency of any problems and the kinds of interventions needed to address them. A foundational issue in ensuring the responsible and accurate use of cognitive testing is to develop and update cognitive norms. The following section examines norms and norming, which are essential to ensuring that evaluation is done responsibly and accurately.

Use of Norms to Interpret Cognitive Test Results

After a tester administers a cognitive test to an individual, such as a measure of memory, the tester has a test score result, also called a "raw score." To transform this raw score into a description of the person's cognition, the tester needs to interpret the raw score. Once interpreted, the score becomes a useful measure of that particular person's cognitive ability.

The key to the interpretation is comparing the score to a standard, a process that is called "norming" (Brooks et al., 2011; Busch et al., 2006; Schretlen et al., 2008). Norming is done for the clinical interpretation of cognitive test results, such as the determination of whether someone has cognitive impairment and, if so, whether it aligns with a pattern seen in a neurodegenerative disease—for example, the amnesia seen in Alzheimer's disease. However, norming is not always appropriate. For example, norming for age in research studies examining how aging contributes to cognition would confound the ability to detect the effects and thus would not be appropriate in that context.

The tester can use the score to inform answers to a test-taker's questions, such as "Do I have normal memory?" or "Do I have a disease that is impairing my memory?" To norm a raw score, the tester finds where the individual's score fits along the distribution of scores of a group of people similar to the individual, called a "normative sample." A group is "similar to the individual" if it resembles the individual in one or more characteristics, typically health, age, gender, race, and years of education.

The need to create groups of people described by these characteristics follows from research observations that these characteristics are associated with cognitive performance in cognitively healthy people. Grouping people based on age is sensible because people experience changes in cognitive ability as they develop from infancy to adulthood. Similarly, because cognitive test performance correlates with education, tests typically group representative normative samples into tiers based on education. Gender and especially ethnicity and race are more complex characteristics by which to categorize people because they encompass a host of implicit but unmeasured environmental, economic, social, and cultural factors, such as the quality of education and childhood development, which are associated with cognitive performance (Romero et al., 2009). Cognitive tests designed to assist in the diagnosis of cognitive impairment or to understand how cognition changes along the life span typically use normative samples that exclude people with conditions that impair cognition. If these people were included in a normative sample, their presumably lower scores would decrease the ability of a test to either detect disease or measure changes that are not the result of disease.

Once normed, a test result has meaning—the performance on the test might be interpreted as "average" or "unimpaired," for example—but this meaning is not absolute. Instead, because of the many characteristics that can be used to group people—some of which, such as race and ethnicity, include other characteristics—a normed score is only a measure of a person's "relative standing." It is relative because its meaning comes from comparing the raw score to the normative group that the tester selected (Brooks et al., 2011). For example, a tester may want to assess the memory performance of a 66-year-old woman with MCI compared to other people with MCI. To do this, the tester compares the woman's score to the scores of a group of people with MCI. The result may show that the woman has memory that is above average for a person with MCI, but when compared to a group of older adults without neurodegenerative disease, her memory is likely to be below average, and when compared to a group of young adults, it is likely to be markedly below average.

Challenges in Developing and Using Norms

The accurate interpretation of an individual's cognitive test score requires quality data from an appropriate normative sample (Brooks et al., 2011). Achieving this presents challenges, especially in the cognitive assessment of older adults (Busch et al., 2006), and these challenges appear both in the design and in the interpretation of the norms.

Developing norms Creating a normative sample for a test requires a sample size large enough to limit errors from common statistical problems related to outliers and skewed distributions. This is particularly important in normative samples of older adults. Older adults, especially those more than 75 years old, have accumulated many of the age-related factors that increase variability in cognitive performance. Although having large sample sizes helps improve normative samples, the size of the normative samples for older adults is often small (Busch et al., 2006).

Excluding people with conditions that impair cognition is particularly important in the design of tests to diagnose cognitive impairment. However, this is especially challenging to do with older adults because they have medical, psychiatric, and neurological diseases, and sensory losses, and they take medications that can affect their cognitive performance. Overzealous exclusion of these people cuts off the lower end of normal performance, creating a distribution that lacks the full range of normative sampling. As a result, higher-functioning people may be categorized toward the low end of the distribution, leading to an overestimate of the prevalence of impaired functioning.

The challenge of determining whether to exclude people having conditions that impair cognition is compounded by changing diagnostic criteria.

For example, many cognitive tests developed for older adults did not exclude persons with MCI because this diagnosis was recognized only relatively recently. As a result, normative samples that formerly were considered to be free of people with impairments included people who would now be considered impaired (Busch et al., 2006). Changing concepts of disease support the need to revisit normative samples periodically to be sure that a given sample still represents the group it is supposed to represent.

An emerging issue in creating normative samples is whether the samples should include individuals who at the time of assessment were normal but subsequently were recategorized as impaired. This poses a particular challenge with the proposed criteria for preclinical stages of neurodegenerative diseases. Neurodegenerative diseases, such as Alzheimer's disease, have a prodromal phase prior to onset of MCI or dementia, and perhaps diagnosis using genetic or biomarker tests might be helpful (Dubois et al., 2014; Sperling et al., 2011). Removing from the normative sample the people who later developed MCI or dementia—a practice that is referred to as robust norming—generally changes the original normative sample. These changes can cause people whose test scores are normed using the original sample to be mistakenly labeled as normal, when in fact they may have low normal or impaired cognition (De Santi et al., 2008; Holtzer et al., 2008; Pedraza et al., 2010). However, this outcome was not seen in a biracial sample of rural older adults with low education (Marcopulos and McLain, 2003), perhaps reflecting the challenges of norming cognition in healthy people who have multiple characteristics associated with low test scores independent of disease.

A final challenge in creating norms is that factors associated with cognitive performance themselves vary or undergo changes, which in turn change their association with cognition. Educational attainment is strongly associated with cognitive performance, but the quality of education is not the same from one state or time period to another. Hence, a 70-year-old in 2015 who reports the same number of years of education as a 70-year-old in 2005 may have a different relative standing.

Using norms When a tester is deciding what is the appropriate representative sample against which to norm an individual's raw cognitive test score, the choice of which sample to use may be obvious, requiring little, if any, judgment. In some cases, however, the individual in question may have characteristics that differ from all of the available samples. Combinations of these differences may become complex—for example, a 75-year-old Latino man who reports a childhood of segregated poverty, learning English at 12 years old, followed by attending college and having a career as a doctor. A normative sample of people with these characteristics may not be available, requiring the tester to judge which group this man most closely resembles.

The failure to address these differences can result in an individual's cognitive performance being misclassified, an error that can have notable consequences for an individual and even a population. California Verbal Learning Tests norms that used a well-educated sample have incorrectly classified more than 30 percent of people as "below average" or "impaired" (Brooks et al., 2011). The much-reported finding that African Americans are at greater risk of developing Alzheimer's disease may in fact reflect the lack of adequate representative samples to norm their cognition instead of a greater prevalence of the disease in this population (Barnes and Bennett, 2014).

One solution to the challenges of developing norms and interpreting them for a particular person is repeat testing over time, such as every year. This allows people to serve as their own normative sample. If serial cognitive assessments become more routine—such as being conducted regularly during Annual Wellness Visits—some adults may receive repeated cognitive testing using the same test battery. Documenting their longitudinal performance might have considerable appeal to patients and their health care providers. However, repeat testing can present its own set of challenges. For example, if an individual repeats a test and the score increases, it might indicate cognitive improvement, or it might indicate enhanced performance as a result of previous exposure to the test. In this latter scenario, stable performance scores could mask declines resulting from aging or disease. In addition, feedback on test performance could affect an individual's performance on subsequent tests. Finally, longitudinal assessment still requires norms so that a tester can determine how much change is expected within the parameters of normal variation as opposed to significant decline.

Future Directions for the Development of Norms

The tester's selection of the "appropriate normative comparison group is one of the most important aspects of neuropsychological assessment, particularly as it pertains to older adults" (Busch et al., 2006, p. 134). It is important in older adults because they are likely to experience diseases that impair cognition, have age-related changes in cognition, and have accumulated a lifetime of exposures and experiences that affect cognition. Most fundamentally, the selection of a comparison group reflects values that shape how society thinks about and therefore defines cognitive aging. Using a normative sample that is entirely free of all diseases (both clinical *and* preclinical), conditions, and risk factors that affect cognition would result in the classification of most age-related changes as being "abnormal," thus embedding the value that most change after development is abnormal. Such decisions need to be addressed directly and with knowledge of their potential implications, such as for the prevalence of disease and the social, cultural, and economic effects. These decisions can be informed by examining how other systems account for aging when using norms. For example, the normative values for hemoglobin, blood glucose, and bone mineral density are not adjusted for age. As a result, more people are diagnosed with diseases such as anemia, diabetes, and osteoporosis, respectively. The committee decided that some cognitive changes are to be expected with aging, and this is reflected in the committee's definition of cognitive aging in Chapter 1.

Public health and health care policy initiatives to preserve cognitive health and prevent cognitive losses require a national investment to develop and update high-quality normative samples that are large and sufficiently representative of the demography of Americans—an investment similar to what the United States has made to discover and validate the biomarkers of neurodegenerative diseases (Weiner et al., 2010). These samples should be followed up in order to assess baseline factors that may affect norms, ways that practice effects influence test results, and the interactions between baseline factors and practice effects. This is especially important as researchers define preclinical stages of neurodegenerative diseases.

Measuring literacy rather than a simple count of the years of education may be especially useful in addressing challenges related to quality of education (Dotson et al., 2008; Manly et al., 2005). As measures are developed for widespread clinical and research application using remote technologies and without the supervision of a trained tester, individual users would benefit from knowing how well the measures are normed for people like them. A clearinghouse that compares how individuals perform on different batteries would be useful for assuring the reliable interpretation of results. This investment will allow testers to readily judge which group is the best comparison group for each person so that individuals can receive meaningful answers to important questions about their cognitive health and so that policy makers will have reliable data to inform the surveillance of the nation's cognitive health and the need for interventions.

RECOMMENDATION

Recommendation 1: *Increase Research and Tools for Assessing Cognitive Aging and Cognitive Trajectories*
The National Institutes of Health, the Centers for Disease Control and Prevention, research foundations, academic research institutions, and private-sector companies should expand research on the trajectories of cognitive aging and improve the tools used to assess cognitive changes and their effects on daily function.

Specific needs include
- Studies using a range of assessments (e.g., neuronal injury biomarkers, neuroimaging, postmortem assessments of neu-

ronal integrity) to explore the physiological and structural basis of cognitive aging;
- Non-human animal studies that examine the mechanisms and clinical correlates of cognitive aging and that are designed to inform human cognitive aging;
- Studies to examine the mechanisms underlying interventions that affect the cognitive trajectory;
- Studies to identify and validate novel tools and measures of function that capture the complexities of real-world tasks and are sensitive to early changes in cognition and function; and
- An update of the norms for cognitive function in older adults (including those in the most advanced age groups) to include the consideration of disease, literacy, language, racial and ethnic diversity, culture, and socioeconomic factors.

REFERENCES

Abrams, L., and J. H. Stanley. 2004. The detection and retrieval of spelling in older adults. In *Advances in psychology research, Vol. 33*, edited by S. P. Shohov. Hauppauge, NY: Nova Science Publishers. Pp. 87-109.

Agarwal, S., J. Driscoll, X. Gabaix, and D. Laibson. 2009. *The age of reason: Financial decisions over the life cycle and implications for regulations*. Washington, DC: Brookings Institution. http://www. brookings. Edu/~/media/Projects/BPEA/Fall%202009/2009b_bpea_agarwal.pdf (accessed February 24, 2015).

Albert, M. S., J. Wolfe, and G. Lafleche. 1990. Differences in abstraction ability with age. *Psychology and Aging* 5(1):94-100.

Albert, M. S., S. T. DeKosky, D. Dickson, B. Dubois, H. H. Feldman, N. C. Fox, A. Gamst, D. M. Holtzman, W. J. Jagust, R. C. Petersen, P. J. Snyder, M. C. Carrillo, B. Thies, and C. H. Phelps. 2011. The diagnosis of mild cognitive impairment due to Alzheimer's disease: Recommendations from the National Institute on Aging-Alzheimer's Association workgroups on diagnostic guidelines for Alzheimer's disease. *Alzheimer's & Dementia* 7(3):270-279.

Allaire, J. C., and M. Marsiske. 1999. Everyday cognition: Age and intellectual ability correlates. *Psychology and Aging* 14(4):627-644.

Alzheimer's Association and CDC (Centers for Disease Control and Prevention). 2013. *The Healthy Brain Initiative: The public health road map for state and national partnerships, 2013-2018*. Chicago, IL: Alzheimer's Association. http://www.cdc.gov/aging/pdf/2013-healthy-brain-initiative.pdf (accessed February 25, 2015).

Amaral, D. G. 1993. Morphological analyses of the brain of behaviorally characterized aged nonhuman primates. *Neurobiology of Aging* 14:671-672.

Anderson, D., C. Seib, and L. Rasmussen. 2014. Can physical activity prevent physical and cognitive decline in postmenopausal women?: A systematic review of the literature. *Maturitas* 79(1):14-33.

Anderson, J. M., B. M. Hubbard, G. R. Coghill, and W. Slidders. 1983. The effect of advanced old age on the neurone content of the cerebral cortex. Observations with an automatic image analyser point counting method. *Journal of the Neurological Sciences* 58(2):235-246.

APA (American Psychiatric Association). 2013. *Diagnostic and statistical manual of mental disorders, 5th ed.* Arlington, VA: American Psychiatric Association.
Ardelt, M. 2004. Wisdom as expert knowledge system: A critical review of a contemporary operationalization of an ancient concept. *Human Development* 47(5):257-285.
Ardelt, M., and O. Hunhui. 2010. Wisdom: Definition, assessment, and its relation to successful cognitive and emotional aging. In *Successful cognitive and emotional aging*, edited by D. Jeste and C. Depp. Washington, DC: American Psychiatric Publishing. Pp. 87-113.
Arnsten, A. F., and P. S. Goldman-Rakic. 1990. Analysis of alpha-2 adrenergic agonist effects on the delayed nonmatch-to-sample performance of aged rhesus monkeys. *Neurobiology of Aging* 11(6):583-590.
Bachevalier, J. 1993. Behavioral changes in aged rhesus monkeys. *Neurobiology of Aging* 14(6):619-621.
Bachevalier, J., L. S. Landis, L. C. Walker, M. Brickson, M. Mishkin, D. L. Price, and L. C. Cork. 1991. Aged monkeys exhibit behavioral deficits indicative of widespread cerebral dysfunction. *Neurobiology of Aging* 12(2):99-111.
Backman, L., B. J. Small, and A. Wahlin. 2001. Aging and memory: Cognitive and biological perspectives. In *Handbook of the psychology of aging, 5th ed.*, edited by J. E. Birren and K. W. Schaie. San Diego, CA: Academic Press. Pp. 348-376.
Ball, K., and C. Owsley. 2003. Driving competence: It's not a matter of age. *Journal of the American Geriatrics Society* 51(10):1499-1501.
Ball, K., C. Owsley, B. Stalvey, D. L. Roenker, M. E. Sloane, and M. Graves. 1998. Driving avoidance and functional impairment in older drivers. *Accident Analysis and Prevention* 30(3):313-322.
Ball, K., D. B. Berch, K. F. Helmers, J. B. Jobe, M. D. Leveck, M. Marsiske, J. N. Morris, G. W. Rebok, D. M. Smith, S. L. Tennstedt, F. W. Unverzagt, and S. L. Willis. 2002. Effects of cognitive training interventions with older adults: A randomized controlled trial. *JAMA* 288(18):2271-2281.
Baltes, P. B., and J. Smith. 1990. Toward a psychology of wisdom and its ontogenesis. In *Wisdom: Its nature, origins, and development*, edited by R. J. Sternberg. New York: Cambridge University Press. Pp. 87-120.
Barense, M. D., M. T. Fox, and M. G. Baxter. 2002. Aged rats are impaired on an attentional set-shifting task sensitive to medial frontal cortex damage in young rats. *Learning and Memory* 9(4):191-201.
Barnes, L. L., and D. A. Bennett. 2014. Alzheimer's disease in African Americans: Risk factors and challenges for the future. *Health Affairs* 33(4):580-586.
Bartus, R. T., R. L. Dean, 3rd, and D. L. Fleming. 1979. Aging in the rhesus monkey: Effects on visual discrimination learning and reversal learning. *Journal of Gerontology* 34(2):209-219.
Baxter, M. G., and M. L. Voytko. 1996. Spatial orienting of attention in adult and aged rhesus monkeys. *Behavioral Neuroscience* 110(5):898-904.
Bell-McGinty, S., K. Podell, M. Franzen, A. D. Baird, and M. J. Williams. 2002. Standard measures of executive function in predicting instrumental activities of daily living in older adults. *International Journal of Geriatric Psychiatry* 17(9):828-834.
Berardi, A., R. Parasuraman, and J. V. Haxby. 2001. Overall vigilance and sustained attention decrements in healthy aging. *Experimental Aging Research* 27(1):19-39.
Birren, J. E. 1970. Toward an experimental psychology of aging. *American Psychologist* 25(2):124-135.
Bizon, J. L., T. C. Foster, G. E. Alexander, and E. L. Glisky. 2012. Characterizing cognitive aging of working memory and executive function in animal models. *Frontiers in Aging Neuroscience* 4:1-19.

Bouras, C., P. R. Hof, P. Giannakopoulos, J. P. Michel, and J. H. Morrison. 1994. Regional distribution of neurofibrillary tangles and senile plaques in the cerebral cortex of elderly patients: A quantitative evaluation of a one-year autopsy population from a geriatric hospital. *Cerebral Cortex* 4(2):138-150.

Brickman, A. M., and Y. Stern. 2009. Aging and memory in humans. In *Encyclopedia of neuroscience, Vol. 1*, edited by L. Squire. Oxford: Academic Press. Pp. 175-180.

Brody, H. 1955. Organization of the cerebral cortex III: A study of aging in the human cerebral cortex. *Journal of Comparative Neurology* 102(2):511-516.

———. 1970. Structural changes in the aging nervous system. *Interdisciplinary Topics in Gerontology* 7:9-21.

Brooks, B., E. S. Sherman, G. Iverson, D. Slick, and E. Strauss. 2011. Psychometric foundations for the interpretation of neuropsychological test results. In *The little black book of neuropsychology: A syndrome-based approach*, edited by M. R. Schoenberg and J. G. Scott. New York: Springer. Pp. 893-922.

Burke, D. M., and M. A. Shafto. 2008. Language and aging. In *The handbook of aging and cognition*, edited by F. I. Craik and T. A. Salthouse. New York: Psychology Press. Pp. 373-443.

Busch, R., G. Chelune, and Y. Suchy. 2006. Using norms in neuropsychological assessment of the elderly. In *Geriatric neuropsychology: Assessment and intervention*, edited by D. K. Attix and K. A. Welsh-Bohmer. New York: Guilford Press. Pp. 133-157.

Carriere, J. S., J. A. Cheyne, G. J. Solman, and D. Smilek. 2010. Age trends for failures of sustained attention. *Psychology and Aging* 25(3):569-574.

Carvalho, A., I. M. Rea, T. Parimon, and B. J. Cusack. 2014. Physical activity and cognitive function in individuals over 60 years of age: A systematic review. *Clinical Interventions in Aging* 9:661-682.

Cavoy, A., and J. Delacour. 1993. Spatial but not object recognition is impaired by aging in rats. *Physiology and Behavior* 53(3):527-530.

CDC (Centers for Disease Control and Prevention). 2013. Self-reported increased confusion or memory loss and associated functional difficulties among adults aged ≥ 60 years—21 states, 2011. *Morbidity and Mortality Weekly Report* 62(18):347-350.

Clay, O. J., V. G. Wadley, J. D. Edwards, D. L. Roth, D. L. Roenker, and K. K. Ball. 2005. Cumulative meta-analysis of the relationship between useful field of view and driving performance in older adults: Current and future implications. *Optometry and Vision Science* 82(8):724-731.

CMS (Centers for Medicare & Medicaid Services). 2013. *Quick reference information: The ABCs of providing the Annual Wellness Visit (AWV)*. http://www.cms.gov/Outreach-and-Education/Medicare-Learning-Network-MLN/MLNProducts/downloads/AWV_chart_ICN905706.pdf (accessed February 23, 2015).

Colon, E. J. 1972. The elderly brain: A quantitative analysis in the cerebral cortex of two cases. *Psychiatria, Neurologia, Neurochirurgia* 75(4):261-270.

Craik, F. I. M., and J. M. Jennings. 1992. Human memory. In *The handbook of aging and cognition*, edited by F. I. Craik and T. A. Salthouse. Hillsdale, NJ: Erlbaum. Pp. 51-110.

Craik, F. I. M., and J. M. McDowd. 1987. Age differences in recall and recognition. *Journal of Experimental Psychology: Learning, Memory, and Cognition* 13:474-479.

Crystal, H., D. Dickson, P. Fuld, D. Masur, R. Scott, M. Mehler, J. Masdeu, C. Kawas, M. Aronson, and L. Wolfson. 1988. Clinico-pathologic studies in dementia: Nondemented subjects with pathologically confirmed Alzheimer's disease. *Neurology* 38(11):1682-1687.

Czaja, S. J., J. Sharit, R. Ownby, D. L. Roth, and S. Nair. 2001. Examining age differences in performance of a complex information search and retrieval task. *Psychology and Aging* 16(4):564-579.

Czaja, S. J., J. Sharit, M. A. Hernandez, S. N. Nair, and D. Loewenstein. 2010. Variability among older adults in internet health information-seeking performance. *Gerontechnology* 9(1):46-55.
Czaja, S. J., J. Sharit, C. C. Lee, S. N. Nair, M. A. Hernandez, N. Arana, and S. H. Fu. 2013. Factors influencing use of an e-health website in a community sample of older adults. *Journal of the American Medical Informatics Association* 20(2):277-284.
Czaja, S. J., P. D. Harvey, and D. Loewenstein. 2014. Development and evaluation of a novel technology-based functional assessment package. Paper presented at Society of Biological Psychiatry 69th Annual Scientific Meeting, New York.
De Santi, S., E. Pirraglia, W. Barr, J. Babb, S. Williams, K. Rogers, L. Glodzik, M. Brys, L. Mosconi, B. Reisberg, S. Ferris, and M. J. de Leon. 2008. Robust and conventional neuropsychological norms: Diagnosis and prediction of age-related cognitive decline. *Neuropsychology* 22(4):469-484.
Denburg, N. L., C. A. Cole, M. Hernandez, T. H. Yamada, D. Tranel, A. Bechara, and R. B. Wallace. 2007. The orbitofrontal cortex, real-world decision making, and normal aging. *Annals of the New York Academy of Sciences* 1121:480-498.
Diehl, M., M. Marsiske, A. L. Horgas, A. Rosenberg, J. S. Saczynski, and S. L. Willis. 2005. The Revised Observed Tasks of Daily Living: A performance-based assessment of everyday problem solving in older adults. *Journal of Applied Gerontology* 24(3):211-230.
Dobson, S. H., K. C. Kirasic, and G. L. Allen. 1995. Age-related differences in adults' spatial task performance: Influences of task complexity and perceptual speed. *Aging and Cognition* 2:19-38.
Dotson, V. M., M. Kitner-Triolo, M. K. Evans, and A. B. Zonderman. 2008. Literacy-based normative data for low socioeconomic status African Americans. *The Clinical Neuropsychologist* 22(6):989-1017.
Dubois, B., H. H. Feldman, C. Jacova, H. Hampel, J. L. Molinuevo, K. Blennow, S. T. DeKosky, S. Gauthier, D. Selkoe, R. Bateman, S. Cappa, S. Crutch, S. Engelborghs, G. B. Frisoni, N. C. Fox, D. Galasko, M. O. Habert, G. A. Jicha, A. Nordberg, F. Pasquier, G. Rabinovici, P. Robert, C. Rowe, S. Salloway, M. Sarazin, S. Epelbaum, L. C. de Souza, B. Vellas, P. J. Visser, L. Schneider, Y. Stern, P. Scheltens, and J. L. Cummings. 2014. Advancing research diagnostic criteria for Alzheimer's disease: The IWG-2 criteria. *Lancet Neurology* 13(6):614-629.
Dumitriu, D., J. Hao, Y. Hara, J. Kaufmann, W. G. Janssen, W. Lou, P. R. Rapp, and J. H. Morrison. 2010. Selective changes in thin spine density and morphology in monkey prefrontal cortex correlate with aging-related cognitive impairment. *The Journal of Neuroscience* 30(22):7507-7515.
Edwards, J. D., L. A. Ross, M. L. Ackerman, B. J. Small, K. K. Ball, S. Bradley, and J. E. Dodson. 2008. Longitudinal predictors of driving cessation among older adults from the ACTIVE clinical trial. *Journals of Gerontology, Series B: Psychological Sciences and Social Sciences* 63(1):6-12.
Eriksson, P. S., E. Perfilieva, T. Bjork-Eriksson, A. M. Alborn, C. Nordborg, D. A. Peterson, and F. H. Gage. 1998. Neurogenesis in the adult human hippocampus. *Nature Medicine* 4(11):1313-1317.
Gazzaley, A. H., M. M. Thakker, P. R. Hof, and J. H. Morrison. 1997. Preserved number of entorhinal cortex layer II neurons in aged macaque monkeys. *Neurobiology of Aging* 18(5):549-553.
Glisky, E. L., S. R. Rubin, and P. S. Davidson. 2001. Source memory in older adults: An encoding or retrieval problem? *Journal of Experimental Psychology: Learning, Memory, and Cognition* 27(5):1131-1146.
Gomez-Isla, T., J. L. Price, D. W. McKeel, Jr., J. C. Morris, J. H. Growdon, and B. T. Hyman. 1996. Profound loss of layer II entorhinal cortex neurons occurs in very mild Alzheimer's disease. *Journal of Neuroscience* 16(14):4491-4500.

Gould, E., A. J. Reeves, M. S. Graziano, and C. G. Gross. 1999. Neurogenesis in the neocortex of adult primates. *Science* 286(5439):548-552.

Graham, C. L., A. E. Scharlach, and J. Price Wolf. 2014. The impact of the "village" model on health, well-being, service access, and social engagement of older adults. *Health Education and Behavior* 41(1 Suppl):9 1s-97s.

Greenwood, P. M., R. Parasuraman, and J. V. Haxby. 1993. Changes in visuospatial attention over the adult lifespan. *Neuropsychologia* 31(5):471-485.

Hara, Y., M. Punsoni, F. Yuk, C. S. Park, W. G. Janssen, P. R. Rapp, and J. H. Morrison. 2012. Synaptic distributions of GluA2 and PKMzeta in the monkey dentate gyrus and their relationships with aging and memory. *Journal of Neuroscience* 32(21):7336-7344.

Henderson, G., B. E. Tomlinson, and P. H. Gibson. 1980. Cell counts in human cerebral cortex in normal adults throughout life using an image analysing computer. *Journal of the Neurological Sciences* 46(1):113-136.

Henry, J. D., M. S. MacLeod, L. H. Phillips, and J. R. Crawford. 2004. A meta-analytic review of prospective memory and aging. *Psychology and Aging* 19(1):27-39.

Herndon, J. G., M. B. Moss, D. L. Rosene, and R. J. Killiany. 1997. Patterns of cognitive decline in aged rhesus monkeys. *Behavioural Brain Research* 87(1):25-34.

Hertzog, C., and B. Rypma. 1991. Age differences in component of mental-rotation task performance. *Bulletin of the Psychonomic Society* 29:209-212.

Hertzog, C., A. F. Kramer, R. S. Wilson, and U. Lindenberger. 2009. Enrichment effects on adult cognitive development: Can the functional capacity of older adults be preserved and enhanced? *Psychological Science in the Public Interest* 9(1):1-65.

HHS (U.S. Department of Health and Human Services). 2014. *Healthy people 2020*. http://www.healthypeople. gov/2020/topicsobjectives2020/overview.aspx?topicid=7 (accessed October 24, 2014).

Holtzer, R., Y. Goldin, M. Zimmerman, M. Katz, H. Buschke, and R. B. Lipton. 2008. Robust norms for selected neuropsychological tests in older adults. *Archives of Clinical Neuropsychology* 23(5):531-541.

Insel, K., D. Morrow, B. Brewer, and A. Figueredo. 2006. Executive function, working memory, and medication adherence among older adults. *The Journals of Gerontology, Series B: Psychological Sciences and Social Sciences* 61(2):102-107.

Jeste, D. V., and A. J. Oswald. 2014. Individual and societal wisdom: Explaining the paradox of human aging and high well-being. *Psychiatry: Interpersonal and Biological Processes* 77(4):317-330.

Johansson, B., S. M. Hofer, J. C. Allaire, M. M. Maldonado-Molina, A. M. Piccinin, S. Berg, N. L. Pedersen, and G. E. McClearn. 2004. Change in cognitive capabilities in the oldest old: The effects of proximity to death in genetically related individuals over a 6-year period. *Psychology and Aging* 19(1):145-156.

Jones, D. N., J. C. Barnes, D. L. Kirkby, and G. A. Higgins. 1995. Age-associated impairments in a test of attention: Evidence for involvement of cholinergic systems. *Journal of Neuroscience* 15(11):7282-7292.

Kaplan, E., H. Goodglass, and S. Weintrab. 1983. *The Boston Naming Test*. Philadelphia, PA: Lea and Febiger.

Katzman, R., R. Terry, R. DeTeresa, T. Brown, P. Davies, P. Fuld, X. Renbing, and A. Peck. 1988. Clinical, pathological, and neurochemical changes in dementia: A subgroup with preserved mental status and numerous neocortical plaques. *Annals of Neurology* 23(2):138-144.

Kemper, S., and R. E. Herman. 2006. Age differences in memory-load interference effects in syntactic processing. *The Journals of Gerontology, Series B: Psychological Sciences and Social Sciences* 61(6):327-332.

Kemper, S., and A. Sumner. 2001. The structure of verbal abilities in young and older adults. *Psychology and Aging* 16(2):312-322.

Kemtes, K. A., and S. Kemper. 1997. Younger and older adults' on-line processing of syntactically ambiguous sentences. *Psychology and Aging* 12(2):362-371.

Kornack, D. R., and P. Rakic. 1999. Continuation of neurogenesis in the hippocampus of the adult macaque monkey. *Proceedings of the National Academy of Sciences of the United States of America* 96(10):5768-5773.

Kramer, A. F., and D. J. Madden. 2008. Attention. In *The handbook of aging and cognition*, 3rd ed., edited by F. I. Craik and T. A. Salthouse. New York: Psychology Press. Pp. 189-249.

Kunzmann, U., and P. B. Baltes. 2003. Wisdom-related knowledge: Affective, motivational, and interpersonal correlates. *Personality and Social Psychology Bulletin* 29(9):1104-1119.

Lachman, M. E., and E. Jelalian. 1984. Self-efficacy and attributions for intellectual performance in young and elderly adults. *Journal of Gerontology* 39(5):577-582.

Lai, Z. C., M. B. Moss, R. J. Killiany, D. L. Rosene, and J. G. Herndon. 1995. Executive system dysfunction in the aged monkey: Spatial and object reversal learning. *Neurobiology of Aging* 16(6):947-954.

Lee, S. W., G. D. Clemenson, and F. H. Gage. 2012. New neurons in an aged brain. *Behavioural Brain Research* 227(2):497-507.

Light, L. L., and E. M. Zelinski. 1983. Memory for spatial information in young and old adults. *Developmental Psychology* 19(6):901-906.

Magnezi, R., Y. S. Bergman, and D. Grosberg. 2014. Online activity and participation in treatment affects the perceived efficacy of social health networks among patients with chronic illness. *Journal of Medical Internet Research* 16(1):e12.

Manly, J. J., N. Schupf, M. X. Tang, and Y. Stern. 2005. Cognitive decline and literacy among ethnically diverse elders. *Journal of Geriatric Psychiatry and Neurology* 18(4):213-217.

Marcopulos, B., and C. McLain. 2003. Are our norms "normal"? A 4-year follow-up study of a biracial sample of rural elders with low education. *The Clinical Neuropsychologist* 17(1):19-33.

Maylor, E. A., G. Smith, S. Della Sala, and R. H. Logie. 2002. Prospective and retrospective memory in normal aging and dementia: An experimental study. *Memory and Cognition* 30(6):871-884.

McArdle, J. 2011. Longitudinal dynamic analyses of cognition in the health and retirement study panel. *Advances in Statistical Analysis* 95(4):453-480.

McDowd, J. M., and R. J. Shaw. 2000. Attention and aging: A functional perspective. In *The handbook of aging and cognition*, edited by T. A. Salthouse and F. I. M. Craik. Mahwah, NJ: Erlbaum. Pp. 221-292.

McEvoy, G. M., and W. F. Cascio. 1989. Cumulative evidence of the relationship between employee age and job performance. *Journal of Applied Psychology* 74:11-17.

McKhann, G. M., D. S. Knopman, H. Chertkow, B. T. Hyman, C. R. Jack, Jr., C. H. Kawas, W. E. Klunk, W. J. Koroshetz, J. J. Manly, R. Mayeux, R. C. Mohs, J. C. Morris, M. N. Rossor, P. Scheltens, M. C. Carrillo, B. Thies, S. Weintraub, and C. H. Phelps. 2011. The diagnosis of dementia due to Alzheimer's disease: Recommendations from the National Institute on Aging-Alzheimer's Association workgroups on diagnostic guidelines for Alzheimer's disease. *Alzheimer's & Dementia* 7(3):263-269.

Mick, P., I. Kawachi, and F. R. Lin. 2014. The association between hearing loss and social isolation in older adults. *Otolaryngology-Head and Neck Surgery* 150(3):378-384.

Mitchell, D. B. 1989. How many memory systems? Evidence from aging. *Journal of Experimental Psychology: Learning, Memory, and Cognition* 15(1):31-49.

Moore, H., P. Dudchenko, J. P. Bruno, and M. Sarter. 1992. Toward modeling age-related changes of attentional abilities in rats: Simple and choice reaction time tasks and vigilance. *Neurobiology of Aging* 13(6):759-772.

Moore, T. L., R. J. Killiany, J. G. Herndon, D. L. Rosene, and M. B. Moss. 2003. Impairment in abstraction and set shifting in aged rhesus monkeys. *Neurobiology of Aging* 24(1):125-134.

Morris, J. C., M. Storandt, D. W. McKeel, Jr., E. H. Rubin, J. L. Price, E. A. Grant, and L. Berg. 1996. Cerebral amyloid deposition and diffuse plaques in "normal" aging: Evidence for presymptomatic and very mild Alzheimer's disease. *Neurology* 46(3):707-719.

Morris, R. G., P. Garrud, J. N. Rawlins, and J. O'Keefe. 1982. Place navigation impaired in rats with hippocampal lesions. *Nature* 297(5868):681-683.

Morrison, J. H., and M. G. Baxter. 2012. The ageing cortical synapse: Hallmarks and implications for cognitive decline. *Nature Reviews Neuroscience* 13(4):240-250.

———. 2014. Synaptic health. *JAMA Psychiatry* 71(7):835-837.

Morrison, J. H., and P. R. Hof. 1997. Life and death of neurons in the aging brain. *Science* 278(5337):412-419.

Moss, M. B., D. L. Rosene, and A. Peters. 1988. Effects of aging on visual recognition memory in the rhesus monkey. *Neurobiology of Aging* 9(5-6):495-502.

Moss, M. B., R. J. Killiany, Z. C. Lai, D. L. Rosene, and J. G. Herndon. 1997. Recognition memory span in rhesus monkeys of advanced age. *Neurobiology of Aging* 18(1):13-19.

Muir, J. L., W. Fischer, and A. Bjorklund. 1999. Decline in visual attention and spatial memory in aged rats. *Neurobiology of Aging* 20(6):605-615.

Newell, F. N., A. Setti, T. Foran, K. Burke, and R. A. Kenny. 2011. Reduced vision impairs spatial cognition in fall-prone older adults. *INSIGHT: Research and Practice in Visual Impairment and Blindness* 4(3):103-111.

Nielsen, K., and A. Peters. 2000. The effects of aging on the frequency of nerve fibers in rhesus monkey striate cortex. *Neurobiology of Aging* 21(5):621-628.

Nilsson, L. G. 2003. Memory function in normal aging. *Acta Neurologica Scandinavica* 179:7-13.

Norris, C. M., D. L. Korol, and T. C. Foster. 1996. Increased susceptibility to induction of long-term depression and long-term potentiation reversal during aging. *The Journal of Neuroscience* 16(17):5382-5392.

O'Donnell, K. A., P. R. Rapp, and P. R. Hof. 1999. Preservation of prefrontal cortical volume in behaviorally characterized aged macaque monkeys. *Experimental Neurology* 160(1):300-310.

Pak, R., S. J. Czaja, J. Sharit, W. A. Rogers, and A. D. Fisk. 2006a. The role of spatial abilities and age in performance in an auditory computer navigation task. *Computers in Human Behavior* 24(6):3045-3051.

Pak, R., W. A. Rogers, and A. D. Fisk. 2006b. Spatial ability subfactors and their influences on a computer-based information search task. *Human Factors* 48(1):154-165.

Parasuraman, R., P. Nestor, and P. Greenwood. 1989. Sustained-attention capacity in young and older adults. *Psychology and Aging* 4(3):339-345.

Pedraza, O., J. A. Lucas, G. E. Smith, R. C. Petersen, N. R. Graff-Radford, and R. J. Ivnik. 2010. Robust and expanded norms for the dementia rating scale. *Archives of Clinical Neuropsychology* 25(5):347-358.

Peters, A. 1996. Age-related changes in oligodendrocytes in monkey cerebral cortex. *Journal of Comparative Neurology* 371:153-163.

Peters, A., D. Leahu, M. B. Moss, and K. J. McNally. 1994. The effects of aging on area 46 of the frontal cortex of the rhesus monkey. *Cerebral Cortex* 4(6):621-635.

Peters, A., J. H. Morrison, D. L. Rosene, and B. T. Hyman. 1998. Are neurons lost from the primate cerebral cortex during normal aging? *Cerebral Cortex* 8(4):295-300.

Petersen, R. C. 2004. Mild cognitive impairment as a diagnostic entity. *Journal of Internal Medicine* 256(3):183-194.

Plude, D. J., W. P. Milberg, and J. Cerella. 1986. Age differences in depicting and perceiving tridimensionality in simple line drawings. *Experimental Aging Research* 12(4):221-225.
Presty, S. K., J. Bachevalier, L. C. Walker, R. G. Struble, D. L. Price, M. Mishkin, and L. C. Cork. 1987. Age differences in recognition memory of the rhesus monkey (Macaca mulatta). *Neurobiology of Aging* 8(5):435-440.
Price, J. L., and J. C. Morris. 1999. Tangles and plaques in nondemented aging and "preclinical" Alzheimer's disease. *Annals of Neurology* 45(3):358-368.
Rapp, P. R. 1990. Visual discrimination and reversal learning in the aged monkey (Macaca mulatta). *Behavioral Neuroscience* 104(6):876-884.
Rapp, P. R., and D. G. Amaral. 1989. Evidence for task-dependent memory dysfunction in the aged monkey. *Journal of Neuroscience* 9(10):3568-3576.
Rapp, P. R., and M. Gallagher. 1996. Preserved neuron number in the hippocampus of aged rats with spatial learning deficits. *Proceedings of the National Academy of Sciences of the United States of America* 93(18):9926-9930.
Rapp, P. R., R. A. Rosenberg, and M. Gallagher. 1987. An evaluation of spatial information processing in aged rats. *Behavioral Neuroscience* 101(1):3-12.
Rapp, P. R., P. S. Deroche, Y. Mao, and R. D. Burwell. 2002. Neuron number in the parahippocampal region is preserved in aged rats with spatial learning deficits. *Cerebral Cortex* 12(11):1171-1179.
Reitan, R. M. 1955. The relation of the trail making test to organic brain damage. *Journal of Consulting Psychology* 19(5):393-394.
Robbins, T. W., and A. F. Arnsten. 2009. The neuropsychopharmacology of fronto-executive function: Monoaminergic modulation. *Annual Review of Neuroscience* 32:267-287.
Robbins, T. W., M. James, A. M. Owen, B. J. Sahakian, A. D. Lawrence, L. McInnes, and P. M. Rabbitt. 1998. A study of performance on tests from the CANTAB battery sensitive to frontal lobe dysfunction in a large sample of normal volunteers: Implications for theories of executive functioning and cognitive aging. Cambridge Neuropsychological Test Automated Battery. *Journal of the International Neuropsychological Society* 4(5):474-490.
Romero, H. R., S. K. Lageman, V. V. Kamath, F. Irani, A. Sim, P. Suarez, J. J. Manly, and D. K. Attix. 2009. Challenges in the neuropsychological assessment of ethnic minorities: Summit proceedings. *The Clinical Neuropsychologist* 23(5):761-779.
Roring, R. W., and N. Charness. 2007. A multilevel model analysis of expertise in chess across the life span. *Psychology and Aging* 22(2):291-299.
Rosene, D. L. 1993. Comparing age-related changes in the basal forebrain and hippocampus of the rhesus monkey. *Neurobiology of Aging* 14(6):669-670.
Rosenzweig, E. S., and C. A. Barnes. 2003. Impact of aging on hippocampal function: Plasticity, network dynamics, and cognition. *Progress in Neurobiology* 69(3):143-179.
Salthouse, T. A. 1984. Effects of age and skill in typing. *Journal of Experimental Psychology: General* 113(3):345-371.
———. 1994. The aging of working memory. *Neuropsychology* 8(4):535-543.
———. 2004. What and when of cognitive aging. *Current Directions in Psychological Science* 13(4):140-144.
Samanez-Larkin, G. R., S. M. Levens, L. M. Perry, R. F. Dougherty, and B. Knutson. 2012. Frontostriatal white matter integrity mediates adult age differences in probabilistic reward learning. *Journal of Neuroscience* 32(15):5333-5337.
Scarmeas, N., and Y. Stern. 2004. Cognitive reserve: Implications for diagnosis and prevention of Alzheimer's disease. *Current Neurology and Neuroscience Reports* 4(5):374-380.
Schaie, K. W. 1983. The Seattle Longitudinal Study: A twenty-one year exploration of psychometric intelligence in adulthood. In *Longitudinal studies of adult psychological development*, edited by K. W. Schaie. New York: Guilford Press. Pp. 64-135.

———. 1994. The course of adult intellectual development. *American Psychologist* 49(4): 304-313.
———. 1996. *Intellectual development in adulthood: The Seattle Longitudinal Study.* New York: Cambridge University Press.
———. 2005. What can we learn from longitudinal studies of adult development? *Research in Human Development* 2(3):133-158.
Scheff, S. W., D. A. Price, F. A. Schmitt, and E. J. Mufson. 2006. Hippocampal synaptic loss in early Alzheimer's disease and mild cognitive impairment. *Neurobiology of Aging* 27(10):1372-1384.
Schinka, J. A. 2010. Use of informants to identify mild cognitive impairment in older adults. *Current Psychiatry Reports* 12(1):4-12.
Schmidt, F. L., and J. E. Hunter. 1998. The validity and utility of selection methods in personnel psychology: Practical and theoretical implications of 85 years of research findings. *Psychological Bulletin* 124(2):262-274.
———. 2004. General mental ability in the world of work: Occupational attainment and job performance. *Journal of Personality and Social Psychology* 86(1):162-173.
Schretlen, D. J., S. M. Testa, J. M. Winicki, G. D. Pearlson, and B. Gordon. 2008. Frequency and bases of abnormal performance by healthy adults on neuropsychological testing. *Journal of the International Neuropsychological Society* 14(3):436-445.
Segev-Jacubovski, O., T. Herman, G. Yogev-Seligmann, A. Mirelman, N. Giladi, and J. M. Hausdorff. 2011. The interplay between gait, falls and cognition: Can cognitive therapy reduce fall risk? *Expert Review of Neurotherapeutics* 11(7):1057-1075.
Sharit, J., and S. J. Czaja. 1999. Performance of a complex computer-based troubleshooting task in the bank industry. *International Journal of Cognitive Ergonomics and Human Factors* 3:1-22.
Sharit, J., M. A. Hernandez, S. J. Czaja, and P. Pirolli. 2008. Investigating the roles of knowledge and cognitive abilities in older adult information seeking on the web. *ACM Transactions on Computer-Human Interaction* 15(1):3.
Shefer, V. F. 1973. Absolute number of neurons and thickness of the cerebral cortex during aging, senile and vascular dementia, and Pick's and Alzheimer's diseases. *Neuroscience and Behavioral Physiology* 6(4):319-324.
Singer, T., P. Verhaeghen, P. Ghisletta, U. Lindenberger, and P. B. Baltes. 2003. The fate of cognition in very old age: Six-year longitudinal findings in the Berlin Aging Study (BASE). *Psychology and Aging* 18(2):318-331.
Smith, T. D., M. M. Adams, M. Gallagher, J. H. Morrison, and P. R. Rapp. 2000. Circuit-specific alterations in hippocampal synaptophysin immunoreactivity predict spatial learning impairment in aged rats. *Journal of Neuroscience* 20(17):6587-6593.
Spaniol, J., D. J. Madden, and A. Voss. 2006. A diffusion model analysis of adult age differences in episodic and semantic long-term memory retrieval. *Journal of Experimental Psychology: Learning, Memory, and Cognition* 32(1):101-117.
Spencer, W. D., and N. Raz. 1995. Differential effects of aging on memory for content and context: A meta-analysis. *Psychology and Aging* 10(4):527-539.
Sperling, R. A., P. S. Aisen, L. A. Beckett, D. A. Bennett, S. Craft, A. M. Fagan, T. Iwatsubo, C. R. Jack, Jr., J. Kaye, T. J. Montine, D. C. Park, E. M. Reiman, C. C. Rowe, E. Siemers, Y. Stern, K. Yaffe, M. C. Carrillo, B. Thies, M. Morrison-Bogorad, M. V. Wagster, and C. H. Phelps. 2011. Toward defining the preclinical stages of Alzheimer's disease: Recommendations from the National Institute on Aging-Alzheimer's Association workgroups on diagnostic guidelines for Alzheimer's disease. *Alzheimer's & Dementia* 7(3):280-292.
Staudinger, U. M. 1999. Older and wiser? Integrating results on the relationship between age and wisdom-related performance. *International Journal of Behavioral Development* 23(3):641-664.

Stilley, C. S., C. M. Bender, J. Dunbar-Jacob, S. Sereika, and C. M. Ryan. 2010. The impact of cognitive function on medication management: Three studies. *Health Psychology* 29(1):50-55.

Stine, E. A. 1990. On-line processing of written text by younger and older adults. *Psychology and Aging* 5(1):68-78.

Stine-Morrow, E. A., M. K. Loveless, and L. M. Soederberg. 1996. Resource allocation in on-line reading by younger and older adults. *Psychology and Aging* 11(3):475-486.

Taha, J., S. J. Czaja, J. Sharit, and D. G. Morrow. 2013. Factors affecting usage of a personal health record (PHR) to manage health. *Psychology and Aging* 28(4):1124-1139.

Techentin, C., D. Voyer, and S. D. Voyer. 2014. Spatial abilities and aging: A meta-analysis. *Experimental Aging Research* 40(4):395-425.

Terry, R. D., R. DeTeresa, and L. A. Hansen. 1987. Neocortical cell counts in normal human adult aging. *Annals of Neurology* 21(6):530-539.

Trott, C. T., D. Friedman, W. Ritter, and M. Fabiani. 1997. Item and source memory: Differential age effects revealed by event-related potentials. *Neuroreport* 8(15):3373-3378.

Tsang, P. S., and T. L. Shaner. 1998. Age, attention, expertise, and time-sharing performance. *Psychology and Aging* 13(2):323-347.

Tsang, R. S., K. Diamond, L. Mowszowski, S. J. Lewis, and S. L. Naismith. 2012. Using informant reports to detect cognitive decline in mild cognitive impairment. *International Psychogeriatrics* 24(6):967-973.

Tucker, A. M., and Y. Stern. 2011. Cognitive reserve in aging. *Current Alzheimer Research* 8(4):354-360.

Verhaeghen, P., and J. Cerella. 2002. Aging, executive control, and attention: A review of meta-analyses. *Neuroscience and Biobehavioral Reviews* 26(7):849-857.

Vincent, S. L., A. Peters, and J. Tigges. 1989. Effects of aging on the neurons within area 17 of rhesus monkey cerebral cortex. *The Anatomical Record* 223(3):329-341.

Waldman, D. A., and B. J. Avolio. 1986. A meta-analysis of age differences in job performance. *Journal of Applied Psychology* 71:33-38.

Wang, M., N. J. Gamo, Y. Yang, L. E. Jin, X. J. Wang, M. Laubach, J. A. Mazer, D. Lee, and A. F. Arnsten. 2011. Neuronal basis of age-related working memory decline. *Nature* 476(7359):210-213.

Weiner, M. W., P. S. Aisen, C. R. Jack, Jr., W. J. Jagust, J. Q. Trojanowski, L. Shaw, A. J. Saykin, J. C. Morris, N. Cairns, L. A. Beckett, A. Toga, R. Green, S. Walter, H. Soares, P. Snyder, E. Siemers, W. Potter, P. E. Cole, and M. Schmidt. 2010. The Alzheimer's Disease Neuroimaging Initiative: Progress report and future plans. *Alzheimer's & Dementia* 6(3):202-211.

Weintraub, S., S. S. Dikmen, R. K. Heaton, D. S. Tulsky, P. D. Zelazo, P. J. Bauer, N. E. Carlozzi, J. Slotkin, D. Blitz, K. Wallner-Allen, N. A. Fox, J. L. Beaumont, D. Mungas, C. J. Nowinski, J. Richler, J. A. Deocampo, J. E. Anderson, J. J. Manly, B. Borosh, R. Havlik, K. Conway, E. Edwards, L. Freund, J. W. King, C. Moy, E. Witt, and R. C. Gershon. 2013. Cognition assessment using the NIH toolbox. *Neurology* 80(11 Suppl 3):S54-S64.

West, M. J. 1993. Regionally specific loss of neurons in the aging human hippocampus. *Neurobiology of Aging* 14:287-293.

Willis, S. L., and M. Marsiske. 1993. *Manual for the Everyday Problems Test.* University Park: Pennsylvania State University.

Willis, S. L., and K. W. Schaie. 1986. Training the elderly on the ability factors of spatial orientation and inductive reasoning. *Psychology and Aging* 1(3):239-247.

Winblad, B., K. Palmer, M. Kivipelto, V. Jelic, L. Fratiglioni, L. O. Wahlund, A. Nordberg, L. Bäckman, M. Albert, O. Almkvist, H. Arai, H. Basun, K. Blennow, M. de Leon, C. DeCarli, T. Erkinjuntti, E. Giacobini, C. Graff, J. Hardy, C. Jack, A. Jorm, K. Ritchie, C. van Duijn, P. Visser, and R. C. Petersen. 2004. Mild cognitive impairment. Beyond controversies, towards a consensus: Report of the International Working Group on Mild Cognitive Impairment. *Journal of Internal Medicine* 256(3):240-246.

Wingfield, A., and M. Grossman. 2006. Language and the aging brain: Patterns of neural compensation revealed by functional brain imaging. *Journal of Neurophysiology* 96(6):2830-2839.

Wingfield, A., P. A. Tun, C. K. Koh, and M. J. Rosen. 1999. Regaining lost time: Adult aging and the effect of time restoration on recall of time-compressed speech. *Psychology and Aging* 14(3):380-389.

Wu, Y., W. Le, and J. Jankovic. 2011. Preclinical biomarkers of Parkinson disease. *Archives of Neurology* 68(1):22-30.

Zacks, R. T., L. Hasher, and K. Z. H. Li. 2000. Human memory. In *The handbook of aging and cognition*, 2nd ed., edited by F. I. Craik and T. A. Salthouse. Mahwah, NJ: Erlbaum. Pp. 293-357.

Zanto, T. P., and A. Gazzaley. 2014. Attention and aging. In *The Oxford handbook of attention*, edited by A. C. Nobre and S. Kastner. Oxford: Oxford University Press. Pp. 927-971.

Zelazo, P. D., F. I. Craik, and L. Booth. 2004. Executive function across the life span. *Acta Psychologica* 115(2-3):167-183.

3

Population-Based Information About Cognitive Aging

While a great deal of research has examined the occurrence, causes, natural history, pathogenesis, and clinical management of dementia, including Alzheimer's disease, less attention has been paid to cognitive aging per se, particularly from a public health perspective. Population-based information about the nature and extent of cognitive aging provides a basis for building public awareness and understanding and can be used to engage individuals and their families in maintaining cognitive health; to inform health care professionals, financial professionals, and others as they educate and advise their older patients and clients; and to guide program development and implementation.

This chapter provides a brief overview of available population-based information about cognitive aging in the United States and discusses challenges and next steps in collecting, analyzing, and disseminating needed information that is not currently available. The chapter addresses the following questions:

- How does a life-course perspective help inform the understanding of cognitive aging?
- What does population-based research show about the cognitive status of older Americans, the amount and types of cognitive change that occur in individuals as they age, and older adults' awareness and perceptions about these changes?
- What are the challenges in collecting population-based information about cognitive aging?
- What additional research is needed in order to increase knowledge about cognitive aging for public health and related purposes?

Although information about cognitive aging is available from a variety of sources, this chapter focuses mainly—although not entirely—on information derived from surveys and studies that have been conducted in representative U.S. population samples, including national, regional, and local populations. The focus on information from U.S. sources is not intended to ignore the important worldwide research literature but rather to maximize the relevance of the information to U.S. programs and policies. Likewise, the focus on surveys and studies conducted in representative population samples is not intended to ignore the important scientific and clinical findings derived from research employing other kinds of samples, including samples of community volunteers and patients in clinical settings, such as physician's offices and health care systems. From a public health perspective however, information based on findings from representative population-based samples is especially relevant and useful.

A major challenge in assembling population-based information about cognitive aging is that most analyses of population data on cognition in older adults have focused on moderate and severe cognitive impairment, dementia, and Alzheimer's disease. This focus has certainly yielded valuable information, such as estimates that 11.2 to 13.9 percent of older Americans have dementia (Kasper et al., 2014; Plassman et al., 2007), including 9.7 to 11.7 percent who have Alzheimer's disease (Hebert et al., 2013; Plassman et al., 2007).[1] But, much less attention has been paid to population data on the less severe cognitive changes experienced by the majority of older adults—changes that may affect important day-to-day activities, such as driving, making financial decisions, and managing medications. The resulting gaps in understanding of the larger picture of changes in cognition with aging underscore the need for population-based information on cognitive aging apart from moderate and severe cognitive impairment, dementia, and Alzheimer's disease.

LIFE-COURSE PERSPECTIVE

In the past few decades, developments in life-course epidemiology have led to a greater understanding of health and disease as they evolve across the life span. Life-course epidemiology studies health in a social, environmental, and cultural context and examines both the factors that affect health and the impact that health has on other outcomes for individuals throughout their lives. A life-course perspective is informative when ap-

---

[1] These and other estimates of the prevalence of dementia and Alzheimer's disease vary because of differences among population-based studies in the definitions of the conditions studied, the tests used to measure them, the age and other characteristics of sample members, and other factors (Brookmeyer et al., 2011; Rocca et al., 2011).

plied to cognitive aging because the cognitive status of older adults reflects not only the changes that occur in older age but also the effects of social and environmental factors and health-related events that occurred earlier in life. A life-course approach emphasizes the role of early brain and cognitive development and the general social and environmental threats and enhancements to that development among infants and children (Hofer and Clouston, 2014). This approach also acknowledges the effects of health-related events and risk factors that occur in adolescence and young and middle adulthood. Examples include head or bodily trauma due to automobile crashes or military combat; major mental illnesses, such as affective disorders, substance abuse, or various psychoses; cerebro-vascular disease risk factors, such as uncontrolled hypertension and lipid disorders; toxic maternal exposures; and physiochemical exposures of hazardous occupations. All of these factors help explain the wide differences in cognitive status observed among individuals as they age. While not all early events and risk factors that can affect cognition in older adults are fully preventable, paying greater attention to the adverse events of human development (such as the physical and social environments associated with poverty or the cognitive decrements associated with severe mental illnesses) may improve clinical and public health interventions and policies and may lead to more optimal human development.

NATURE AND EXTENT OF COGNITIVE AGING IN THE UNITED STATES

In order to understand cognitive aging in the context of whole communities and populations, it is necessary to carry out studies of representative samples of those populations. Many ongoing and completed surveys and studies conducted with samples of national, regional, and local populations in the United States include items that measure cognition and cognition-related factors. Some survey items measure survey respondents' cognition directly, resulting in what is sometimes referred to as *objective* information about cognition. Other survey items measure survey respondents' awareness and perceptions about their cognition, resulting in what is often referred to as *subjective* information about cognition. Box 3-1 provides examples of these two kinds of survey items.

A recent review identified more than 40 U.S. surveys and studies that have used valid and reliable measures of cognition in adults age 50 and older (Bell et al., 2014). Approximately half of these surveys and studies have been conducted in representative samples of national, regional, or local populations. Some of the surveys and studies use only a few items, including validated brief mental status tests or items drawn from those tests, to measure cognition directly. Others use more extensive batteries of

> **BOX 3-1**
> **Survey Items Used to Measure Cognition**
>
> **Direct Measures of Cognition**
> These survey items often use standardized cognitive tests that ask the respondent to answer questions intended to measure various components of cognition, such as memory, orientation, executive function, vocabulary, and reasoning. Memory is often measured by asking a respondent to listen to a list of words and then repeat all of the words remembered (*immediate word recall*). After a specified time interval, the respondent is again asked to repeat all of the words remembered (*delayed word recall*). Orientation may be measured by asking a respondent for the current day, month, year, and day of the week and the name of the current president. Other commonly used survey items ask respondents to name common objects, such as scissors; to name as many different animals as they can in a minute or two; to complete one or more partial sentences; to count backward from 100 by 7s; and to identify a missing number in a series of numbers. (See Box 2-1 in Chapter 2 for additional information about commonly used cognitive tests.)
>
> **Measures of Awareness and Perceptions About Cognition**
> These survey items may ask respondents to rate their memory (excellent, very good, good, fair, or poor) or ask whether they have difficulty remembering, concentrating, making decisions, or learning something new. Respondents may be asked whether they have noticed changes in their thinking ability or whether their memory is better, the same, or worse than at a specified time in the past. Similarly, they may be asked whether they have experienced confusion or memory loss and whether it is happening more often or getting worse. Related measures include how an individual feels about and adapts to these perceived changes in cognitive function.

neuropsychological tests. Many also measure respondents' awareness and perceptions about their own cognition. Still others measure respondents' awareness and perceptions about their cognition but do not measure cognition directly.

Table 3-1 provides descriptive information about five ongoing surveys and studies that are being conducted in nationally representative U.S. samples. These surveys and studies are used as examples throughout this chapter to illustrate the kinds of information about cognitive aging that are being or could be collected in population-based research. Other surveys and studies that are being or have been conducted in the United States also provide information about cognitive aging. For example, the Established Populations for Epidemiologic Studies of the Elderly (EPESE), which was conducted in four states, provides information about the proportion of adults age 65 years and older who had errors on a brief cognitive test (Cornoni-Huntley et al., 1986, 1990). Appendix B lists not only the surveys and studies shown in Table 3-1 but also many of these other research efforts.

TABLE 3-1 Selected Surveys and Studies Conducted in Representative Samples of the U.S. Population That Collect Information About Cognition in Adults

	Behavioral Risk Factor Surveillance System (BRFSS)	Health and Retirement Study (HRS)	Midlife in the United States Study (MIDUS)	National Health and Aging Trends Study (NHATS)	National Health and Nutrition Examination Survey (NHANES)
Primary sponsoring agency	CDC	NIA and SSA	NIA	NIA	NCHS
Conducted by	State health departments	University of Michigan	University of Wisconsin–Madison	Johns Hopkins University	NCHS
Sample size	About 500,000 annually	More than 26,000 every 2 years	7,100 (MIDUS I) 4,300 (MIDUS II)	8,200 in 2011	About 5,000 annually
Sample criteria	Age: 18 years and older	Age: 50 years and older	Age: 25 to 74 years (MIDUS I) Age: 32 to 84 years (MIDUS II)	Age: 65 years and older Medicare enrollee	All ages
Includes nursing home residents	No	Yes	No	Yes	No
Measures cognition directly	No	Yes	Yes	Yes	Yes
Measures awareness and perceptions about cognition	Yes	Yes	Yes	Yes	Yes
Collects information about sample person's cognition from a proxy/informant	No	Yes	No	Yes	Yes

continued

TABLE 3-1 Continued

	Behavioral Risk Factor Surveillance System (BRFSS)	Health and Retirement Study (HRS)	Midlife in the United States Study (MIDUS)	National Health and Aging Trends Study (NHATS)	National Health and Nutrition Examination Survey (NHANES)
Collects longitudinal information about cognition	No	Yes, every 2 years	Yes (MIDUS II and a subsample from MIDUS I)	Yes, annually	No
Conducted in person, by telephone, other	Telephone	In-person and telephone interviews with survey subject and a proxy	Telephone and self-administered questionnaire	In-person interviews with the survey subject or a proxy respondent	In-person interviews and health examinations in mobile centers
Asks about activities of daily living (ADLs)	Dressing and bathing only	All 5 ADLs	Dressing and bathing only	All 5 ADLs	Dressing, bathing, transferring from bed to chair, and eating
Asks about instrumental activities of daily living (IADLs)	Shopping only	All 7 IADLs	No	Shopping, food preparation, laundry, managing finances, managing medications	Shopping, food preparation, laundry, housekeeping, managing finances, managing medications
Asks about other physical activity limitations	Walking and climbing stairs	Walking, climbing stairs, crouching, stooping, kneeling, lifting, getting up from a chair	Walking, climbing stairs, stooping, kneeling, lifting	Walking, climbing stairs, kneeling, lifting	Walking, climbing stairs, crouching, stooping, kneeling, lifting, getting up from a chair
Asks about race/ethnicity	Yes	Yes	Yes	Yes	Yes
Asks about veteran status	"ever served in the military"	"ever served in the military"	No	Yes	Yes

TABLE 3-1 Continued

	Behavioral Risk Factor Surveillance System (BRFSS)	Health and Retirement Study (HRS)	Midlife in the United States Study (MIDUS)	National Health and Aging Trends Study (NHATS)	National Health and Nutrition Examination Survey (NHANES)
Asks about physical activity and exercise	Yes	Yes	Yes	Yes	Yes
Asks about cardiovascular risk factors: hypertension, diabetes, smoking	Yes	Yes	Yes	Yes	Yes
Asks about social engagement	No	Yes	Yes	Yes	Asks about difficulty participating in social activities or lack of such participation

NOTES:
Activities of daily living (ADLs): bathing, dressing, transferring from bed to chair, using the toilet, and eating. Instrumental activities of daily living (IADLs): using the telephone, shopping, food preparation, laundry, housekeeping, managing finances, and managing medications. Other physical activities: includes walking, climbing stairs, crouching, stooping, kneeling, lifting, and getting up from a chair. MIDUS III: The next phase of the Midlife in the United States Study, MIDUS III, began data collection in 2013. Interviews about cognition will be conducted with 2,680 sample members (MIDUS, 2011e).

Abbreviations:
CDC = Centers for Disease Control and Prevention; MIDUS I = Midlife in the United States, Baseline Study; MIDUS II = Midlife in the United States, Follow-up Study; NCHS = National Center for Health Statistics; NIA = National Institute on Aging; SSA = Social Security Administration.

SOURCES:
BRFSS items come from the 2014 questionnaire, BRFSS: Behavioral Risk Factor Surveillance System (CDC, 2013b).
The HRS items come from the 2014 questionnaire, HRS: Health and Retirement Study (HRS, 2014a, 2015).
MIDUS items come from the MIDUS I and II phone interview questionnaires and the self-administered questionnaires: MIDUS I (MIDUS, 2011b); MIDUS II (MIDUS, 2011c,d,e).
NHATS items come from the 2011, 2012, and 2013 questionnaires, NHATS: National Health and Aging Trends Study (NHATS, 2014a,d,e,f).
NHANES items come from the 2013/2014 questionnaire, NHANES: National Health and Nutrition Examination Survey (CDC, 2014b,c).

As shown in Table 3-1, the sample sizes for the five ongoing surveys and studies range from 5,000 participants annually for the National Health and Nutrition Examination Survey (NHANES) up to about 500,000 for the Behavioral Risk Factor Surveillance System (BRFSS). NHANES includes people of all ages, while BRFSS and the Midlife in the United States (MIDUS) study include adults age 18 years and older and 24 years and older, respectively. The Health and Retirement Study (HRS) includes adults age 50 years and older, while the National Health and Aging Trends Study (NHATS) includes adults age 65 years and older. Four of the five surveys and studies shown in Table 3-1 measure respondents' cognition directly, and all five include survey items to assess respondents' awareness and perceptions about their cognition.

Like all nationally representative research, these surveys and studies have limitations in their breadth and depth of coverage. The five studies described in Table 3-1 cover numerous health and social topics, but none is dedicated solely to cognition. The breadth of topics they cover enhances their value for researching potential correlations between cognition and other factors of interest from a public health perspective. All five collect information about race and ethnicity, and four of the five collect information about veteran status. All five ask about medical conditions, such as hypertension, heart disease, diabetes, and stroke, and other factors related to cognitive aging as discussed in Chapters 4A and 4B—for instance, physical activity and exercise, smoking, and social engagement. All five also ask about various functional activities that may be affected as part of cognitive aging. At the same time, the breadth of topics covered in the surveys and studies necessarily limits the depth of information specifically about cognitive aging. Moreover, nationally representative surveys and studies often have too few people with similar characteristics to assess regional or local variations with the precision needed to inform public health decisions or explore less common minority, nationality, or language groups. These more in-depth questions usually require targeted surveys or expanded samples or subsamples in national surveys.

A brief overview of the information available about cognitive aging from these existing surveys and studies is presented below. Information is provided about three aspects of cognitive aging: cognitive status at a point in time, cognitive changes that occur in individuals as they age, and older adults' self-reported awareness and perceptions regarding these changes.

Although some researchers are familiar with the available information about cognitive aging from these and other surveys and studies, the information is generally not presented in formats, language, and media that are accessible to most older adults; to health care and financial professionals and others who work with older adults; to the staff of government and private-sector organizations that plan, implement, and evaluate public health programs; and to other non-research audiences. If reformatted and stated in language that is meaningful to these audiences, this information could help to increase public awareness and understanding, answer questions and address concerns of older adults and their families, assist health care and financial professionals and others in educating and advising their older patients and clients, and guide program development and implementation.

Information About Cognitive Status at a Point in Time

Research that directly measures cognition can provide a snapshot of the cognitive status of individuals at a single point in time. Such snapshots reveal differences between people of different ages or who differ on other characteristics; such differences are often referred to as *inter-individual* differences. Three of the studies shown in Table 3-1—MIDUS, the HRS, and NHATS—have provided information about inter-individual differences in cognitive status.

Midlife in the United States (MIDUS) Study

The MIDUS study examines a variety of factors that play a role in age-related variations in health and well-being (see Table 3-1; MIDUS, 2011a). The first phase of the study, MIDUS I, conducted from 1995 to 1996, assembled a sample of 7,108 individuals ages 24 to 75 years; cognition was measured directly in only a subsample of 302 individuals (Agrigoroaei and Lachman, 2011). The second phase of the study, MIDUS II, was conducted from 2004 to 2006, and cognition was measured in 4,268 of the original sample members, who were then ages 32 to 84 years (Lachman et al., 2014). Figure 3-1 shows the average scores for all MIDUS II sample members on tests of two components of cognition: episodic memory, including immediate and delayed recall, and executive functioning. The figure shows lower average scores on tests of episodic memory and executive function for individuals in each successive 5-year age group.

Figure 3-2, based on data from the MIDUS II study sample, shows a steady decline by age on each of the seven tests of various components of cognition (Lachman and Tun, 2008). The pattern differed somewhat from test to test, but the decline was steady in all. As in Figure 3-1, this figure reflects differences between individuals of different ages rather than changes in cognition in the same individuals over time.

Health and Retirement Study (HRS)

The HRS examines changes in many characteristics of adults age 50 years and older as they transition from work to retirement and older age

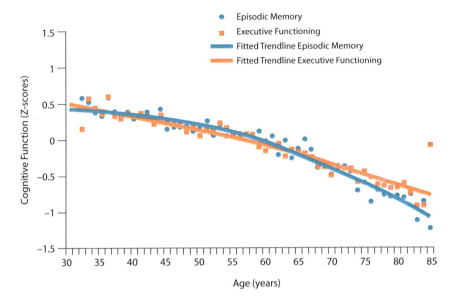

FIGURE 3-1 Differences in cognitive functioning by age, Midlife in the United States Study II (MIDUS II), N = 4,268, United States, 2004–2006.
NOTE: The use of Z-scores, shown on the vertical axis, enables data from different tests to be shown on the same scale. The dots represent the average scores of individuals by year of age. The solid lines are trend lines developed by statistical methods to show average trends in the data.
SOURCE: Lachman et al., 2014. Reprinted by permission of Sage Publications.

(see Table 3-1; HRS, 2014a). As discussed earlier, analyses of data from many existing surveys and studies often focus on moderate and severe cognitive impairment, dementia, and Alzheimer's disease rather than on the less severe cognitive changes that are the topic of this Institute of Medicine report. Figure 3-3 provides one example of findings from such an analysis, using data from the 2002 HRS. The figure shows the proportions of men and women age 65 years and older who had moderate or severe memory impairment according to tests that measured immediate and delayed recall as well as the much larger proportions of these men and women who had no memory impairment or only mild memory impairment. Sample members were considered to have had moderate memory impairment if they remembered four or fewer words out of 20 on immediate- and delayed-recall tests. They were counted as having severe memory impairment if they remembered two or fewer words on the tests.

The original graph from which Figure 3-3 was adapted appeared in *Older Americans 2000: Key Indicators of Well-Being*, a publicly available federal government report (FIFARS, 2004). That graph showed only the

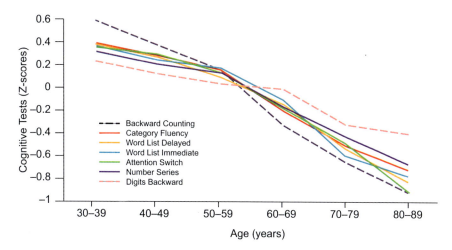

FIGURE 3-2 Differences in cognitive functioning by age based on different cognitive tests, Midlife in the United States Study II (MIDUS II), N = 4,268, United States, 2004–2006.
NOTE: The use of Z-scores, shown on the vertical axis, allows data from different tests to be shown on the same scale.
SOURCE: Lachman and Tun, 2008, revised and reformatted; Lachman, 2014. Published with permission from Sage Publications.

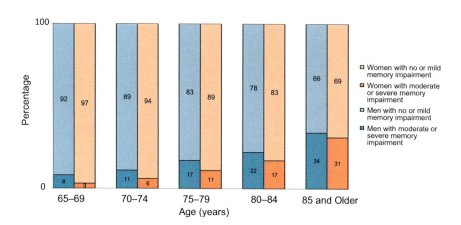

FIGURE 3-3 Proportions of people age 65 and older with moderate or severe memory impairment versus no or mild memory impairment, Health and Retirement Study, United States, 2002.
SOURCE: Adapted from FIFARS, 2004.

lower parts of the bars, which represented the proportions of men and women who had moderate or severe memory impairment. The extension of the bars in Figure 3-3 is intended to call attention to the large numbers of men and women age 65 years and older who are left out when the analyses focus only on moderate or severe impairment—in this case, proportions ranging from 92 percent of men and 97 percent of women age 65 to 69 years to 66 percent of men and 69 percent of women age 85 years and older.

Figure 3-3 is informative with respect to the extent of moderate and severe memory impairment in the older population and the way that the proportion of older adults with these conditions increases with increasing age. Even with the extended bars, however, the figure provides no information about variations in memory within the large proportions of older adults who did not have moderate or severe memory impairment. Yet some—and perhaps many—of the people who are shown as having no memory impairment or only mild memory impairment are likely to have experienced changes in memory and other cognitive functions that concern them and affect their day-to-day activities.

The HRS findings on global cognition, including memory and other cognitive functions, are often reported in four categories: normal, plus three categories of cognitive impairment as defined for the particular study. Using these categories, data for the HRS study population in 2002 show that 3.5 percent of the subjects who were age 70 years and older had "mild cognitive impairment," 5.2 percent had "moderate" or "severe cognitive impairment," and 91.3 percent had "normal cognitive function" (Langa et al., 2008). As is true for Figure 3-3, these proportions are informative with respect to the extent of cognitive impairment in older adults and are encouraging in the sense that the great majority of older adults do not have cognitive impairment as measured by the tests and scoring procedures used for study. However, no information is provided about variations in cognition in the very large proportion of the sample categorized as having "normal cognitive function."

National Health and Aging Trends Study (NHATS)

NHATS examines changes in the daily life and activities of adults of age 65 years and older (see Table 3-1; NHATS, 2014c). NHATS findings about cognition are often reported in three categories: probable dementia, possible dementia, and no dementia (Kasper et al., 2013). NHATS data for more than 7,600 sample members indicate that in 2011, 11.2 percent had probable dementia, and 10.6 percent had possible dementia, leaving 78.2 percent with no dementia (Kasper et al., 2014). Like the HRS figures, these NHATS figures are informative with respect to the extent of probable and possible dementia and encouraging in the sense that the great majority of older adults do not have these conditions. Yet, as with the HRS data, the NHATS figures provide no information about variations in cognitive function among the majority of older adults categorized as having no dementia.

*Challenges and Opportunities for Point-in-Time
Data Collection and Analysis*

In these surveys and studies, the focus on moderate and severe cognitive impairment and on probable and possible dementia undoubtedly reflects the high level of interest in dementia and dementia-related conditions among researchers, policy makers, and the public as well as the relatively lower level of interest to date in the less severe changes in cognition that are the focus of this report. People with less severe cognitive changes are variously categorized as having "normal cognitive function," "mild cognitive impairment," or "no dementia." The implications of these terms and categories are unclear with respect to cognitive abilities, impairments, and needs for information and assistance among the large number of adults so categorized. Raw data from the HRS, NHATS, and other surveys and studies could be used to discriminate more finely between these individuals. As discussed later in this chapter, the challenge will be to create operational definitions of meaningful categories for analyzing the raw data and reporting survey findings. Establishing these definitions would allow further differentiation of cognitive functioning among the vast majority of elders and enable the development of needed, population-based information about cognitive aging.

A few studies and surveys have tested methods to identify older adults who have a high level of cognition even at very old ages, thus enabling the creation of a category of cognition that has been referred to as "successful cognitive aging," a term this report does not use (see Chapter 1). One study tested several identification methods in a sample of 560 community-dwelling adults age 65 years and older (Negash et al., 2011). One method classified "successful agers" as those individuals with scores above the sample average on tests of four components of cognition. A second method compared the sample members' scores on tests of four components of cognition with the scores of adults ages 24 to 35 years and identified as "successful agers" the older adults who had scores at a specified level above the average for the younger adults. Both of these methods identified more sample members as "successful agers" than did a third method, which identified older adults with scores in the top 10 percent on a composite measure of the four components. Each of these methods could be used to create useful new categories of cognition within the current undifferentiated categories "normal cognitive function" and "no dementia." The three methods identified some of the same individuals, but many individuals were identified by only one or two of the methods, illustrating the difficulties facing those who aim to create meaningful categories for analyzing and reporting survey findings about cognition.

Information About Changes in Cognition Over Time

Many surveys that directly measure sample members' cognition are longitudinal; that is, they interview the same individuals more than once—and often numerous times—over a period of years. About three-quarters of the 40 U.S. surveys and studies identified by Bell and colleagues (2014) and 3 of the 5 surveys and studies included in Table 3-1 are longitudinal. Data from these studies could be used to describe changes in cognition for individuals over time. Depending on the cognitive functions measured in each survey, information could be provided about changes in global cognitive function as well as about particular components of cognition, such as memory, orientation, executive function, vocabulary, and reasoning. Information also could be gleaned about rates of change in cognitive performance, including the proportions of individuals whose cognition improves, stays the same, or declines over time.

As discussed in Chapters 1 and 2, the patterns and trajectories of cognitive change in individuals over time are extremely varied. Figure 2-1 in Chapter 2 shows data from the HRS on changes in cognitive scores over time in a representative sample of adults who had taken the cognitive tests in two or more waves of the study (McArdle, 2011). The figure illustrates the extensive variation among older adults in their patterns and trajectories of cognitive aging. It also shows the substantial variation between sample members at each age, something that is difficult to appreciate when only the average scores are presented. Furthermore, it shows that even though the average scores declined steadily over time, the scores for some individuals improved or at least stayed the same from one test time to a later one.

Other longitudinal studies conducted in representative samples of regional and local populations and in non-representative community samples have reported the proportions of older adults whose cognition stayed the same or declined over various time periods. All of these studies started with samples of individuals who were functioning at a relatively high level. A study of 2,733 generally healthy men and women ages 70 to 79 years found that after 4 years, 36 percent of the sample members had maintained the same level of cognitive functioning, 48 percent had experienced a minor decline in cognitive functioning, and 16 percent had had a major decline (Yaffe et al., 2010). Among the 2,509 sample members who were still participating in the study after 8 years, cumulative results show that 30 percent had maintained their level of cognitive functioning, 53 percent had a minor decline, and 16 percent had a major decline (Yaffe et al., 2009).

As could be expected, studies that lasted longer found lower proportions of sample members whose cognition had stayed the same over the study period. A 15-year study of 9,704 women age 65 years and older found that 9 percent maintained the same level of cognition functioning until the end of the study, 58 percent had a minor decline, and 33 percent had a major decline (Barnes et al., 2007). Similarly, a 9-year study of 322 women ages 70 to 80 years found that 49 percent had declined to predesignated levels of impairment in one or more components of cognition by the end of the study, with 37 percent having declined in executive function, 28 percent in immediate recall, 26 percent in delayed recall, and 21 percent in psychomotor speed (Carlson et al., 2009).

As part of the Mayo Clinic Study of Aging, which is conducted in a representative sample of a regional population, researchers measured changes over time in the cognitive trajectories of 1,390 adults ages 71 to 89 years (Machulda et al., 2013). All of the sample members were classified as cognitively unimpaired at the beginning of the study. Figure 3-4 shows the changes in the cognitive trajectories for global cognition in those sample members who were tested at least twice (and up to five times) over the course of the 5-year study. Of the 1,390 sample members, 947 (68 percent) remained cognitively unimpaired, 397 (29 percent) developed diagnosable mild cognitive impairment (MCI), and 46 (3 percent) developed dementia. Trajectories for sample members who developed MCI or dementia started out lower and had a somewhat steeper rate of decline when compared either with all sample members or with those who remained cognitively unimpaired. The researchers called attention to the fact that both the entire sample and the cognitively unimpaired sample—but not the sample that developed MCI or dementia—showed improvements in scores of cognition between the first and the second visits. They attribute the improvements to practice effects and note that all three groups showed improvements in scores on memory between the first and second visits (Machulda et al., 2013). (For further discussion about practice effects, see Chapter 2 and Thorgusen and Suchy, 2014.)

Self-Reported Awareness and Perceptions About Changes in Cognition

Surveys and studies that measure individuals' awareness and perceptions about their cognition can provide insight into older adults' thinking about changes in their own cognition and into how those changes affect their functioning. Each of the five nationally representative surveys and studies described in Table 3-1 includes one or more questions designed to measure respondents' awareness and perceptions of change in their cognition. At least four other ongoing surveys and studies conducted in nation-

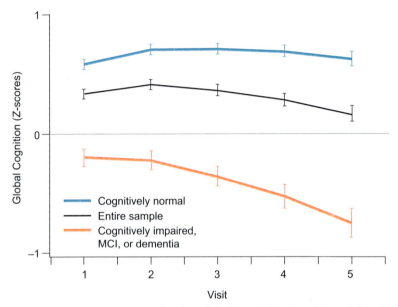

FIGURE 3-4 Cognitive trajectories for global cognition in older adults, Mayo Clinic Study of Aging, N = 1,390.
NOTE: MCI = mild cognitive impairment. The middle (black) line represents changes in cognitive trajectories for the sample as a whole. The lower (orange) line represents changes in trajectories for individuals who developed MCI or dementia during the study, and the top (blue) line represents changes in trajectories for individuals who remained cognitively unimpaired at the end of the study.
SOURCE: Machulda et al., 2013. Reprinted with permission of Taylor & Francis, Ltd.

ally representative samples also include one or more such questions[2] as do many regional and local surveys and studies. These surveys and studies use terms, such as "thinking," "remembering," "forgetting," "confusion," "memory loss," and "serious difficulty concentrating, remembering, or making decisions," to refer to cognition in their questions.

BRFSS conducts annual surveys to collect information about personal health behaviors and risk factors for mortality and morbidity (see Table 3-1; CDC, 2013a). BRFSS surveys are conducted by individual states, with administrative support and funding from the Centers for Disease Control and Prevention (CDC). The surveys include three types of questions: core questions, optional modules, and state-added questions. States are required to use the core questions in their state BRFSS surveys, but they can choose

---

[2] American Community Survey, Medicare Current Beneficiary Survey, Medicare Expenditure Panel Survey, and National Health Interview Survey.

whether to use any of the optional modules and whether to add questions of their own. In 2007, the CDC's Healthy Aging Program developed a set of 10 questions, referred to as the Optional Impact of Cognitive Impairment Module (CDC, 2007), to collect information about survey respondents' awareness and perceptions about their cognition (CDC, 2014a). The CDC and the Alzheimer's Association encouraged states to use this optional module and provided financial support for its use and for analysis of the resulting data.

Findings from 21 states that used the 2007 optional module in their 2011 BRFSS surveys show that among adult respondents age 60 years and older, 12 percent reported increased confusion or memory loss in the preceding 12 months, and that in that group more than a third also reported increased functional difficulties. The proportion of respondents reporting increased confusion or memory loss was higher among respondents who were 85 years or older, who were Hispanic, who had less than a high school education, or who reported that they were disabled (CDC, 2013c).

In 2014, the CDC and the states developed a new six-item optional module, the 2015 Cognitive Decline Module, to replace the 2007 module. As shown in Box 3-2, the new model asks respondents whether they have noticed changes in their cognition in the previous year and whether any such changes have affected their day-to-day functioning or resulted in the need for help with these activities. Some states are including the new module in their 2015 BRFSS survey, and it is hoped that many states will eventually do so.

Over at least the past four decades, questions have been raised about the validity of self-reported information about cognition. Research conducted in the United States and other countries has attempted to determine whether individuals' reports of cognitive decline, usually referred to as "subjective memory complaints," reflect true decline or other factors. Many studies have found subjective memory complaints to be associated with depression, other psychological distress, and personality characteristics such as conscientiousness, self-esteem, and neuroticism (Blazer et al., 1997; Kahn et al., 1975; O'Connor et al., 1990; Pearman and Storandt, 2004). Some researchers have concluded that these factors are the main driver of subjective memory complaints (see, e.g., Pearman and Storandt, 2004). Others have been persuaded that subjective memory complaints indicate real cognitive impairment and may also predict future cognitive decline (see, e.g., Geerlings et al., 1999; Jonker et al., 1996, 2000).

Research on the association between subjective memory complaints and current and future cognitive status as measured with objective tests has resulted in complex and sometimes contradictory findings. Among studies that have measured the association between subjective memory complaints and current cognitive status, those studies conducted in community samples

> **BOX 3-2**
> **Introduction and Questions in the 2015**
> **BRFSS Cognitive Decline Module**
>
> **Interviewer Introduction:** The next few questions ask about difficulties in thinking or remembering that can make a big difference in everyday activities. This does not refer to occasionally forgetting your keys or the name of someone you recently met, which is normal. This refers to confusion or memory loss that is happening more often or getting worse, such as forgetting how to do things you've always done or forgetting things that you would normally know. We want to know how these difficulties impact you.
>
> 1. During the past 12 months, have you experienced confusion or memory loss that is happening more often or is getting worse?
> 2. During the past 12 months, as a result of confusion or memory loss, how often have you given up day-to-day household activities or chores you used to do, such as cooking, cleaning, taking medications, driving, or paying bills?
> 3. As a result of confusion or memory loss, how often do you need assistance with these day-to-day activities?
> 4. When you need help with these day-to-day activities, how often are you able to get the help that you need?
> 5. During the past 12 months, how often has confusion or memory loss interfered with your ability to work, volunteer, or engage in social activities outside the home?
> 6. Have you or anyone else discussed your confusion or memory loss with a health care professional?
>
> SOURCE: CDC, 2014a.

have often found a stronger association than those conducted in clinical samples (Jonker et al., 2000). Studies that include individuals with various levels of cognitive impairment have generally found a stronger association between subjective memory complaints and current cognitive status in individuals with no or very mild cognitive impairment than in individuals with more cognitive impairment (Lerner et al., 2015; Turvey et al., 2000). Similarly, studies that include individuals with depressive symptoms have generally found a stronger association between subjective memory complaints and current cognitive status in individuals with fewer depressive symptoms than in individuals with more depressive symptoms (Hohman et al., 2011; Jungwirth et al., 2004). One analysis of data from a nationally representative community sample of 5,444 individuals age 70 years and older found a substantial association between individuals' reports about their own cognition and their scores on objective tests of cognition (Turvey et al., 2000). The association was weaker, however, for sample members whose cognitive test scores were in the lowest quarter of test scores, 57 percent of whom reported their memory was good, very good, or excellent. Likewise, the association was weaker for sample members with depressive symptoms.

Age, level of education, and other socio-demographic factors have also been found to affect the association between subjective memory complaints and current cognitive status in older adults. For example, three studies found substantial associations between subjective memory complaints and scores on objective tests of cognition in the young-old sample members (individuals under ages 75 or 80 in the study samples) but not in the older-old sample members (Fritsch et al., 2014; Hohman et al., 2011; Lerner et al., 2015).

Associations between subjective memory complaints and scores on objective tests of cognition may also depend on the specific complaints, the number of complaints, and the components of cognition measured (Amariglio et al., 2011; Riedel-Heller et al., 1999). An analysis of data from a large—but not population-based—study of almost 17,000 women of ages 70 to 81 years found that some subjective memory complaints, such as difficulty finding one's way around familiar streets, were more highly associated than other complaints with scores on objective tests of cognition (Amariglio et al., 2011). The complaint of forgetting things from one second to the next was not associated with cognitive status, but sample members who had many subjective memory complaints were more likely to score low on the cognitive test than those with fewer complaints.

Older adults' awareness and perceptions about changes in their own cognition are important because awareness and perceptions can affect the likelihood that they will hear and respond to messages about lifestyle and other factors that could improve their cognitive health and reduce the negative effects of cognitive aging. Gaining an increased understanding about the variations among older adults in their awareness and perceptions about changes in their own cognition could help health care and financial professionals and others who work with older adults individualize the education and advice that they provide to their patients and clients. Similarly, population-based information about older adults' awareness and perceptions about changes in their cognition could help public- and private-sector agencies at the national, state, and local levels develop and deliver messages and programs that match the array of perceptions about cognitive aging in the populations they serve.

Furthermore, the results of recent longitudinal studies generally support earlier findings of associations between subjective memory complaints and future cognitive decline (Glodzik-Sobanska et al., 2007; Kryscio et al., 2014; Reid and MacLullich, 2006; Reisberg et al., 2010; Slavin et al., 2010; Wang et al., 2004). These studies are generally conducted with samples of people who do not show any cognitive impairment on objective tests, suggesting that subjective memory complaints may represent very early awareness of changes in cognition that are too subtle to detect with objective cognitive tests (Petersen, 2014).

Given the complexity of findings about the association of subjective memory complaints and current cognitive status based on objective cognitive tests, and given the still early stage of research on the association of subjective memory complaints and future cognitive impairment, caution is needed in the dissemination of findings from population-based surveys and studies that measure self-reported changes in cognition, such as BRFSS. Reported findings must clearly discriminate between self-reported findings and those findings that are based on objective cognitive tests. Reported findings must also avoid language implying that findings based on self-report represent respondents' cognitive status as measured with objective tests. In this context, it is also important to acknowledge that some—and perhaps many—people may be aware of changes in their own cognition but are not willing to report their awareness on a survey for various reasons, including stigma. As discussed in Chapter 2, age, ethnicity, culture, level of education, and other factors associated with familiarity and comfort in testing situations can affect responses to research questions. Thus, reviews of findings from surveys and studies that measure self-reported cognitive status and cognitive changes in older adults' awareness and perceptions about changes in cognition must acknowledge the many factors that could lead to underreporting.

CHALLENGES TO INCREASING POPULATION-BASED INFORMATION ABOUT COGNITIVE AGING

At least five important challenges will have to be addressed in creating a system that will effectively collect, analyze, and disseminate population-based information about cognitive aging, particularly for public health purposes. These challenges are the development of (1) operational definitions of cognitive aging; (2) standards and procedures for ensuring representative, population-based samples; (3) cognitive tests and survey questions relevant for cognitive aging; (4) efficient modes of testing that maximize respondent participation and the accuracy of findings; and (5) methods for the appropriate use of proxy respondents and the incorporation of proxy responses into the available information about cognitive aging.

Although the availability of improved population-based information about cognitive aging is likely to be useful for research and public policy purposes, the primary objectives in creating a system to collect, analyze, and disseminate this information are to:

- increase public awareness and understanding about cognitive aging;
- engage individuals and their families in maintaining cognitive health across the life span;
- inform health care professionals, financial professionals, and others in how to educate and advise their older patients about cognitive aging; and
- guide the planning, implementation, and evaluation of programs and initiatives to maintain cognitive health and reduce the negative effects of cognitive aging for older adults, their families, and their communities.

Developing Operational Definitions of Cognitive Aging

While many population-based surveys and studies collect or use data on cognition in older persons (Bell et al., 2014), relatively little attention has been given to developing operational definitions that would allow for population-based estimates of the nature and extent of cognitive aging. As described in this chapter, findings about cognition from nationally representative surveys and studies, such as the HRS and NHATS, are often reported in categories that emphasize moderate and severe cognitive impairment and dementia. These categories reflect the current high level of interest in dementia and dementia-related conditions among researchers, policy makers, and the public, but they leave out the kinds of cognitive changes that are experienced by the majority of older adults—changes that are troubling to many older adults and that may affect important day-to-day functions, such as driving, making financial decisions, and managing medications.

Developing operational definitions of cognitive aging is challenging because aging is an ongoing process with wide variation among individuals. As discussed in Chapter 2, the current understanding about the boundaries between the various levels of cognition in older adults is incomplete. Uncertainty about these boundaries and the current lack of agreed-upon standards or norms that could be used to translate individuals' raw scores on cognitive tests into meaningful categories are major barriers to the development of a system of population-based surveillance. It remains to be determined whether acceptable boundaries and thresholds can be identified.

The comprehensive characterization of cognitive aging used by the committee in this report (see Chapter 1) has not yet been translated into explicit operational definitions and criteria that could be applied in surveys and studies conducted in population-based, volunteer, or clinical samples. The current lack of standardized and explicit diagnostic and categorization criteria impedes the conduct and interpretation of epidemiologic studies. Comprehensive population-based surveys and studies require operational definitions in order to compare findings across studies and population segments and to determine any time trends. Once consensus definitions are developed, it will be important to determine the optimal interval between surveys in a study cohort for determining rates of cognitive aging over time.

Operational definitions of cognitive aging will require, among other considerations, a standardized set of cognitive scales and tests. Many population studies use similar cognitive items and tap similar cognitive domains (such as memory, executive function, and orientation), but variations in item and scale origin and structure may make comparisons among them difficult.

Newer test development initiatives based on modern test theory aim to increase the standardization of cognitive testing across studies, improve the reliability and validity of cognitive tests, and increase the efficiency in the number of test items. Item response theory, for example, has been used in the development of the National Institutes of Health (NIH) Patient-Reported Outcomes Measurement Information System (PROMIS) self-report cognitive function scales (Cella et al., 2010) and the NIH Toolbox Assessment of Neurological and Behavioral Function®. Item response modeling is designed to measure the underlying traits that are producing performance on a test (Wilson et al., 2006a,b) and has the practical advantages of allowing the aggregation of items measuring common constructs and also allowing item banking for computer adaptive testing targeted to the individual (Becker et al., 2014; Gershon et al., 2014). Both the PROMIS cognitive scales and the NIH Toolbox® cognitive battery were originally designed to meet research needs, but they may also be useful in developing operational definitions and criteria for population-based surveillance.

Ensuring the Representativeness of Population-Based Samples

Another important challenge in conducting population-based research on cognitive aging is that the sampling frame may not represent the population. In general, participation rates for national and regional surveys have been declining (Galea and Tracy, 2007). It is quite plausible that people having different levels of cognitive function may differ in their likelihood of participating in such surveys, and some individuals, because of illness or a refusal to participate, may not be testable even in special clinical settings. The impact of such selective non-participation can be understood if important characteristics of the sampling frame sources are available, such as from a Medicare beneficiary sample, but this information is frequently not easily accessible. Significant levels of survey non-response can lead to uncertainty and potential bias in survey findings.

Among the most important demographic characteristics in population surveys are race and ethnicity. Racial disparities in late-life cognitive performance are well documented (see, e.g., Sisco et al., 2014). While some of these disparities can be statistically explained by variation in individual or family socioeconomic status (SES) or disadvantages in the childhood social environment (Cheng et al., 2014), there may be important differences between how SES correlates with cognitive status and how it correlates with the changes in cognitive status over time (Yaffe et al., 2009; Zahodne et al., 2011). Furthermore, other factors—for example, test bias and reading levels—may account for part of the variation among racial groups, particularly between whites and African Americans (see, e.g., Fyffe et al., 2011; Mehta et al., 2004). These factors are often not well studied, particularly with respect to adjusting findings for racial and ethnic variation. More work is needed when planning and executing research to assess cognitive aging across population groups known to have systematic variation in cognitive performance.

Each of the five surveys and studies in Table 3-1 includes questions about race and ethnicity. As noted earlier, however, nationally representative surveys and studies often have an insufficient sample size to explore less common minority, nationality, or language groups with the precision needed to affect public health decisions; understanding these groups in any detail usually requires separately targeted surveys or expanded samples or subsamples.

Other important issues affecting the representativeness of population-based surveys and studies pertain to the inclusion of individuals with serious co-morbid medical or mental health conditions and individuals living in nursing homes and assisted living facilities. These individuals are more likely to have higher-than-average levels of cognitive impairment. Even those who do not have diagnosable MCI or dementia are likely to have age-related cognitive changes that affect their day-to-day functioning.

Including Relevant Cognitive Tests and Survey Questions About Cognition

As noted earlier, cognitive test results vary, depending on the specific test used. This is important because the cognitive tests used in existing population-based surveys and studies vary widely, in part because of the amount of time they allocate for cognitive assessment. Furthermore, many of the cognitive tests used in national surveys are oriented to assessing or at least screening for major dementia-related conditions, using validated mental status scales and instruments. Some of these instruments lack the ability to detect and evaluate variations at the higher end of cognitive performance, and additional, more sensitive instruments to measure cognition in the high functioning range may be needed. Still, within surveys and studies that address cognitive aging, the ability to identify MCI and dementia is important so that those individuals can be excluded from the analysis of cognitive aging, as characterized in Chapter 1.

Additional test-related issues include identifying the best measures of change in cognition and determining the time intervals that are most appropriate for monitoring change. Questions about cognition must be as comprehensible as possible across a broad range of literacy levels, and responses may need to be interpreted differently for people who have different primary languages or racial and ethnic backgrounds. Furthermore, the contribution of practice effects, when individuals are given the same tests or test items on two or more different occasions, need clarification.

As noted in Chapters 1 and 2, any definition of cognitive aging must consider the functional impact of such aging on individuals and on the people in their social environment. However, much more research is needed to identify the physical, mental, and social functions that may be affected by cognitive aging, and these alterations may differ substantially among individuals for any number of reasons. Existing population-based surveys and studies include questions about activities of daily living (such as bathing and dressing) and instrumental activities of daily living (IADLs), and several IADLs—notably money and medication management—have been described as "cognitive IADLs." It is also important to capture, to the extent possible, how cognitive changes affect other complex tasks with practical relevance, such as tasks that take place within work, family, or other social environments (Czaja and Sharit, 2003). The BRFSS Cognitive Decline module (CDC, 2014a) includes questions about the areas in which a person needs the most help, such as whether the person's confusion or memory loss has interfered with his or her ability to work, volunteer, or engage in social activities. Likewise, the HRS and NHATS include questions that link cognitive decline with problems with various activities such as "being able to work familiar machines," "learning to use a new tool, appliance, or gadget," and "being able to follow a story in a book or on TV" (HRS, 2014b; NHATS, 2014b).

Selecting Efficient Modes of Testing

It is important to select efficient modes of testing that maximize respondent participation and the accuracy of findings. Existing surveys and studies of cognition generally rely on in-person and telephone interviews, and some of them use printed or online self-assessments completed by the respondent at home. Newer modes of online testing are also being used. The choice of survey modes will be dictated at least in part by cost considerations. In-person interviews, which are the most costly mode of testing, can allow the self-report of cognitive symptoms, consequent dysfunction, the use of self- or family-directed remedies, relevant co-morbidity, and the use and outcomes of consultation in formal medical care. Such information is critical and would be difficult to collect for individuals, family caregivers, and other family members in any other way.

Using Proxy Respondents and Responses

Many existing population-based surveys and studies that measure cognition include questions that are asked of proxy respondents, who are usually family members and other informants, in addition to or instead of those questions for the older adults themselves. In some surveys, the proxy respondent answers questions only if the sample person is not able to, while in other surveys both the proxy respondent and the sample person answer the questions.

Population-based surveillance of cognitive aging might profitably include proxy respondents as a matter of routine whenever they are available. They may provide different and more detailed information than the index respondent. It is unclear, however, to what extent proxy respondents are needed in the case of respondents with cognitive changes that do not reach the level of MCI or dementia. It is also likely that there will be differences in the responses given by the older adult, by a family member, or by other proxy respondents. These differences have been studied for many years among people with dementia but have received less attention with respect to people with less severe cognitive change.

NEXT STEPS AND RECOMMENDATION

As noted in this chapter, a substantial amount of community and population research has been conducted on cognitive performance among older persons. The problem of cognitive aging, which is increasing in public health importance, underscores the need for a more robust surveillance system. While much of the research on representative geographic samples has focused on the detection and assessment of moderate and severe dementia-related conditions, investigative and public interest in cognitive aging is also rapidly increasing. Studies on volunteer research populations have provided important scientific findings, but from a public health perspective, a more complete view is needed of the nature and extent of cognitive aging in older adults. The committee concludes, therefore, that a more extensive surveillance approach is warranted, which will require careful planning and pretesting. The committee offers the following vision for the next steps for such a program.

Build on Current Surveys and Related Data Sources

Because of both the costs and the complexity of surveillance for cognitive aging, it may be useful to share resources and questionnaire space with other ongoing national surveys and studies. Many relevant items are already in place, and collaborations with existing surveys should prove worthwhile. Surveys conducted with representative samples of regional and local populations can also contribute to the understanding of cognitive aging.

Some of the categories used to report information about cognition in surveys and studies conducted with representative regional and local population samples are the same from survey to survey, and some vary. Some surveys (e.g., the HRS and NHATS) use categories that reflect a strong emphasis on dementia and predementia conditions. Other regional and local research obtains detailed information about cognition as an outcome, a control variable, or a predictor of other study outcomes (McArdle et al., 2007). This detailed information is rarely reported, however. Instead, it is often converted to statistics, which are essential for research but which cannot be used to increase understanding of cognitive aging in non-research audiences.

Perhaps the most important question remaining is whether existing population data accurately characterize, in terms of the prevalence and incidence of cognitive aging, the overall cognitive status of a community or nation. Accepting existing cognitive measures as indicators of age-related changes would enable the development of score thresholds and ancillary rules or algorithms to define population rates. However, as discussed earlier, providing community-wide information about cognitive aging rates requires more research as well as the specification of well-considered operational definitions of cognitive aging. Only then could even provisional rates of population cognitive aging rates be estimated. Additional logistical and practical questions, include

- How inclusive does a population sample have to be? How can adequate representation of racial, ethnic, and non-English-speaking minority individuals be assured? Should those who may be cognitively impaired and residing in institutional settings be included? How would incomplete participation rates, as well as information from proxy respondents, be handled?
- What battery of cognitive tests should be included? How should co-existing cognitive conditions such as MCI or Alzheimer's disease be excluded, and by what means would dementia-related illnesses be determined?

- How would the test battery be standardized? Would this be based on statistical distributions, such as percentiles? How would a composite cognitive index be constructed? Would there be adjustment for educational attainment or other factors known to alter cognitive performance? Would designation of cognitive aging require evidence of physical or social dysfunction?
- How would self-reported cognitive symptoms be integrated with cognitive test scores?
- What modes of testing would be acceptable, and would mixed modes be credible?
- How would individuals with serious co-morbid medical or mental conditions be surveyed and counted?

Expand the Types of Data Collected and Examine Other Approaches to Data Collection

Ongoing or periodic surveillance for cognitive aging may include data collection from sources other than personal interviews and test results. For example, analyses of de-identified data from large health systems' electronic health records may provide useful information in many cognitive and related clinical domains, as is occurring in other areas of surveillance. Sales data for drugs or other products used for the prevention or management of cognitive impairment may provide useful insights into population and professional concerns. Similarly, it may be useful to monitor secondary effects of cognitive aging from public records, such as police reports of persons getting lost and automobile crash rates among older persons. Financial transactions, such as mispaid bills, aberrant fund transfers, and unsuitable transactions, are another ecologically valid means of surveillance at both the individual and the population level, although confidentiality and privacy concerns would need to be addressed.

Disseminating Information to Survey Participants

Whatever the established protocols for routine surveillance programs, the emotional sensitivity of finding evidence for any level of clinical impairment during a cognitive assessment may raise the issue of whether test results should be returned to the surveillance participants for possible medical consultation. Individuals have different views on the desirability of receiving this information (Dawson et al., 2006), and providing cognitive test results without a clinical interpretation should be done cautiously, particularly when the results label a person as cognitively impaired. A sensible response to requests for results would be to also provide participants with information about how to discuss cognitive concerns with their health care provider.

Widely Disseminate Information to the General Public

As discussed in this chapter, existing U.S. surveys and other studies collect substantial amounts of information about cognition in older adults. Although some researchers are familiar with the available information about cognition, it is generally not presented in formats and media that are accessible to most older adults, health care professionals and others who work with older adults, administrative and program staff of government and private-sector organizations, and other non-research audiences. To make the information understandable and meaningful to these audiences will require significant reformatting and clear explanations of complex concepts. Terms will have to be defined in lay language, and methodological practices, such as the use of Z-scores to standardize results from different cognitive tests, will have to be explained or replaced. One of the biggest challenges in communicating meaningful and useful information about cognitive aging to the general public will be providing easy-to-understand explanations about the relationship between changes in cognition that older adults may experience and their risk of developing MCI or dementia, a relationship that is still not well understood. Increased understanding about cognitive aging could help increase public awareness, answer questions and address concerns of older adults and their families, improve the information advice health care and financial professionals and others provide to their older patients and clients, and help public health agencies and other public and private organizations create effective programs to reduce cognitive impairment and improve cognitive health in older adults.

RECOMMENDATION

Recommendation 2: *Collect and Disseminate Population-Based Data on Cognitive Aging*
The Centers for Disease Control and Prevention (CDC), state health agencies, and other relevant government agencies, as well as nonprofit organizations, research foundations, and academic research institutions, should strengthen efforts to collect and disseminate population-based data on cognitive aging. These efforts should identify the nature and extent of cognitive aging throughout the population, including high-risk and underserved populations, with the goal of informing the general public and improving relevant policies, programs and services.

Specifically, expanded cognitive aging data collection and dissemination efforts should include

- A focus on the cognitive health of older adults as separate from dementia or other clinical neurodegenerative diseases.

- The development of operational definitions of cognitive aging for use in research and public health surveillance and also the development of a process for periodic reexamination. Analyses of existing longitudinal datasets of older persons should be used to inform these efforts.
- Expanded data collection efforts and further analyses of representative surveys involving geographically diverse and high-risk populations. These efforts should include cognitive testing when standardized, feasible, and clinically credible and also self-reports of perceptions or concerns regarding cognitive aging, personal and social adaptations, and self-care and other management practices.
- Longitudinal assessments of changes in cognitive performance and risk behaviors in diverse populations.
- Inclusion of cognition-related questions in the core instrument of the Behavioral Risk Factor Surveillance System, rather than an optional module.
- Exploration of other available relevant data on cognitive health such as health insurance claims data, sales and marketing data for cognition-related products and treatments, data on financial and banking transactions as well as on financial fraud and scams, and data on automobile insurance claims.
- Active dissemination of data on cognitive aging in the population. An annual or biennial report to the U.S. public should be issued by the CDC or other federal agency on the nature and extent of cognitive aging in the U.S. population.

REFERENCES

Agrigoroaei, S., and M. E. Lachman. 2011. Cognitive functioning in midlife and old age: Combined effects of psychosocial and behavioral factors. *The Journals of Gerontology, Series B: Psychological Sciences and Social Sciences* 66B(S1):i130-i140.

Amariglio, R. E., M. K. Townsend, F. Grodstein, R. A. Sperling, and D. M. Rentz. 2011. Specific subjective memory complaints in older persons may indicate poor cognitive function. *Journal of the American Geriatrics Society* 59:1612-1617.

Barnes, D. E., J. A. Cauley, L. Y. Lui, H. A. Fink, C. McCulloch, K. L. Stone, and K. Yaffe. 2007. Women who maintain optimal cognitive function into old age. *Journal of the American Geriatrics Society* 55(2):259-264.

Becker, H., A. Stuifbergen, H. Lee, and V. Kullberg. 2014. Reliability and validity of PROMIS cognitive abilities and cognitive concerns scales among people with multiple sclerosis. *International Journal of MS Care* 16(1):1-8.

Bell, J. F., A. L. Fitzpatrick, C. Copeland, G. Chi, L. Steinman, R. L. Whitney, D. C. Atkins, L. L. Bryant, F. Grodstein, E. Larson, R. Logsdon, and M. Snowden. 2014. Existing data sets to support studies of dementia or significant cognitive impairment and comorbid chronic conditions. *Alzheimer's & Dementia* (September 4).

Blazer, D. G., J. C. Hays, G. G. Fillenbaum, and D. T. Gold. 1997. Memory complaint as a predictor of cognitive decline: A comparison of African American and White elders. *Journal of Aging and Health* 9(2):171-184.

Brookmeyer, R., D. A. Evans, L. Hebert, K. M. Langa, S. G. Heeringa, B. L. Plassman, and W. A. Kukull. 2011. National estimates of the prevalence of Alzheimer's disease in the United States. *Alzheimer's & Dementia* 7(1):61-73.

Carlson, M. C., Q. L. Xue, J. Zhou, and L. P. Fried. 2009. Executive decline and dysfunction precedes declines in memory: The Women's Health and Aging Study II. *The Journals of Gerontology, Series A: Biological Sciences and Medical Sciences* 64A(1):110-117.

CDC (Centers for Disease Control and Prevention). 2007. Behavioral Risk Factor Surveillance System (BRFSS) Optional Impact of Cognitive Impairment Module. http://www.cdc.gov/aging/pdf/impact_of_cognitive_impairment_ module.pdf (accessed February 26, 2015).

———. 2013a. *BRFSS: About BRFSS.* http://www.cdc.gov/brfss/about/index.htm (accessed December 19, 2014).

———. 2013b. *2014 Behavioral risk factor surveillance system questionnaire.* http://www.cdc.gov/brfss/questionnaires/pdf-ques/2014_BRFSS.pdf (accessed January 12, 2015).

———. 2013c. Self-reported increased confusion or memory loss and associated functional difficulties among adults aged ≥ 60 years—21 states, 2011. *Morbidity and Mortality Weekly Report* 62(18):347-350.

———. 2014a. *Behavioral Risk Factor Surveillance System (BRFSS) 2015 Cognitive Decline Module.* http://www.cdc.gov/aging/healthybrain/brfss-faq.htm (accessed December 19, 2014).

———. 2014b. *National Health and Nutrition Examination Survey.* http://www.cdc.gov/nchs/nhanes.htm (accessed December 19, 2014).

———. 2014c. *NHANES 2013–2014.* http://wwwn.cdc.gov/nchs/nhanes/search/nhanes13_14.aspx (accessed January 12, 2015).

Cella, D., W. Riley, A. Stone, N. Rothrock, B. Reeve, S. Yount, D. Amtmann, R. Bode, D. Buysse, S. Choi, K. Cook, R. Devellis, D. DeWalt, J. F. Fries, R. Gershon, E. A. Hahn, J. S. Lai, P. Pilkonis, D. Revicki, M. Rose, K. Weinfurt, and R. Hays, and PROMIS Cooperative Group. 2010. The Patient-Reported Outcomes Measurement Information System (PROMIS) developed and tested its first wave of adult self-reported health outcome item banks: 2005–2008. *Journal of Clinical Epidemiology* 63(11):1179-1194.

Cheng, E. R., H. Park, S. A. Robert, M. Palta, and W. P. Witt. 2014. Impact of county disadvantage on behavior problems among U.S. children with cognitive delay. *American Journal of Public Health* 104(11):2114-2121.

Cornoni-Huntley, J., D. B. Brock, A. Ostfeld, J. O. Taylor, R. B. Wallace, and M. E. Lafferty. 1986. *Established populations for epidemiologic studies of the elderly: Resource data book.* Vol. I. Bethesda, MD: National Institute on Aging.

Cornoni-Huntley, J., D. G. Blazer, M. E. Lafferty, D. F. Everett, D. B. Brock, and M. E. Farmer. 1990. *Established populations for epidemiologic studies of the elderly.* Vol. II. Bethesda, MD: National Institute on Aging.

Czaja, S. J., and J. Sharit. 2003. Practically relevant research: Capturing real world tasks, environments, and outcomes. *Gerontologist* 43(Suppl. 1):9-18.

Dawson, E., K. Savitsky, and D. Dunning. 2006. "Don't tell me, I don't want to know": Understanding people's reluctance to obtain medical diagnostic information. *Journal of Applied Psychology* 36(3):751-768.

FIFARS (Federal Interagency Forum on Aging-Related Statistics). 2004. *Indicator 17: Memory impairment.* http://www.agingstats.gov/agingstatsdotnet/Main_Site/Data/2004_Documents/healthstatus.aspx#Indicator17 (accessed December 19, 2014).

Fritsch, T., M. J. McClendon, M. S. Wallendal, T. F. Hude, and J. D. Larsen. 2014. Prevalence and cognitive bases of subjective memory complaints in older adults: Evidence from a community sample. *Journal of Neurodegenerative Diseases.* http://www.hindawi.com/journals/jnd/2014/176843 (accessed March 23, 2015).

Fyffe, D. C., S. Mukherjee, L. L. Barnes, J. J. Manly, D. A. Bennett, and P. K. Crane. 2011. Explaining differences in episodic memory performance among older African Americans and Whites: The roles of factors related to cognitive reserve and test bias. *Journal of the International Neuropsychological Society* 17(4):625-638.

Galea, S., and M. Tracy. 2007. Participation rates in epidemiologic studies. *Annals of Epidemiology* 17(9):643-653.

Geerlings, M. I., C. Jonker, L. M. Bouter, H. J. Ader, and B. Schmand. 1999. Association between memory complaints and incident Alzheimer's disease in elderly people with normal baseline cognition. *American Journal of Psychiatry* 156(4):531-537.

Gershon, R. C., K. F. Cook, D. Mungas, J. J. Manly, J. Slotkin, J. L. Beaumont, and S. Weintraub. 2014. Language measures of the NIH Toolbox Cognition Battery. *Journal of the International Neuropsychology Society* 20(6):642-651.

Glodzik-Sobanska, L., B. Reisberg, S. De Santi, J. S. Babb, E. Pirraglia, K. E. Rich, M. Brys, and M. J. de Leon. 2007. Subjective memory complaints: Presence, severity and future outcome in normal older subjects. *Dementia and Geriatric Cognitive Disorders* 24(3):177-184.

Hebert, L. E., J. Weuve, P. A. Scherr, and D. A. Evans. 2013. Alzheimer disease in the United States (2010-2050) estimated using the 2010 census. *Neurology* 80:1778-1783.

Hofer, S. M., and S. Clouston. 2014. Commentary: On the importance of early life cognitive abilities in shaping later life outcomes. *Research in Human Development* 11(3):241-246.

Hohman, T. J., L. L. Beason-Held, and S. M. Resnick. 2011. Cognitive complaints, depressive symptoms, and cognitive impairment: Are they related? *Journal of the American Geriatrics Society* 59(10):1908-1912.

HRS (Health and Retirement Study). 2014a. *Health and Retirement Study: A longitudinal study of health, retirement, and aging.* http://hrsonline.isr.umich.edu (accessed December 18, 2014).

———. 2014b. *HRS 2014—Section D: Cognition.* http://hrsonline.isr.umich.edu/modules/meta/2014/core/qnaire/online/04hr14D.pdf (accessed December 19, 2014).

———. 2015. *Biennial interview questionnaires.* http://hrsonline.isr.umich.edu/index.php?p=qnaires (accessed January 12, 2015).

Jonker, C., L. J. Launer, C. Hooijer, and J. Lindeboom. 1996. Memory complaints and memory impairment in older individuals. *Journal of the American Geriatrics Society* 44(1):44-49.

Jonker, C., M. I. Geerlings, and B. Schmand. 2000. Are memory complaints predictive for dementia? A review of clinical and population-based studies. *International Journal of Geriatric Psychiatry* 15:983-991.

Jungwirth, S., P. Fischer, S. Weissgram, W. Kirchmeyr, P. Bauer, and K. H. Tragl. 2004. Subjective memory complaints and objective memory impairment in the Vienna–Transdanube aging community. *Journal of the American Geriatrics Society* 52(2):263-268.

Kahn, R. L., S. H. Zarit, N. M. Hilbert, and G. Niederehe. 1975. Memory complaint and impairment in the aged. The effect of depression and altered brain function. *Archives of General Psychiatry* 32(2):1569-1573.

Kasper, J. D., V. A. Freedman, and B. C. Spillman. 2013. *Classification of persons by dementia status in the National Health and Aging Trends Study: Technical paper #5.* Baltimore, MD: Johns Hopkins University School of Public Health. http://www.nhats.org/scripts/documents/NHATS_Dementia_Technical_Paper_5_Jul2013.pdf (accessed January 7, 2015).

———. 2014. *Disability and care needs of older Americans by dementia status: An analysis of the 2011 National Health and Aging Trends Study*. Washington, DC. http://aspe.hhs.gov/daltcp/reports/2014/NHATS-DS.pdf (accessed December 19, 2014).

Kryscio, R. J., E. L. Abner, G. E. Cooper, D. W. Fardo, G. A. Jicha, P. T. Nelson, C. D. Smith, L. J. Van Eldik, L. Wan, and F. A. Schmitt. 2014. Self-reported memory complaints: Implications from a longitudinal cohort with autopsies. *Neurology* 83(15):1359-1365.

Lachman, M. E. 2014. *Monitoring cognitive functioning: National Survey of Midlife in the United States (MIDUS)*. http://www.iom.edu/~/media/Files/Activity%20Files/Aging/Cognitive%20aging/10-APR-2014/Margie%20Lachman.pdf (accessed December 18, 2014).

Lachman, M. E., and P. A. Tun. 2008. Cognitive testing in large-scale surveys: Assessment by telephone. In *Handbook of Cognitive Aging: Interdisciplinary Perspectives*, edited by S. Hofer and D. Alwin. Thousand Oaks, CA: Sage Publishers.

Lachman, M. E., S. Agrigoroaei, P. A. Tun, and S. L. Weaver. 2014. Monitoring cognitive functioning: Psychometric properties of the brief test of adult cognition by telephone. *Assessment* 21(4):404-417.

Langa, K. M., E. B. Larson, J. H. Karlawish, D. M. Cutler, M. U. Kabeto, S. Y. Kim, and A. B. Rosen. 2008. Trends in the prevalence and mortality of cognitive impairment in the United States: Is there evidence of a compression of cognitive morbidity? *Alzheimer's & Dementia* 4(2):134-144.

Lerner, J., S. Kogler, C. Lamm, D. Moser, S. Klug, G. Pusswald, P. Dal-Bianco, W. Pirker, and E. Auff. 2015. Awareness of memory deficits in subjective cognitive decline, mild cognitive impairment, Alzheimer's disease and Parkinson's disease. *International Psychogeriatrics* 27(3):357-366.

Machulda, M. M., V. S. Pankratz, T. J. Christianson, R. J. Ivnik, M. M. Mielke, R. O. Roberts, D. S. Knopman, B. F. Boeve, and R. C. Petersen. 2013. Practice effects and longitudinal cognitive change in normal aging vs. incident mild cognitive impairment and dementia in the Mayo Clinic Study of Aging. *The Clinical Neuropsychologist* 27(8):1247-1264.

McArdle, J. 2011. Longitudinal dynamic analyses of cognition in the Health and Retirement Study panel. *Advances in Statistical Analysis* 95(4):453-480.

McArdle, J. J., G. G. Fisher, and K. M. Kadlec. 2007. Latent variable analyses of age trends of cognition in the Health and Retirement Study, 1992-2004. *Psychology and Aging* 22(3):525-545.

Mehta, K. M., E. M. Simonsick, R. Rooks, A. B. Newman, S. K. Pope, S. M. Rubin, and K. Yaffe. 2004. Black and white differences in cognitive function test scores: What explains the difference? *Journal of the American Geriatrics Society* 52(12):2120-2127.

MIDUS (Midlife Development in the United States). 2011a. *History and overview of MIDUS*. http://www.midus.wisc.edu/scopeofstudy.php (accessed February 22, 2015).

———. 2011b. *National Survey of Midlife Development in the United States (MIDUS I), 1995–1996*. http://www.midus.wisc.edu/midus1/index.php (accessed January 12, 2015).

———. 2011c. *Project 1-MIDUS II, 2004–2006*. http://www.midus.wisc.edu/midus2/project1 (accessed Feburary 22, 2015).

———. 2011d. *MIDUS II cognitive test battery, Brief Test of Adult Cognition by Telephone (BTACT)*. http://www.midus.wisc.edu/midus2/project3/BTACT_FORM_A_rev2_12.pdf (accessed February 22, 2015).

———. 2011e. *MIDUS data timelines*. http://www.midus.wisc.edu/data/timeline.php (accessed January 13, 2015).

Negash, S., G. E. Smith, S. Pankratz, J. Aakre, Y. E. Geda, R. O. Roberts, D. S. Knopman, B. F. Boeve, R. J. Ivnik, and R. C. Petersen. 2011. Successful aging: Definitions and prediction of longevity and conversion to mild cognitive impairment. *American Journal of Geriatric Psychiatry* 19(6):581-588.

NHATS (National Health and Aging Trends Study). 2014a. *NHATS at a glance.* http://www.nhats.org/scripts/default.htm (accessed January 6, 2015).
———. 2014b. *NHATS Round 3: Section GG—Cognition.* http://nhats.org/scripts/instruments/017_CG_Round3.pdf (accessed December 19, 2014).
———. 2014c. *NHATS: National Health and Aging Trends Study.* http://nhats.org (accessed December 18, 2014).
———. 2014d. *Round 1 data collection instruments.* http://www.nhats.org/scripts/data CollInstr.htm (accessed January 12, 2015).
———. 2014e. *Round 2 data collection instruments.* http://www.nhats.org/scripts/data CollInstrR2.htm (accessed January 12, 2015).
———. 2014f. *Round 3 data collection instruments.* http://www.nhats.org/scripts/data CollInstrR3.htm (accessed January 12, 2015).
O'Connor, D. W., P. A. Pollitt, M. Roth, P. B. Brook, and B. B. Reiss. 1990. Memory complaints and impairment in normal, depressed, and demented elderly persons identified in a community survey. *Archives of General Psychiatry* 47(3):224-227.
Pearman, A., and M. Storandt. 2004. Predictors of subjective memory in older adults. *The Journals of Gerontology, Series B: Psychological Sciences and Social Sciences* 59(1):P4-P6.
Petersen, R. C. 2014. Presentation to the IOM Committee on Public Health Dimensions of Cognitive Aging, Washington, DC, September 26.
Plassman, B. L., K. M. Langa, G. G. Fisher, S. G. Heeringa, D. R. Weir, M. B. Ofstedal, J. R. Burke, M. D. Hurd, G. G. Potter, W. L. Rodgers, D. C. Steffens, R. J. Willis, and R. B. Wallace. 2007. Prevalence of dementia in the United States: The Aging, Demographics, and Memory Study. *Neuroepidemiology* 29:125-132.
Reid, L. M., and A. M. J. MacLullich, 2006. Subjective memory complaints and cognitive impairment in older people. *Dementia and Geriatric Cognitive Disorders* 2(5-6):471-485.
Reisberg, B., M. B. Shulman, C. Torossian, L. Leng, and W. Zhu. 2010. Outcome over seven years of healthy adults with and without subjective cognitive impairment. *Alzheimer's & Dementia* 6(1):11-24.
Riedel-Heller, S. G., H. Matschinger, A. Schork, and M. C. Angermeyer. 1999. Do memory complaints indicate the presence of cognitive impairment? Results of a field study. *European Archives of Psychiatry and Clinical Neurosciences* 249:197-204.
Rocca, W. A., R. C. Peterson, D. S. Knopman, L. E. Hebert, D. A. Evans, K. S. Hall, S. Gao, F. W. Unverzagt, K. M. Langa, E. B. Larson, and L. R. White. 2011. Trends in the incidence and prevalence of Alzheimer's disease, dementia and cognitive impairment in the United States. *Alzheimer's & Dementia* 7(1):80-93.
Sisco, S., A. L. Gross, R. A. Shih, B. C. Sachs, M. M. Glymour, K. J. Bangen, A. Benitez, J. Skinner, B. C. Schneider, and J. J. Manly. 2014. The role of early-life educational quality and literacy in explaining racial disparities in cognition in late life. *The Journals of Gerontology, Series B: Psychological Sciences and Social Sciences* (February 28).
Slavin, M. J., H. Brodaty, N. A. Kochan, J. D. Crawford, J. N. Troller, B. Draper, and P. S. Sachdev. 2010. Prevalence and predictors of "subjective cognitive complaints" in the Sydney Memory and Ageing Study. *American Journal of Geriatric Psychiatry* 18(8):701-710.
Thorgusen, S., and Y. Suchy. 2014. Contributions of learning and novelty to practice effects in older adults. Abstract from poster presentation given at the 34th Annual Conference of the National Academy of Neuropsychology in Fajardo, Puerto Rico. November 12-15. *Archives of Clinical Neuropsychology* 29(6):509.
Turvey, C. L., S. Schultz, S. Arndt, R. B. Wallace, and R. Herzog. 2000. Memory complaint in a community sample aged 70 and older. *Journal of the American Geriatrics Society* 48(11):1435-1441.

Wang, L., G. van Belle, P. K. Crane, W. A. Kukull, J. D. Bowen, W. C. McCormick, and E. B. Larson. 2004. Subjective memory deterioration and future dementia in people aged 65 and older. *Journal of the American Geriatrics Society* 52(12):2045-2051.

Wilson, M., D. D. Allen, and J. C. Li. 2006a. Improving measurement in health education and health behavior research using item response modeling: Introduction to item response modeling. *Health Education Research* 21(Suppl 1):i4-i18.

———. 2006b. Improving measurement in health education and health behavior research using item response modeling: Comparison with the classical test theory approach. *Health Education Research* 21(Suppl 1):i19-i32.

Yaffe, K., A. J. Fiocco, K. Lindquist, E. Vittinghoff, E. M. Simonsick, A. B. Newman, S. Satterfield, C. Rosano, S. M. Rubin, H. N. Ayonayon, and T. B. Harris. 2009. Predictors of maintaining cognitive function in older adults: The Health ABC study. *Neurology* 72(23):2029-2035.

Yaffe, K., K. Lindquist, E. Vittinghoff, D. Barnes, E. M. Simonsick, A. Newman, S. Satterfield, C. Rosano, S. M. Rubin, H. N. Ayonayon, and T. Harris. 2010. The effect of maintaining cognition on risk of disability and death. *Journal of the American Geriatrics Society* 58(5):889-894.

Zahodne, L. B., M. M. Glymour, C. Sparks, D. Bontempo, R. A. Dixon, S. W. MacDonald, and J. J. Manly. 2011. Education does not slow cognitive decline with aging: 12-year evidence from the Victoria Longitudinal Study. *Journal of the International Neuropsychological Society* 17(6):1039-1046.

4A

Risk and Protective Factors and Interventions: Lifestyle and Physical Environment

The brain is subject to a lifetime of demands and exposures, both beneficial and deleterious. Given the importance to the public's health of preventing individuals' cognitive impairment and promoting their cognitive health, it is important to develop an in-depth understanding of these various beneficial and deleterious factors to guide prevention and remediation efforts. Risk and protective factors include all of the personal lifestyle, behavioral, social, medical, and genetic characteristics of an individual or environment that are associated with, respectively, decreases or increases in cognitive function. There is wide variability in cognitive functioning levels among individuals, and risk and protective factors may affect a person's long-term cognitive trajectory in varying ways. Most of the interventions that have been developed to date focus on prevention efforts, although some remediation efforts are also being explored.

This and the next two chapters explore risk and protective factors and interventions organized into discussions of lifestyle factors and the physical environment (Chapter 4A), medical and physical factors (Chapter 4B), and general approaches to remediation (Chapter 4C). Details of the organization are provided in Table 4A-1. This chapter begins with an overview of some of the opportunities and challenges associated with examining the risk and protective factors for cognitive aging and determining the effectiveness of interventions. Subsequent sections in Chapters 4A and 4B focus on specific risk or protective factors. Each discussion provides an overview of observational and intervention studies, followed by a summary comment on the strength of the evidence. Chapter 4C discusses interventions that are not specific to any one risk factor, and it also provides the committee's

TABLE 4A-1 Risk and Protective Factors and Interventions Discussed in the Report

Lifestyle and Physical Environment (Chapter 4A)	Health and Medical Factors (Chapter 4B)	General Approaches (Chapter 4C)
• Physical activity and exercise • Education and intellectual engagement • Social isolation, loneliness, and social engagement • Diet • Vitamins • Alcohol • Smoking • Substance abuse • Physical environment—air pollution and occupational exposures • Stress	• Medications • Cerebrovascular and cardiovascular disease and risk factors • Delirium and hospitalization • Major surgery and general anesthesia • Thyroid disorders • Chronic kidney disease • Cancer • Depression • Traumatic brain injury • Hearing and visual loss • Sleep • Genetic factors	• Cognitive stimulation and training • Arts • Pharmacologics, nootropics, and supplements • Trans-cranial direct current stimulation • Multi-domain trials

NOTES: A number of other topics are relevant to this discussion, including early childhood factors: developmental conditions, childhood exposures; environmental exposures, including to trace metals or pesticides; elder abuse and neglect; psychological factors, including resilience, anxiety, mental illness, posttraumatic stress disorder; atrial fibrillation; chronic liver disease; chronic lung disease; diseases affecting the brain (infections, inflammatory conditions, neoplasm, and neurodegenerative diseases); lifelong learning (education during adulthood); specific medications, such as aspirin and nonsteroidal anti-inflammatory drugs, cholinesterase inhibitors, memantine, and prednisone and corticosteroids; and gonadal steroids (e.g., estrogen, testosterone). These areas represent important gaps in our knowledge and will be important to explore through future investigation.

recommendations on actions needed to better prevent, delay, or attenuate cognitive aging.

ISSUES IN STUDYING RISK AND PROTECTIVE FACTORS AND INTERVENTIONS

This report uses a health promotion approach because such an approach is applicable to broad community-based populations and also applicable across the life span. Efforts to promote cognitive health should begin early to have maximal benefit. Discussions about prevention become complex because cognitive aging is not a disease but rather is a highly variable process of cognitive change as individuals get older.

Further complicating discussions of risk and protective factors for cognitive aging is the intertwined and not fully understood nature of the relationship between medical conditions that may result in short-term cognitive decline (e.g., stroke, delirium, and medications that compromise cognition) and cognitive aging over time. Although some individuals with acute decline may return to their baseline level of cognitive functioning, others may make only a limited recovery, and still others may find that their cognitive function does not improve at all; the long-term impacts of acute cognitive decline on cognitive aging are not fully understood. Furthermore, much of the literature on medical-related risk factors has focused on neurodegenerative diseases and less research on these factors has been devoted to cognitive aging per se.

One of the overriding issues in assessing the role of risk factors as correlates or determinants of cognitive aging is the socioeconomic status (SES) of the individual or the group of interest (Deary, 2012). SES is often measured by an individual's social status, educational attainment, occupational level, and income. Importantly, it is one of the strongest correlates of cognitive status, performance, and outcomes, and these associations persist across the life span (Kuh et al., 2014). SES is also correlated with many other health states and outcomes, including those related to infant and childhood developmental outcomes, and thus it is an important consideration—both as a determinant and a confounder of associations—in any analysis and interpretation of cognitive aging studies of risk and intervention programs (Wong and Edwards, 2013). In many instances, SES is likely to be a surrogate for various environmental and genetic exposures, which, if possible, should be identified.

Because of the limited number of available studies of any type on cognitive aging, the committee decided to include the wide range of available studies but also to note the challenges and limitations of the studies where relevant. Although often the available studies evaluate cognitive outcomes with only short-term follow-up and do not examine long-term cognitive aging trajectories, the committee determined that since the short-term cognitive effects are potentially preventable, they should be noted in this report.

In compiling the evidence for each of the relevant factors and interventions, the committee did not conduct new systematic reviews of primary evidence. It based its assessments on existing systematic reviews, updated literature reviews, original articles, clinical guidelines, and input from experts. The goal was to create a synthesis of the evidence that would be sufficient to guide recommendations on important risk factors and on the interventions to address them. While this report's focus is on cognitive aging, some of the included studies addressed the outcomes of cognitive impairment, dementia, and Alzheimer's disease.

One major effort to evaluate recent studies that have examined modifiable risk factors for cognition and dementia reviewed 247 studies published between January 1990 and October 2012, each of which included at least

300 generally healthy people and used either a cross-sectional or a prospective (longitudinal) study design (Beydoun et al., 2014a). The authors considered all cognitive outcomes, including global and domain-specific cognitive outcomes, cognitive decline, prevalent and incident mild cognitive impairment (MCI), dementia, and Alzheimer's disease. A variety of modifiable risk factors was considered, including education, physical activity, and nutrition. The committee drew on this comprehensive review when summarizing the available evidence on modifiable risk factors, but also examined other reviews pertinent to individual risk factors as well as primary studies. The committee recognized a number of methodological challenges, which are described in subsequent sections.

Interpreting Observational Studies

Observational studies are designed to collect data from people regarding their risk factors and cognitive abilities without experimenting upon them by, for example, giving them either an active intervention (such as a pill or exercise) or a placebo. While hundreds of observational studies have been published on risk factors for cognitive decline and dementia or Alzheimer's disease, it is often difficult to draw firm conclusions from them. The studies differ in many ways, having various strengths and limitations, and their findings are often inconsistent. The following factors affect the interpretation of the evidence about the risk factors for cognitive aging and the ability to draw conclusions from that evidence:

- *Age range:* Ideally, an evaluation of risk factors for cognitive aging would include representative populations of adults followed from young adulthood to very late life. Many studies include only cross-sectional (one-time) examinations or short follow-up periods, and their conclusions are inherently limited.
- *Measures of cognitive changes:* As noted in Chapter 2, there are many challenges in measuring cognitive change with age, including the wide variety and large number of available assessment measures. Instruments are needed that eliminate or minimize cultural or race/ethnicity bias. Methods that account for practice effects are important to utilize. Because baseline information is critical and the focus is on change across time in varying cognitive domains (see Chapter 2), it is useful to have multiple measurements conducted at various points across the life span in order to more fully inform conclusions on risk and protective factors.
- *Study outcomes:* Study outcomes need to measure effects on cognitive aging and outcomes other than the development of diseases.

Cognitive aging can occur in the adult population without the eventual development of disease. In many existing studies, cognitive outcomes are often combined (e.g., both cognitive decline and dementia) or poorly specified. For this report, cognitive decline was the most relevant study outcome; however, when no studies reporting cognitive decline were available, the committee chose to use dementia outcomes (in some sections) with full recognition of the limitations of this approach.

- *Confounding:* Sometimes risk and protective factors may be associated with cognitive outcomes because of the influence of other factors that have not been or that cannot be accounted for in the study. Such "confounding" is a major impediment to determining whether a causal association exists between a risk factor and a cognitive outcome.

Because of these issues, it is difficult to firmly establish in many cases whether a risk factor is causing cognitive changes with age or whether changing the risk factor would alter the course of cognitive function. Despite these limitations, the overviews of observational studies provide the best currently available evidence on risk factors that may be modifiable and that have been studied sufficiently to help produce reasonable recommendations on risk factors now; these overviews of observational studies also point to important avenues for future research. The committee acknowledges that the list of risk and protective factors is not exhaustive; rather, it is heavily weighted toward factors that are reasonably common, are potentially preventable, and have a substantial evidence base.

Interpreting Intervention Studies

Intervention studies have the potential to provide strong evidence for behavior change or other interventions that could mitigate the risk factors associated with cognitive aging. The synergistic effects of various components of an intervention (e.g., the social component of a physical activity intervention) also add to the opportunities and the challenges of understanding cognitive aging. As discussed in Chapter 4C, a number of intervention studies are examining the effects of multicomponent interventions.

The evidence base for cognitive aging–related interventions has many gaps, some of which are noted here. First, for many interventions, well-designed rigorous studies, including randomized controlled trials (RCTs), have not been conducted. In some situations where interventions are known to be beneficial, a true control (i.e., non-intervention group) is often not ethical.

Second, studies have not used consistent outcome measures. Because each specific task or measure is subject to measurement error, cognitive change should be assessed using several tasks or measures in order to reduce error variance and converge on important constructs. Some studies have used multidimensional measures of cognition or dementia (e.g., the Mini-Mental State Examination [MMSE]), whereas others have examined only specific tasks (e.g., the digit–symbol substitution test), and still others have used structural or functional brain changes (e.g., total brain or hippocampal volume, or activation of brain regions as cognitive tasks are performed) as proxies for cognitive decline. As a result, the clinical meaning of changes associated with particular interventions is still uncertain.

Moreover, the time frames for administration of interventions and for the assessment of their effects vary widely. Some interventions have looked at short-term outcomes, whereas others have looked for changes decades after the intervention. A problem shared by intervention trials and prospective observational studies is that individuals often improve at taking cognitive tests over time because of "learning effects," which can mask declines in cognition. Furthermore, it is unclear whether cognitive interventions translate into real-life behavior changes that can be sustained over time.

Additionally, much remains to be learned about the biological mechanisms by which a given intervention affects cognition and also the psychological factors (e.g., control beliefs, changes in self-efficacy, or the acquisition of cognitive strategies) by which positive change can be sustained.

Finally, there are various costs of some interventions aimed at improving cognition that must be taken into account, including costs in time, money, and even the safety of the individual. Although some lifestyle changes (e.g., physical activity) may have significant benefits beyond cognition, others (e.g., transcranial direct current stimulation) have the potential for harm, even when no such harm has not been identified in short-term studies. The monetary cost of some interventions (e.g., dietary supplements) also must be considered. Indeed, the diversion of resources to pay for ineffective rather than effective treatments is an important public health consideration.

PHYSICAL ACTIVITY AND EXERCISE

Physical activity is strongly linked to healthy aging and remaining independent, and it has been associated with helping individuals maintain their physical and cognitive function throughout life and also with older adults developing fewer chronic conditions (Lee at el., 2012; NIH, 2014b). Conversely, ample evidence suggests that low levels of physical activity are associated with an increased risk of developing a number of diseases including stroke, hypertension, type 2 diabetes, osteoporosis, and a variety of cancers including colon and breast cancer (Lee et al., 2012).

Evidence from Observational Studies

The relationship between physical activity and cognitive heath has been studied over decades. In the 1970s Spirduso and colleagues compared the performance of younger and older individuals, both athletes and non-athletes, on a series of reaction time and movement tasks (Spirduso, 1975; Spirduso and Clifford, 1978) and observed that older athletes outperformed older non-athletes on many of these tasks. These results, and others, led to a multitude of cross-sectional studies that generally found older high-fit individuals to perform better than low-fit adults on a number of perceptual, cognitive, and motor tasks (Abourezk and Toole, 1995; Clarkson-Smith and Hartley, 1990). Longitudinal observational studies have also generally found a relationship between physical activity and cognitive health outcomes. For example, Zhu and colleagues (2014) found that a graded exercise measure of cardiorespiratory fitness predicted performance on a variety of cognitive tasks 25 years after the original measurement, even after accounting for differences in participants' race, sex, age, and education.

Several recently published systematic reviews (Anderson et al., 2014; Beydoun et al., 2014b; Blondell et al., 2014), as well as many qualitative reviews (Ahlskog et al., 2011; Bherer et al., 2013; Bielak, 2010; Lautenschlager et al., 2012), have reiterated these findings. A 2014 review included 21 prospective studies on physical activity and cognitive decline and 26 prospective studies on physical activity and dementia (Blondell et al., 2014). A meta-analysis was conducted on these studies, and as shown in Figure 4A-1, the majority showed benefit, with the overall finding that physically active adults had a 35 percent lower risk of cognitive decline (relative risk [RR] = 0.65; 95% confidence interval [CI] 0.55–0.76) than those who were inactive.

Studies with the highest-quality, longest follow-ups, and with a greater number of adjustments for differences between study designs, have yielded findings about the value of exercise that are more conservative but still in the protective direction (Blondell et al., 2014). In the Study of Osteoporotic Fracture, women who reported more physical activity at any time in their life course (adolescence and at age 30 years, 50 years, or in later life) had lower risk of cognitive impairment than inactive women; the association was especially strong for women who had been active teenagers (Middleton et al., 2010). In a recent systematic review, 21 of 24 prospective studies found an association between physical activity and cognitive outcomes, and all four of the cross-sectional reports included did so as well (Beydoun et al., 2014b).

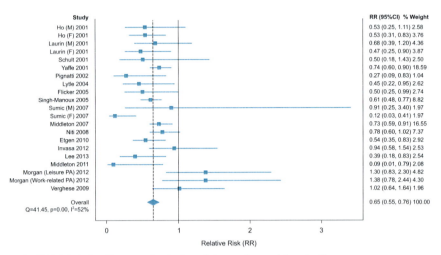

FIGURE 4A-1 Studies on physical activity and cognitive decline.
SOURCE: Blondell et al., 2014.

Evidence from Intervention Studies

A substantial number of intervention studies have reported that physical activity and exercise have a benefit on cognition. For example, in one early randomized trial, three groups of older adults (an aerobic exercise group, a strength and flexibility group, and a non-exercising control group) were tested on a variety of cognitive tasks before and after the 4-month intervention. The aerobic exercise group demonstrated performance improvements on a number of cognitive tasks[1] (Dustman et al., 1984). In an effort to examine the specificity of exercise's effects on cognition, Kramer and colleagues (1999) conducted a 6-month intervention trial with 124 older adults. Subjects were randomized to two groups, a walking group (aerobic) and a toning and stretching (non-aerobic) control group. The primary questions addressed were whether performance on tasks that had components of executive control processes would be improved for the walkers but not for the stretching group and whether non–executive control processes would show equivalent improvements for both exercise groups. The walking group improved to a significantly greater extent than the ton-

---

[1] These tasks included the critical flicker fusion test (the point at which the viewer perceives a flickering light source is a steady, continuous one, used as a measure of the brain's processing capacity), the digit symbol substitution test (which measures memory and processing speed), and the Stroop test (which also tests memory, processing, and executive brain functions) (Cohn et al., 1984; Rikli and Edwards, 1991).

ing and stretching group in skills that involve aspects of executive brain function. Other interventions have often, but not always, found aerobic exercise interventions to have beneficial effects on cognition (Blumenthal et al., 1991; Madden et al., 1989).

A series of meta-analyses (Angevaren et al., 2008; Colcombe and Kramer, 2003; Smith et al., 2010b) has helped to clarify this literature. In general, these meta-analyses have found modest effect sizes for the exercise–cognition relationship. Some of the meta-analyses have also examined the moderating effects of various factors. For example, Colcombe and Kramer (2003) found that the relationship between exercise and cognition had larger benefits for executive tasks than for other cognitive processes (but also had benefits across different dimensions of cognition). They also found the exercise–cognition relationship to be influenced by gender, intervention duration, age, and exercise type. Women showed larger benefits than men. Combined aerobic and strength programs showed greater benefits than aerobic programs alone. People older than 65 years showed more benefits than those from 55 to 65 years of age, and exercise sessions longer than 30 minutes showed larger cognitive benefits than shorter ones.

More recently, behavioral assessments of physical activity and exercise effects have been augmented with human neuroimaging studies, particularly studies using functional magnetic resonance imaging (fMRI). To briefly summarize this expanding literature, intervention studies have found that increases in aerobic fitness are associated with increased volume in a number of brain regions—in particular, the frontal and hippocampal areas, which generally show a decrease in volume during adult aging (Colcombe et al., 2006; Erickson et al., 2010). However, other studies have found structural changes in the brain to be associated with increased physical activity, regardless of exercise type (both aerobic and non-aerobic activity) (Ruscheweyh et al., 2011; Voss et al., 2013a). Furthermore, studies using fMRI have found that as participants' aerobic fitness improves, there are changes in certain patterns of brain activation that are known to predict increased performance on executive function and processing speed tasks (Colcombe et al., 2004; Rosano et al., 2010). The fMRI studies have also found increased functional connectivity among brain regions that are known to contribute to better executive function and memory after 4 to 12 months of aerobic exercise interventions (Burdette et al., 2010; Voss et al., 2010).

Animal research conducted over the past couple of decades complements these studies by revealing the underlying molecular and cellular mechanisms that are associated with exercise-related improvements in cognition. This literature is extensive and several thorough reviews can be consulted for details (Cotman and Berchtold, 2002; Vaynman and Gomez-Pinilla, 2005; Voss et al., 2013b).

Summary

A consensus is emerging in the scientific community that physical activity can slow or attenuate cognitive decline and improve cognitive function in middle-aged and older adults. Possible mechanisms include indirect effects, such as aerobic exercise optimizing vascular health throughout life and reducing the burden of cerebrovascular disease, as well as direct effects on slowing neurodegenerative processes and improving the body's own neuroprotective neurotrophic factors and neuroplasticity (Ahlskog et al., 2011). This increasing body of literature has prompted several panels to recommend minimum levels of physical activity on a daily and weekly basis (Haskell et al., 2007; HHS, 2014a,b). Although the evidence is strong that physical activity and exercise can positively affect cognitive aging, many unanswered questions need to be addressed in future research, such as:

- Do different modes of exercise produce different cognitive benefits?
- Can different exercise parameters (e.g., intensity, duration, interaction with other lifestyle factors) optimize cognition and brain health benefits?
- To what extent do genetic differences, particularly in genes related to cognition, moderate the effects of exercise on cognition?
- Is there an optimal period of life in which to begin exercise to reap the largest cognitive benefits?
- Are the effects of exercise synergistic with other lifestyle factors?
- How best can individuals be helped to start and sustain appropriate regular physical activity throughout their lives?

EDUCATION AND INTELLECTUAL ENGAGEMENT

Educational attainment is a well-known demographic characteristic that is correlated with peak cognitive ability, and inversely correlated with cognitive decline and dementias, including Alzheimer's disease. Low literacy and low educational attainment often reflect, in part, adverse early life conditions that may have deleterious effects on cognitive abilities throughout life. Educational attainment is one of the easiest and most consistently evaluated measures of SES. However, the challenge with studies on education and cognitive aging is clarifying the cause and effect (EClipSE Collaborative Members et al., 2010). Many midlife and older adults are involved in a wide variety of intellectual activities that extend beyond traditional education, including taking college or enrichment courses, reading, learning new languages or musical instruments, and doing crossword puzzles or other types of efforts to learn more or challenge themselves. The extent and impact of these efforts on cognitive aging is not fully known (ACE and MetLife, 2007).

Higher levels of education may allow older people to perform better on cognitive tests (Meng and D'Arcy, 2012) and may provide a buffer against cognitive decline. This finding is consistent with the concept of "cognitive reserve." As noted in Chapter 2, cognitive reserve is a theoretical concept proposing that certain lifetime experiences, including education, degree of literacy, and occupational attainment, increase the flexibility, efficiency, and capacity of brain networks, thereby allowing individuals with higher cognitive reserve to sustain greater levels of brain pathology before showing clinical impairment (for a review of cognitive reserve, see Stern, 2009). Supporting the concept of cognitive reserve, cross-sectional studies of nondemented and demented individuals have reported greater levels of brain atrophy among individuals with higher cognitive reserve than among those with lower cognitive reserve and similar levels of cognitive functioning, suggesting that the effects of atrophy on cognition are reduced in individuals with higher reserve (Arenaza-Urquijo et al., 2013; Liu et al., 2012; Querbes et al., 2009; Reed et al., 2010; Sole-Padulles et al., 2009). In older adults without dementia, studies suggest that education is strongly associated with cognitive performance globally, as well as in many specific domains, but that it is not associated with the rate of cognitive decline (Singh-Manoux et al., 2011; Zahodne et al., 2011). Thus, cognitive reserve appears to delay the onset of the clinical signs of dementia, including Alzheimer's disease, while in cognitively healthy people, it is associated with higher cognitive performance throughout life but no difference in the rate of cognitive decline with aging.

Cross-sectional studies of older adults have also shown positive relationships between literacy and cognitive performance even after adjusting for level of education (Albert and Teresi, 1999; Federman et al., 2009; Jefferson et al., 2011). Two longitudinal studies evaluated the association between literacy and cognitive decline in aging and found that, even after controlling for education, individuals with lower literacy showed greater declines in memory, language, and executive functioning (Manly et al., 2003, 2005). Furthermore, literacy has been shown to help explain difference between black and white older adults in both cognitive performance and rates of cognitive decline, again after controlling for education (Mehta et al., 2004; Sachs-Ericsson and Blazer, 2005).

More highly educated people also typically have lower risk of cardiovascular disease and engage in healthier behaviors; these differences can translate into more favorable cognitive trajectories during adulthood (Hendrie et al., 2006). However, race/ethnicity, country of origin, cultural diversity, and language fluency also relate to educational attainment and the ability to score well on cognitive tests, making it extremely difficult to disentangle the influence of these various factors. In a systematic review, 18 of 27 prospective studies and 21 out of 25 cross-sectional studies found that lower educational attainment was associated with worse cognitive outcomes (Beydoun et al., 2014a).

Some studies have addressed the impact of intellectual engagement and lifelong learning on cognitive outcomes. Such studies often record individuals' self-report of intellectually challenging activities at one point in time and compare the number and frequency of these activities with measures of cognition or the diagnosis of neurodegenerative disorders years later. In a study of 294 older adults, Wilson and colleagues (2013) found that greater cognitive activity in early life (e.g., reading books, visiting a library, writing letters, etc.) was associated with a lower rate of cognitive decline later in life. This relationship (increased activity early in life associated with decreased rate of cognitive decline at a later time) remained when cognitive declines associated with neuropathology were removed from the equation. These results might be viewed as an example of cognitive reserve—that is, an enhancement of cognition either earlier in life or in late life that serves as a protective factor with aging (Stern, 2012; see Chapter 2). In examining data on intellectual engagement and lifelong learning efforts (midlife and later life) in participants of the Mayo Clinic Study of Aging (a longitudinal population-based study of cognitive aging in Olmsted County, Minnesota), researchers found that intellectually related efforts may have protective effects on cognitive aging (Geda et al., 2011; Vemuri et al., 2014). There are also ongoing studies comparing cognitive training and cognitive engagement activities (Stine-Morrow et al., 2014). The challenges of studies in this area include the many different types of activities that individuals engage in, the varying extent to which these activities are engaged in by individuals, and the long-term nature of follow-up. Many of these studies are observational, and while they are important in establishing the relationship between cognitively stimulating activities and cognitive decline or age-related neurodegenerative diseases, they do not establish causality.

Summary

Education is one of the most consistent and influential personal characteristics influencing cognitive function throughout life (Beydoun et al., 2014a; Hendrie et al., 2006). Much remains to be learned about the extent to which there is a cognitive reserve and, if so, what are its physiological mechanisms. As educational levels become more uniform in advanced societies, indicators of the quality of education, especially literacy, may become better predictors of cognitive function. The available evidence emphasizes the importance of both early life education and maintaining cognitive function over the life span for peak cognitive capacities. Research is also showing that intellectual engagement and lifelong learning are associated with positive cognitive outcomes, although there is still much to be learned regarding the specific activities, duration of efforts, and other factors that influence cognitive outcomes.

SOCIAL ISOLATION, LONELINESS, AND SOCIAL ENGAGEMENT

Evidence from Observational Studies

Social Isolation and Loneliness

Loneliness can be defined as the emotional state caused by unfulfilled social and intimacy needs (Luanaigh and Lawlor, 2008). The concept of loneliness is distinct from being alone, or social isolation, which is usually defined as living alone, not having a partner, and having few social supports (Steptoe et al., 2013). The perception of loneliness is strongly related to depression (Luanaigh and Lawlor, 2008). Cacioppo and Hawkley (2009) have described a number of possible mechanisms connecting loneliness with decline in cognition, including (1) stress and activation of the hypothalamic–pituitary–adrenal axis with possible increased inflammatory responses in the brain; (2) less neuroplasticity in those older individuals who lack interaction with others, resulting in less ability to compensate for age-related neurodegenerative changes; (3) lower cognitive stimulation because of social isolation; (4) increased cognitive demand due to chronic surveillance for and protection from threats; (5) increased depression and decreased physical activity; (6) reduced quality and quantity of social interactions; and (7) diminished sleep quality resulting in impaired learning.

Several studies have shown that social isolation and loneliness are associated with declines in global cognition, psychomotor processing speed, and delayed visual memory (O'Luanaigh et al., 2012); with cognitive decline (Shankar et al., 2013; Tilvis et al., 2004); Alzheimer's disease (Holwerda et al., 2014; Wilson et al., 2007); and other physical problems, including sleep disruption, blood pressure, inflammation, and heart disease. Some evidence suggests that loneliness is more detrimental than social isolation (Holwerda et al., 2014) and that poorly educated people are affected more than those who are more educated (Shankar et al., 2013). Cognitive declines may lead to lower social engagement, creating a downward spiral of social isolation and loneliness.

Social Engagement

A growing and diverse body of evidence has evaluated whether social engagement, social activities, social support, and social strain are related to cognitive decline with age. The measures of social activity in this research vary widely, with some including lifestyle activities that require both physical and cognitive effort. One example is the Life Complexity Inventory used originally in the Seattle Longitudinal Study (Schaie, 1996). This scale is constructed by combining scores for the frequency of various activities, including going to parties, volunteering, going to dances, playing cards, visiting others, attending church, and speaking with friends and family on the phone (Brown et al., 2012). Despite the diversity of measures used in the various studies, some consistent patterns are emerging. First, social activity, including social contacts and social support, is usually associated with improved cognitive abilities at baseline or at any single point in time (Barnes et al., 2013; Bielak, 2010; Brown et al., 2012; Seeman et al., 2011). However, some studies have found that higher cognitive measures predicted greater social engagement (Bielak, 2010; Brown et al., 2012). This leaves open the possibility that people with higher cognitive abilities choose to be more socially engaged, on average, than those with lower cognitive abilities (Gow et al., 2012). Second, social engagement is generally related to some cognitive domains—including speed of processing and various aspects of memory—but not to all (Gow et al., 2012). Third, increases in social activity are associated with higher levels of cognition, at least in some studies (Brown et al., 2012; Carlson et al., 2009; Stine-Morrow et al., 2008). Fourth, there can be negative associations between social engagement and cognitive outcomes, particularly when those activities cause social strain or stress (Seeman et al., 2011; Tun et al., 2013). For example, a study of grandparenting by postmenopausal women found that working memory and processing speed were positively associated with spending time with grandchildren 1 day per week, while poorer cognition was associated with minding grandchildren several days per week, a situation that prompted feelings of greater demand (Burn et al., 2014). Fifth, there may be gender differences in associations between social engagement and cognitive aging. For women, there is evidence that social engagement relates to better cognitive abilities (Thomas, 2011). The phenomenon of older adults with cognitive declines relinquishing social engagement has also been observed in studies that did not report results by gender (e.g., Small et al., 2012). This large and evolving evidence base lends support to the value of social activity for maintaining cognitive health and suggests the importance of using many possible approaches to increasing social engagement.

Evidence from Intervention Studies

Very few intervention studies have examined the effects of socialization alone on cognition. The majority of these have been small pilot studies (e.g., Carlson et al., 2009) involving people with dementia or else they have been multimodal—that is, they combined socialization with physical activity or cognitive stimulation (e.g., Kamegaya et al., 2014). One such study did find a small improvement from a social interaction intervention as compared with other activities or no intervention. A study conducted in Shanghai by Mortimer and colleagues (2012) randomized adults 60 to 79 years of age (40 men and 80 women) without dementia to one of four groups (tai chi, social interaction, walking, or no interaction). The socialization group met with a group leader and assistant for 1 hour three times per week at the local community center. Cognitive measures included a neuropsychological battery at baseline, 20 weeks, and 40 weeks. MRI scans were obtained pre- and post-intervention. Increases in brain volume were seen in the tai chi and social intervention groups, and the social group also improved on measures of verbal fluency.

The Experience Corps is a multimodal social services program that trains older volunteers to work in schools as tutors and mentors.[2] A pilot study of Experience Corps, which randomized participants to placements in elementary schools for 15 hours per week or to a waiting list (control group), demonstrated improvements in executive function and memory in the elementary school volunteers but declines in control group members (Carlson et al., 2009). Older adults at increased risk for cognitive impairment showed intervention-specific short-term gains in executive functioning and in the activity of prefrontal cortical regions, as demonstrated through fMRI (Carlson et al., 2009).

Summary

Although evidence from some epidemiological and observational studies indicates that increases in social activity and social engagement may be associated with higher levels of cognition (Bielak, 2010; Brown et al., 2012; Carlson et al., 2009; Stine-Morrow et al., 2008), evidence from RCTs is needed before recommendations can be made for specific social interaction interventions. Social engagement is often integral to other activities, such as physical activity or participation in the arts, that also have shown cognitive benefits (see Chapter 4C), and fostering social activity in older adults likely has multiple benefits.

---

[2]The Experience Corps trains and places volunteers in elementary schools for an academic year and covers three areas: general literacy support, library support, and conflict resolution. It is designed to bolster memory and executive functions of the volunteers by reading with children, problem solving, and working with team members and through various program activities (Rebok et al., 2004).

DIET

Various dietary patterns have been studied in the hope of identifying nutritional approaches to preserving brain function and preventing cognitive decline. Among these are diets characterized by a higher intake of fruits and vegetables and a lower intake of meat, including the Mediterranean diet and the DASH (Dietary Approaches to Stop Hypertension) diet.

Mediterranean diets, based on the dietary patterns prominent in countries bordering the Mediterranean Sea, emphasize:

- a high consumption of fruits, vegetables, cereals, and legumes;
- a moderate consumption of fish and alcohol, especially red wine; and
- a low consumption of saturated fats (with olive oil as the main source) and dairy products (with yogurt and cheese as the main sources).

The DASH diet emphasizes vegetables, fruits, and fat-free or low-fat dairy products. It includes whole grains, fish, poultry, beans, seeds, nuts, and vegetable oil, and it limits sodium, sweets, sugary beverages, and red meats. In terms of nutrition content, DASH is low in saturated and transfats and rich in potassium, calcium, magnesium, fiber, and protein (NIH, 2014a).

Evidence from Observational Studies

A 2010 review cited two studies in which the Mediterranean diet was associated with a decreased risk of cognitive decline (Feart et al., 2009; Plassman et al., 2010; Scarmeas et al., 2009), but it concluded that the quality of the available evidence was low at that time. In two more recent studies, Cache County and Health ABC, global cognitive function scores were found to be significantly higher among those who most adhered to the Mediterranean diet than among those who followed it the least (p = 0.001), and these differences were consistent over an extended follow-up (Koyama et al., 2014; Wengreen et al., 2013). Similar findings were seen for the DASH diet.

By contrast, a study of 6,174 women age 65 years and older who were participating in the Women's Health Study found no associations between the Mediterranean diet and changes in global cognition and verbal memory scores over 5 years (Samieri et al., 2013). In that study, better average global cognition scores were associated with whole-grain intake, and less cognitive decline was seen among those with higher intake of monosaturated versus saturated fats. In Sweden, a 5-year study of 194 older adults without cognitive impairment found that the Mediterranean diet, particularly a low intake of red meat, was associated with better cognitive performance and larger total brain volumes (Titova et al., 2013). Finally, in a study of 2,326 adults in their 70s who were followed for 8 years (38 percent of whom were African American), the Mediterranean diet was associated with slower cognitive decline in African Americans but not in white Caucasians (Koyama et al., 2014). A recent review of 11 observational epidemiologic studies and 1 RCT found that most (9 of 12 studies) indicated that a stricter adherence to the Mediterranean diet was associated with better cognitive function, slower cognitive decline, and a lower risk of developing Alzheimer's disease (Lourida et al., 2013).

People who follow the Mediterranean diet may differ in a number of ways from those who do not, including in such areas as genetic factors, education, SES, physical activity, and other behavioral and cultural characteristics related to cognition. Long-term RCTs that attempt to change people's dietary patterns are difficult and expensive, yet many scientists have called for these in order to more firmly determine whether the Mediterranean diet can actually slow cognitive aging.

The intake of n-3 fatty acids is one aspect of the Mediterranean diet that has received a great deal of attention. These n-3 fatty acids are found in fish that have a high fat content, such as salmon. Fatty acids in the n-3 and n-6 categories are labeled "essential" because the human body does not produce them; food and supplements with these fatty acids are needed to avoid nutritional deficiencies (Beydoun et al., 2014a). Fatty-acid levels in brain cell membranes have been shown to reflect dietary intake (Beydoun et al., 2014a; Haag, 2003), and it has been postulated that n-3 fatty acid intake can increase neurotransmission and the density of neurotransmitter receptors for acetylcholine and dopamine, which in turn can improve learning and memory (Beydoun et al., 2014a; Haag, 2003). A review of five prospective studies concluded that cognitive decline might be reduced by n-3 fatty acid intake but the quality of the evidence was rated low, in part because a single RCT found no such association (Plassman et al., 2010). Seven of 18 prospective studies and five cross-sectional studies found associations between n-3 fatty acid measures and cognitive outcomes (Beydoun et al., 2014a). No cross-sectional or longitudinal associations between the plasma levels of two n-3 fatty acids (docosahexaenoic acid and eicosapentaenoic acid) and seven domains of cognitive function (fine motor speed, verbal memory, visual memory, spatial ability, verbal knowledge, verbal fluency, and working memory) were found in 2,157 U.S. women 65 years old and older who were examined annually over about 6 years of follow-up (Ammann et al., 2013). One study of 390 older adults obtained measures of lifetime fish intake, including both current intakes and reported intake in childhood, and also measured levels of n-3 fatty acid in red blood cell membranes, and all of these measures were correlated with performance on several cognitive speed constructs (Danthiir et al., 2014). However, in 86 older adults who were followed for 4 years (average age = 86 years), higher plasma levels of n-3 fatty acids were associated with less decline in executive function per year of aging, although not with verbal memory or global cognition (Bowman et al., 2013).

Evidence from Intervention Studies

Little intervention evidence supports the benefit of a Mediterranean or DASH diet for cognitive function. However, two secondary analyses of dietary intervention trials for cardiovascular disease outcomes did report positive results. In one, people following the DASH diet combined with a behavioral weight management program exhibited greater improvements in executive function memory learning and in psychomotor speed, and participants following the DASH diet alone exhibited better psychomotor speed than did those in a control group following their usual diet (Smith et al., 2010a). In a Spanish trial comparing two Mediterranean diets (supplemented with either extra-virgin olive oil or mixed nuts) versus a low-fat control diet, those following Mediterranean diets had higher scores on some tests (MMSE and Clock Drawing Test) after 6.5 years of nutritional intervention (Martinez-Lapiscina et al., 2013). However, several potential limitations of these studies must be noted: sample sizes were small, few outcomes were measured, and the populations may not be representative.

Summary

Based on observational studies and limited clinical trials, dietary interventions such as the DASH and Mediterranean diets appear to have promise but their efficacy and effectiveness need to be confirmed in additional clinical trials and community-based studies. While interesting and promising in some studies, the evidence regarding their effects on cognitive aging is too inconclusive to warrant recommendations for dietary change. Yet the evidence summarized here provides some justification for individual choices to eat less meat and more nuts and legumes, whole grains, and monosaturated fats, such as olive oil, to preserve cognitive health. These food choices are consistent with current dietary guidelines for Americans (USDA, 2014).

VITAMINS

Despite widespread publicity about the benefits of vitamins and supplements for brain health and the large expenditures made on these products for a wide variety of reasons (in 2012, $32.5 billion was spent on dietary supplements, including $13.1 billion for vitamin- and mineral-containing supplements [NIH, 2013]), the evidence for supplements enhancing cognition or preventing decline is limited. Much of the published literature is based on cross-sectional or longitudinal observational studies and few RCTs. In addition, methodological differences among the published studies hinder conclusions. These differences include variable doses of the nutrient, different timings of the intervention (e.g., midlife versus late life), different lengths of follow-up, variable adherence (for prospective studies), and variations in recall (for retrospective studies). The evidence base is further complicated by the fact that the same nutrient may have different effects when it is delivered as a supplement from when it is obtained through increased dietary intake. Similarly, foods and beverages may have other components (e.g., polyphenols in coffee) that may be at least partly responsible for an effect attributed to a particular item (e.g., caffeine). Moreover, supplements are not regulated by the Food and Drug Administration and may not be pure and may not contain consistent doses of the active ingredients.

Antioxidants

Antioxidants inhibit the oxidation of other molecules. Oxidation produces free radicals that damage organ systems, including the brain (Christen, 2000; Nunomura et al., 2006). Vitamins C and E, flavonoids, and betacarotene are antioxidants that commonly occur in food and that are also available as supplements. Of particular interest to researchers has been vitamin E—a potent antioxidant that has beneficial effects on a variety of brain structures and functions (e.g., beta-amyloid deposition, loss of neurons, neuroinflammation) associated with cognitive decline in animal and laboratory studies (Nunomura et al., 2006).

Several recent systematic reviews of prospective and cross-sectional studies have found no strong evidence that dietary intakes of antioxidants preserves cognition (Beydoun et al., 2014a; Crichton et al., 2013; Rafnsson et al., 2013). However, in the National Institute on Aging (NIA) systematic review, 9 of 21 prospective studies and 2 of 6 cross-sectional studies did find positive associations between antioxidant intakes, especially vitamin E, and cognitive outcomes (Beydoun et al., 2014a).

A large RCT of vitamin E within the Women's Health Initiative demonstrated no overall benefit, except for women with a low dietary intake of the vitamin (Kang et al., 2006). Moreover, high doses of vitamin E may increase the overall risk of mortality (particularly at doses higher than 400 international units per day, IU/d) (Miller et al., 2005). Finally, a recent systematic review of cross-sectional and longitudinal studies found little or mixed evidence supporting the intake of vitamin E, vitamin C, flavonoids, or carotenoids as a way to improve cognitive function (Crichton et al., 2013).

B Vitamins and Homocysteine

Elevated homocysteine, a sulfur amino acid in the blood, has been consistently associated with increased risk of heart disease and stroke, although it is not known to what extent these associations are explained by poor kidney function which allows homocysteine to build up in the blood (He et al., 2014; Humphrey et al., 2008). Homocysteine levels increase with age (as do markers of kidney function aging) but intervention trials show that homocysteine levels in the blood can be lowered by supplemental intake of B6 and B12 vitamins and folate (Clarke et al., 2014).

Recently, Canadian researchers conducted an evidence-based review to determine the answers to several important questions about homocysteine and vitamin B12 in relation to cognitive decline and dementia (OHTAC, 2013). What seems most clear from this effort is that homocysteine is consistently, though not universally, associated with poor cognitive outcomes. In the NIA systematic review, 12 of 19 prospective studies and 11 of 14 prospective studies found higher homocysteine levels to be associated with poor cognitive outcomes (Beydoun et al., 2014a). However, associations between B vitamin intake and blood levels of B vitamins and cognitive health are inconclusive, with the Canadian report concluding that B12 supplementation did not appreciably change cognitive function or decline based on moderately strong evidence (OHTAC, 2013).

In a small clinical trial among people with mild B12 deficiency, supplementation did not improve cognition (Eussen et al., 2006).

Folate

Folate supplementation has not produced improved cognitive benefit among people in general (Malouf and Grimley Evans, 2008; Wald et al., 2010), although some benefit has been shown among those who have folic acid insufficiency as indicated by high homocysteine levels at baseline (Durga et al., 2007).

Vitamin D

Several prospective epidemiologic studies have shown associations of low serum vitamin D levels with lower global cognition and a more rapid functional decline (Annweiler and Beauchet, 2014; Bartali et al., 2014; Slinin et al., 2012; Wilson et al., 2014), although this association may not be relevant for African Americans, who in general have lower serum vitamin D levels than white Caucasians (Schneider et al., 2014). In a recent review of 10 epidemiologic studies, the serum level for vitamin D most clearly demarcating insufficiency for cognitive health was found to be around 10 nanograms/milliliter (Annweiler and Beauchet, 2014). It is less clear whether and to what extent vitamin D supplements would improve cognition or prevent its decline in older populations. Moreover, high levels of serum 25-hydroxyvitamin D, especially among those taking vitamin D supplements, are associated with cognitive impairment on a battery of attention tests, suggesting that the benefit may be confined to middle-range serum levels (Granic et al., 2014).

In the Women's Health Initiative Memory Study, women randomized to receive 1,000 mg of calcium carbonate and 400 IU/d of vitamin D3 did not show differences in performance (attention and working memory, working memory, word knowledge, spatial ability, verbal fluency, verbal memory, figural memory, or fine motor speed) over 7.8 years (Rossom et al., 2012). An RCT of vitamin D (5,000 IU/d of cholecalciferol) in young adults demonstrated no significant changes compared to placebo on measures related to working memory, response inhibition, or cognitive flexibility (Dean et al., 2011). Hopefully, future large RCTs testing vitamin D supplements will shed light on this question (Rossom et al., 2012).

Summary

The medical literature does not convincingly support any vitamin supplement intervention to prevent cognitive decline. There is evidence to support the replacement of folate among older people who are folate-deficient, as evidenced by high homocysteine levels, but not for the supplementation of older persons who are not deficient. Whether it is worthwhile to screen for these deficiencies in general populations remains an unanswered question. To date, the U.S. Preventive Services Task Force has not issued recommendations regarding such screenings.

ALCOHOL

Excessive alcohol consumption has detrimental effects on judgment and reaction times and can cause long-term cognitive damage (Bartley and Rezvani, 2012). The reasons for this include altered nutrition; the consequences of excessive alcohol consumption, such as cirrhosis; interactions with medications and other substances; and alcohol-associated injuries, such as those sustained in vehicular crashes. Furthermore, high levels of alcohol intake may be associated with psychiatric comorbidity, which also may have adverse cognitive consequences. Compared to either abstinence or excessive alcohol consumption, moderate drinking in adulthood—generally less than two drinks per day and in most populations much less than this—is associated with various health benefits such as the avoidance of heart disease and a lower mortality risk (Jayasekara et al., 2014; Roerecke and Rehm, 2012), although consideration needs to be given to baseline cognitive function (Krahn et al., 2003). This J- or U-shaped relationship between alcohol consumption and some health outcomes has been postulated to extend to cognitive aging and dementia. Possible mechanisms for the lower rates of cognitive and other impairments associated with moderate alcohol intake include decreased cardiovascular risk, improved lipid levels, the antioxidant properties of flavonoids found in red wine, lower platelet aggregation, improved insulin sensitivity, reduced inflammation, and possibly a direct effect of alcohol on cognitive function through acetylcholine release in the hippocampus that may improve learning and memory (Beydoun et al., 2014a; Peters et al., 2008a). Moderate, controlled intake may also be a behavioral indicator of personal control regarding risky behaviors. A 2008 systematic review examined 23 studies involving adults age 65 years and older (20 prospective and 3 case-control studies nested in a cohort) and found a nonsignificant pooled relative risk for cognitive decline (RR = 0.89; 0.67–1.17) (Peters et al., 2008a). In the NIA systematic review, 8 of 18 prospective studies found the J- or U-shaped association between moderate alcohol consumption and cognitive outcomes, as did 9 of 12 cross-sectional studies (Beydoun et al., 2014a).

Observational evidence suggests that light to moderate alcohol consumption is not a risk factor for the loss of cognitive function and may even be a protective factor throughout adulthood. However, the evidence base is insufficient to recommend an amount of alcohol intake, if any, that would be beneficial for cognition, particularly across the life span. Excessive alcohol consumption has well-established cognitive harms (Peters et al., 2008a).

SMOKING

Smoking is a strong risk factor for heart disease, stroke, cancer, lung disease, and many other chronic conditions (CDC, 2008). Its relationship to cognitive outcomes is complex. Given that smoking increases the risk of stroke, it would be expected also to increase the risk of vascular dementia and cognitive decline. However, the nicotine in cigarettes increases the release of acetylcholine, which improves attention and information processing (Beydoun et al., 2014a). Moreover, deficits in the cholinergic system are involved in Alzheimer's disease, and thus it has been suggested that smoking can delay Alzheimer's disease (Beydoun et al., 2014a). The death rate of smokers is three times that of non-smokers, and their life expectancy is shortened by approximately 10 years (Jha et al., 2013). Thus, it may be that the lower incidence of Alzheimer's disease among smokers is an artifact of their earlier deaths from other causes. Furthermore, systematic reviews have found that current smokers have an increased age-specific risk of Alzheimer's disease, vascular dementia, and other dementias (Peters et al., 2008b), while these risks were not significantly increased among former smokers.

In the NIA systematic review, 16 of 29 prospective studies observed associations between smoking and poorer cognitive outcomes, while four studies found associations with some outcomes or in some subgroups, and nine studies found no associations or associations in which smokers had better cognitive outcomes than non-smokers (Beydoun et al., 2014a). Only two of seven cross-sectional studies found associations of smoking with poorer cognitive outcomes. Several large studies have found associations with cognitive decline, dementia, and Alzheimer's disease in heavy smokers, but not in lighter smokers (Beydoun et al., 2014a).

To the committee's knowledge, no intervention trials have been conducted that manipulate smoking initiation or smoking cessation and then examine the effects on cognitive outcomes.

The evidence linking smoking to cognitive outcomes is mixed and inconclusive. Given the many health problems of aging smokers and the relationship of smoking to coronary disease, stroke, and dementias, there are ample reasons for current smokers to quit, despite the uncertainty about the cognitive benefits.

SUBSTANCE ABUSE

Evidence from Observational Studies

Several substances commonly abused in Western societies have been suggested as contributing to cognitive impairment, including cannabis, particularly in teenagers and young adults (Becker et al., 2014; Jacobus and Tapert, 2014; Thames et al., 2014). Much of this impairment comes during the acute and post-acute phases of use (Crane et al., 2013), and evidence suggests that among adolescents who stop using cannabis, there are no residual cognitive effects (Hooper et al., 2014). Also, little evidence suggests that cannabis use has an adverse impact on cognitive performance among older adults (van Holst and Schilt, 2011).

Methamphetamine is a highly addictive and neurotoxic psychostimulant that in experimental animals produces long-lasting memory deficits (North et al., 2013). However, in humans, the long-term effects of chronic methamphetamine use on cognition are less clear. In a review of this drug as a cause of cognitive decline in humans, the findings were judged to be mixed (Dean et al., 2013), and some cognitive decrements could be attributed to other factors or to variation in study designs. In one large study of chronic methamphetamine users, lifetime use was not related to cognitive functioning per se, but it was related to psychiatric comorbidity and the use of other substances, such as crack cocaine (Herbeck and Brecht, 2013).

Chronic opiate use has been associated with poorer cognitive performance in human studies (Darke et al., 2012; Terrett et al., 2014; van Holst and Schilt, 2011), but, as above, several problems arise in interpreting this research, including the presence of psychiatric comorbidity and neurotoxic exposures. A systematic review of the impact of methadone, an opioid congener used in the treatment of opiate addiction, suggested that impaired cognitive function was correlated with its use (Wang et al., 2013).

While all of these substances have proved neurotoxic, producing adverse neurodevelopmental effects in both animal models and humans, there is a dearth of information on long-term cognitive performance in older adults who were former substance abusers. Hospitalizations for substance abuse among older persons have recently increased (Wu and Blazer, 2011), but available data—limited primarily to hospital claims data—so far do not suggest increased cognitive comorbidity as a result (Wu et al., 2013).

Further research is needed to better understand the long-term cognitive consequences of substance abuse and the changes in cognitive function that are associated with the treatment of drug addictions. If long-term adverse effects emerge, they would provide added impetus for drug abuse prevention at all ages and possible special preventive and therapeutic approaches for those with drug abuse histories.

PHYSICAL ENVIRONMENT

Older people experience a number of general as well as occupational exposures that may adversely affect cognitive performance. The role of potentially adverse exposures that occur early in life on cognitive trajectories is often uncertain, in part because of the challenges of performing the critical research needed, but also because of the multiple confounding exposures and experiences that occur across a lifetime. However, middle-aged and older individuals may also have continuing environmental exposures that may alter their cognitive performance. Some of the more common and potentially important exposures are described here.

Air Pollution

Growing evidence indicates that general, ambient air pollution is associated with decrements in cognitive performance among middle-aged and older adults (Ailshire and Clarke, 2014; Ailshire and Crimmins, 2014; Fonken et al., 2011; Gatto et al., 2014). However, because most air pollution is a complex mixture of gaseous and particulate components, it is difficult to attribute the effect to a specific factor. Most epidemiological studies assess the level of particulate matter less than 2.5 microns in diameter as the index of exposure (Ailshire and Crimmins, 2014). Higher levels of air pollution are sometimes accompanied by adverse climatic conditions, such as extremely high temperatures, which also can have adverse health effects (Gold and Mittleman, 2013). Air pollutants may have other important, if indirect, effects on cognitive function through their contributions to the development of cardiopulmonary conditions, including ischemic heart disease, stroke, lung conditions (Gold and Mittleman, 2013; Shah et al., 2013), and other chronic illnesses (see Chapter 4B). Taken together, such effects provide an argument for the environmental control of air pollution in general and for the prevention of exposures among older adults.

Occupational Exposures

For many years, occupational environmental exposures of various types have been suspected of having adverse cognitive consequences. This is a large and complex literature on this subject, and only certain exposures will be discussed here. As in the assessment of other risk factors, cognitive decrements associated with occupational exposures have been easier to demonstrate with concurrent exposure—and less research having been done on the long-term consequences, especially as they may affect older adults (Genuis and Kelln, 2015).

One important set of work-related chemical exposures that has been the subject of substantial research is exposure to organophosphate pesticides. Most but not all reviews of this topic suggest that job-related exposures do lead to cognitive decrements in late life (Blanc-Lapierre et al., 2013). Animal models also suggest that continued later-life exposure may be harmful (Levin et al., 2010), but no important human evidence is available.

The neurotoxic effects of lead exposure have been known for centuries, and the effect of lead on children has been a prominent public health issue. Studies of occupational lead exposure find that decrements in cognitive performance caused by earlier job-related exposure extend into late mid-life and that among older adults higher levels of lead in the bone are correlated with worse cognitive performance (Khalil et al., 2009). Lead exposure is one of those environmental and occupational exposures that will require ongoing attention and preventive interventions in the future.

Another category of occupational exposures that has received research attention is exposure to organic solvents. While these substances' acute and subacute toxic effects have been demonstrated, their late-life cognitive decrements due to chronic exposures have not been firmly established, although there is some evidence suggesting that there are long-term cognitive changes (Berr et al., 2010). For example, long-lasting neuropsychiatric symptoms associated with heavy solvent exposure have been found among tile layers (Nordling Nilson et al., 2007), although a subsequent analysis of the data from Berr and colleagues (2010) found that the cognitive effects appeared only among individuals with lesser educational attainment (Sabbath et al., 2012), suggesting that not all individuals are equally at risk from a given exposure.

While knowledge about the effects of occupational exposures on cognitive performance is an extremely important area for prevention, research on these effects is always challenging: many similar chemical and other exposures occur simultaneously; industrial processes and consequent exposures change with advances in production; exposed workers may be subject to other factors, occupational or non-occupational, that could lead to cognitive decrements; some studies use clinical dementia or specific neurodegenerative diseases as outcomes rather than cognitive aging; and workers in jobs with substantial occupational chemical exposures may have lower levels of education, itself an important risk factor for cognitive change in later life. Despite the uncertainties, one clear message is that whenever workers may be exposed to a substance for which there is reasonable evidence of neurotoxicity, effective exposure prevention programs should be enforced in the workplace at all times to protect both younger and older workers. Furthermore, it would be prudent for any comprehensive cognitive health program to screen older adults for non-occupational exposures to these same neurotoxic chemicals, such as exposures through hobby or recreational activities.

Other potential workplace exposures—such as might occur in workplaces relying heavily on computers and information and communications technologies—can lead to stress, mental health symptoms, and, at least potentially, alterations in cognitive function (Salanova et al., 2013; Thomee et al., 2010). However, it is also possible that the technological features of a job can reduce job stress and demand (Day et al., 2012). Whether technology-related job stress leads to cognitive functional change remains uncertain.

Noise can also be a factor in occupational settings. Environmental noise from traumatic and non-traumatic sources indisputably causes hearing impairment (Gourevitch et al., 2014). Hearing impairment from various causes, including age-related hearing loss, has been associated with reduced cognitive performance (see Chapter 4B). The cognitive performance of older adults experiencing higher levels of ambient noise may be affected indirectly, if it is distracting or reduces concentration (Jahncke, 2012) or interrupts normal sleep patterns (Muzet, 2007). The committee is not aware of any intervention trials that have examined cognitive outcomes after manipulating noise levels.

A more general question is whether occupations, when they are challenging, have a protective effect and lead to more cognitive engagement.

While a number of observational studies of this question have been conducted, the results are decidedly mixed, and many of the studies do not show any clear effect of type of occupation on brain function (Finkel et al., 2009; Gow et al., 2014; Jorm et al., 1998).

STRESS

With the publication of Hans Selye's letter to the journal *Nature* in 1936, the concept of "stress" became a subject of interest to researchers (Szabo et al., 2012). Early on, stress was defined non-specifically as the response of the body to a noxious stimulus, which later became known as "general adaptation syndrome" (Szabo et al., 2012). As the American Institute of Stress notes, "Stress is not a useful term for scientists because it is such a highly subjective phenomenon that it defies definition. And if you can't define stress, how can you possibly measure it?" (AIS, 2014). Thus, it is not surprising that the evidence relating stress to cognitive outcomes has been compiled in diverse ways and has produced results that are inconsistent and difficult to interpret. The "distress" encountered daily comes in many forms—from traffic congestion to the experience of having a bad boss to the death of a loved one—and it raises the question, "Does stress cause cognitive decline?" For this reason, the committee briefly addresses stress here, even though the current evidence base raises more questions than it answers.

Selye's original experiments were done with mice, and indeed a number of studies have assessed the effects of experimental stressors on cognition in laboratory settings. For example, it is known that in both monkeys and rodents, stress affects the pyramidal neurons in the prefrontal cortex, the same neurons that are affected by aging. The interactive effects of stress and aging in the rodent model were recently reviewed in detail (McEwen and Morrison, 2013).

In epidemiological studies, stress is frequently defined in terms of stressful life events (poor parenting in early life, divorce, loss of a job, or death of a loved one), and perceived stress is measured by various validated scales, or personality traits that make some people more vulnerable to stress than others. Finnish boys separated from their parents during World War II were found to have lower cognitive scores in several domains at age 60, with longer separations linked to greater deficits (Pesonen et al., 2007). The death of a child is a major life stressor associated with a faster rate of cognitive decline in later life (Comijs et al., 2011; Greene et al., 2014), especially when the loss occurred among parents who were young adults or had no subsequent children (Greene et al., 2014). However, the number and subjective ratings of stressful life events in the Cache County Study were associated only inconsistently with cognitive decline; stronger associations between stressful life events and cognitive decline were found in younger participants and those with less education (Tschanz et al., 2013). In the Longitudinal Aging Study Amsterdam, the death of a child or grandchild was associated with faster cognitive decline, and having experienced fewer major life events was associated with better cognitive function (Comijs et al., 2011).

Similarly, perceived daily stress has also been associated with greater memory problems among adults with cognitive decline (Rickenbach et al., 2014). Greater levels of perceived stress were also associated with lower initial cognitive performance and faster rates of decline among 6,207 older adults followed for almost 7 years in the Chicago Health and Aging Project (Aggarwal et al., 2014). Perceived social strain has been shown to elevate levels of cortisol (Friedman et al., 2012), a stress hormone and a marker of activation of the hypothalamic–pituitary–adrenal axis. Chronic activation of this axis has been associated with poor health outcomes, including cardiovascular disease, which could also further contribute to cognitive decline and dementia (Kremen et al., 2012).

Few intervention trials have been carried out with the goal of preserving cognition by modifying perceived stress or attempting to reduce stress responses during or after major life events. In a recent review of 12 studies of meditation and mindfulness and cognition in older people, 6 of which were randomized trials, meditation and mindfulness seemed to have benefits for a number of cognitive domains, but the trials were small and susceptible to bias (Gard et al., 2014). Major life events, as well as perceived stress and mild worry, have been associated with decreased cognitive performance and faster cognitive decline in several recent studies. Interventions that reduce the perceptions of stress or responses to it, such as meditation and mindfulness, may be helpful but require further study.

REFERENCES

Abourezk, T., and T. Toole. 1995. Effect of task complexity on the relationship between physical fitness and reaction time in older women. *Journal of Aging and Physical Activity* (3):251-260.

ACE (American Council on Education) and MetLife Foundation. 2007. *Framing new terrain: Older adults and higher education.* http://plus50.aacc.nche.edu/documents/older_adults_and_higher_education.pdf (accessed on February 26, 2015).

Aggarwal, N. T., R. S. Wilson, T. L. Beck, K. B. Rajan, C. F. Mendes de Leon, D. A. Evans, and S. A. Everson-Rose. 2014. Perceived stress and change in cognitive function among adults 65 years and older. *Psychosomatic Medicine* 76(1):80-85.

Ahlskog, J. E., Y. E. Geda, N. R. Graff-Radford, and R. C. Petersen. 2011. Physical exercise as a preventive or disease-modifying treatment of dementia and brain aging. *Mayo Clinic Proceedings* 86(9):876-884.

Ailshire, J. A., and P. Clarke. 2014. Fine particulate matter air pollution and cognitive function among U.S. older adults. *The Journals of Gerontology, Series B: Psychological Sciences and Social Sciences* 70(2):322-328.

Ailshire, J. A., and E. M. Crimmins. 2014. Fine particulate matter air pollution and cognitive function among older U.S. adults. *American Journal of Epidemiology* 180(4):359-366.

AIS (American Institute of Stress). 2014. *What is stress?* http://www.stress.org/what-is-stress (accessed December 5, 2014).

Albert, S. M., and J. A. Teresi. 1999. Reading ability, education, and cognitive status assessment among older adults in Harlem, New York City. *American Journal of Public Health* 89(1):95-97.

Ammann, E. M., J. V. Pottala, W. S. Harris, M. A. Espeland, R. Wallace, N. L. Denburg, R. M. Carnahan, and J. G. Robinson. 2013. Omega-3 fatty acids and domain-specific cognitive aging: Secondary analyses of data from WHISCA. *Neurology* 81(17):1484-1491.

Anderson, D., C. Seib, and L. Rasumssen. 2014. Can physical activity prevent physical and cognitive decline in postmenopausal women? A systematic review of the literature. *Maturitas* 79(1):14-33.

Angevaren, M., G. Aufdemkampe, H. J. Verhaar, A. Aleman, and L. Vanhees. 2008. Physical activity and enhanced fitness to improve cognitive function in older people without known cognitive impairment. *The Cochrane Database of Systematic Reviews* (2):Cd005381.

Annweiler, C., and O. Beauchet. 2014. Vitamin D in older adults: The need to specify standard values with respect to cognition. *Frontiers in Aging Neuroscience* 6:72.

Arenaza-Urquijo, E. M., J. L. Molinuevo, R. Sala-Llonch, C. Sole-Padulles, M. Balasa, B. Bosch, J. Olives, A. Antonell, A. Llado, R. Sanchez-Valle, L. Rami, and D. Bartres-Faz. 2013. Cognitive reserve proxies relate to gray matter loss in cognitively healthy elderly with abnormal cerebrospinal fluid amyloid-beta levels. *Journal of Alzheimer's Disease* 35(4):715-726.

Barnes, D. E., W. Santos-Modesitt, G. Poelke, A. F. Kramer, C. Castro, L. E. Middleton, and K. Yaffe. 2013. The mental activity and exercise (MAX) trial: A randomized controlled trial to enhance cognitive function in older adults. *JAMA Internal Medicine* 173(9):797-804.

Bartali, B., E. Devore, F. Grodstein, and J. H. Kang. 2014. Plasma vitamin d levels and cognitive function in aging women: The Nurses' Health Study. *Journal of Nutrition, Health, and Aging* 18(4):400-406.

Bartley, P. C., and A. H. Rezvani. 2012. Alcohol and cognition–Consideration of age of initiation, usage patterns and gender: A brief review. *Current Drug Abuse Reviews* 5(2):87-97.

Becker, M. P., P. F. Collins, and M. Luciana. 2014. Neurocognition in college-aged daily marijuana users. *Journal of Clinical and Experimental Neuropsychology* 36(4):379-398.

Berr, C., M. N. Vercambre, S. Bonenfant, A. S. Manoux, M. Zins, and M. Goldberg. 2010. Occupational exposure to solvents and cognitive performance in the GAZEL cohort: Preliminary results. *Dementia and Geriatric Cognitive Disorders* 30(1):12-19.

Beydoun, M. A., H. A. Beydoun, A. A. Gamaldo, A. Teel, A. B. Zonderman, and Y. Wang. 2014a. Epidemiologic studies of modifiable factors associated with cognition and dementia: Systematic review and meta-analysis. *BMC Public Health* 14:643.

Beydoun, M. A., A. A. Gamaldo, H. A. Beydoun, T. Tanaka, K. L. Tucker, S. A. Talegawkar, L. Ferrucci, and A. B. Zonderman. 2014b. Caffeine and alcohol intakes and overall nutrient adequacy are associated with longitudinal cognitive performance among U.S. adults. *Journal of Nutrition* 144(6):890-901.

Bherer, L., K. I. Erickson, and T. Liu-Ambrose. 2013. A review of the effects of physical activity and exercise on cognitive and brain functions in older adults. *Journal of Aging Research* 657508.

Bielak, A. A. 2010. How can we not "lose it" if we still don't understand how to "use it"? Unanswered questions about the influence of activity participation on cognitive performance in older age. A mini-review. *Gerontology* 56(5):507-519.

Blanc-Lapierre, A., G. Bouvier, A. Gruber, K. Leffondre, P. Lebailly, C. Fabrigoule, and I. Baldi. 2013. Cognitive disorders and occupational exposure to organophosphates: Results from the PHYTONER study. *American Journal of Epidemiology* 177(10):1086-1096.

Blondell, S. J., R. Hammersley-Mather, and J. L. Veerman. 2014. Does physical activity prevent cognitive decline and dementia?: A systematic review and meta-analysis of longitudinal studies. *BMC Public Health* 14:510.

Blumenthal, J. A., C. F. Emery, D. J. Madden, S. Schniebolk, M. Walsh-Riddle, L. K. George, D. C. McKee, M. B. Higginbotham, F. R. Cobb, and R. E. Coleman. 1991. Long-term effects of exercise on psychological functioning in older men and women. *Journal of Gerontology* 46(6):P352-P361.

Bowman, G. L., H. H. Dodge, N. Mattek, A. K. Barbey, L. C. Silbert, L. Shinto, D. B. Howieson, J. A. Kaye, and J. F. Quinn. 2013. Plasma omega-3 PUFA and white matter mediated executive decline in older adults. *Frontiers in Aging Neuroscience* 5:92.

Brown, C. L., L. E. Gibbons, R. F. Kennison, A. Robitaille, M. Lindwall, M. B. Mitchell, S. D. Shirk, A. Atri, C. R. Cimino, A. Benitez, S. W. Macdonald, E. M. Zelinski, S. L. Willis, K. W. Schaie, B. Johansson, R. A. Dixon, D. M. Mungas, S. M. Hofer, and A. M. Piccinin. 2012. Social activity and cognitive functioning over time: A coordinated analysis of four longitudinal studies. *Journal of Aging Research* 287438.

Burdette, J. H., P. J. Laurienti, M. A. Espeland, A. Morgan, Q. Telesford, C. D. Vechlekar, S. Hayasaka, J. M. Jennings, J. A. Katula, R. A. Kraft, and W. J. Rejeski. 2010. Using network science to evaluate exercise-associated brain changes in older adults. *Frontiers in Aging Neuroscience* 2:23.

Burn, K. F., V. W. Henderson, D. Ames, L. Dennerstein, and C. Szoeke. 2014. Role of grandparenting in postmenopausal women's cognitive health: Results from the Women's Healthy Aging Project. *Menopause* 21(10):1069-1074.

Cacioppo, J. T., and L. C. Hawkley. 2009. Perceived social isolation and cognition. *Trends in Cognitive Sciences* 13(10):447-454.

Carlson, M. C., K. I. Erickson, A. F. Kramer, M. W. Voss, N. Bolea, M. Mielke, S. McGill, G. W. Rebok, T. Seeman, and L. P. Fried. 2009. Evidence for neurocognitive plasticity in at-risk older adults: The Experience Corps program. *The Journals of Gerontology, Series A: Biological Sciences and Medical Sciences* 64(12):1275-1282.

CDC (Centers for Disease Control and Prevention). 2008. Smoking-attributable mortality, years of potential life lost, and productivity losses—United States, 2000–2004. *Morbidity and Mortality Report* 57(45):1226-1228.

Christen, Y. 2000. Oxidative stress and Alzheimer disease. *American Journal of Clinical Nutrition* 71(2):621s-629s.

Clarke, R., D. Bennett, S. Parish, S. Lewington, M. Skeaff, S. J. Eussen, C. Lewerin, D. J. Stott, J. Armitage, G. J. Hankey, E. Lonn, J. D. Spence, P. Galan, L. C. de Groot, J. Halsey, A. D. Dangour, R. Collins, and F. Grodstein. 2014. Effects of homocysteine lowering with B vitamins on cognitive aging: Meta-analysis of 11 trials with cognitive data on 22,000 individuals. *American Journal of Clinical Nutrition* 100(2):657-666.

Clarkson-Smith, L., and A. A. Hartley. 1990. Structural equation models of relationships between exercise and cognitive abilities. *Psychology and Aging* 5(3):437-446.

Cohn, N. B., R. E. Dustman, and D. C. Bradford. 1984. Age-related decrements in Stroop color test performance. *Journal of Clinical Psychology* 40(5):1244-1250.

Colcombe, S., and A. F. Kramer. 2003. Fitness effects on the cognitive function of older adults: A meta-analytic study. *Psychological Science* 14(2):125-130.

Colcombe, S. J., A. F. Kramer, E. McAuley, K. I. Erickson, and P. Scalf. 2004. Neurocognitive aging and cardiovascular fitness: Recent findings and future directions. *Journal of Molecular Neuroscience* 24(1):9-14.

Colcombe, S. J., K. I. Erickson, P. E. Scalf, J. S. Kim, R. Prakash, E. McAuley, S. Elavsky, D. X. Marquez, L. Hu, and A. F. Kramer. 2006. Aerobic exercise training increases brain volume in aging humans. *The Journals of Gerontology, Series A: Biological Sciences and Medical Sciences* 61(11):1166-1170.

Comijs, H. C., T. N. van den Kommer, R. W. Minnaar, B. W. Penninx, and D. J. Deeg. 2011. Accumulated and differential effects of life events on cognitive decline in older persons: Depending on depression, baseline cognition, or ApoE epsilon4 status? *Journals of Gerontology: Series B, Psychological Sciences and Social Sciences* 66(Suppl 1):i111-i120.

Cotman, C. W., and N. C. Berchtold. 2002. Exercise: A behavioral intervention to enhance brain health and plasticity. *Trends in Neurosciences* 25(6):295-301.

Crane, N. A., R. M. Schuster, P. Fusar-Poli, and R. Gonzalez. 2013. Effects of cannabis on neurocognitive functioning: Recent advances, neurodevelopmental influences, and sex differences. *Neuropsychology Review* 23(2):117-137.

Crichton, G. E., J. Bryan, and K. J. Murphy. 2013. Dietary antioxidants, cognitive function and dementia—A systematic review. *Plant Foods for Human Nutrition* 68(3):279-292.

Danthiir, V., D. Hosking, N. R. Burns, C. Wilson, T. Nettelbeck, E. Calvaresi, P. Clifton, and G. A. Wittert. 2014. Cognitive performance in older adults is inversely associated with fish consumption but not erythrocyte membrane n-3 fatty acids. *Journal of Nutrition* 144(3):311-320.

Darke, S., S. McDonald, S. Kaye, and M. Torok. 2012. Comparative patterns of cognitive performance amongst opioid maintenance patients, abstinent opioid users and non-opioid users. *Drug and Alcohol Dependence* 126(3):309-315.

Day, A., S. Paquet, N. Scott, and L. Hambley. 2012. Perceived information and communication technology (ICT) demands on employee outcomes: The moderating effect of organizational ICT support. *Journal of Occupational Health Psychology* 17(4):473-491.

Dean, A. C., S. M. Groman, A. M. Morales, and E. D. London. 2013. An evaluation of the evidence that methamphetamine abuse causes cognitive decline in humans. *Neuropsychopharmacology* 38(2):259-274.

Dean, A. J., M. A. Bellgrove, T. Hall, W. M. Phan, D. W. Eyles, D. Kvaskoff, and J. J. McGrath. 2011. Effects of vitamin D supplementation on cognitive and emotional functioning in young adults—a randomised control trial. *PLoS ONE* 6(11):e25966.

Deary, I. J. 2012. Intelligence. *Annual Review of Psychology* 63:453-482.

Durga, J., M. P. van Boxtel, E. G. Schouten, F. J. Kok, J. Jolles, M. B. Katan, and P. Verhoef. 2007. Effect of 3-year folic acid supplementation on cognitive function in older adults in the FACIT trial: A randomised, double blind, controlled trial. *Lancet* 369(9557):208-216.

Dustman, R. E., R. O. Ruhling, E. M. Russell, D. E. Shearer, H. W. Bonekat, J. W. Shigeoka, J. S. Wood, and D. C. Bradford. 1984. Aerobic exercise training and improved neuropsychological function of older individuals. *Neurobiology of Aging* 5(1):35-42.

EClipSE Collaborative Members, C. Brayne, P. G. Ince, H. A. Keage, I. G. McKeith, F. E. Matthews, T. Polvikoski, and R. Sulkava. 2010. Education, the brain and dementia: Neuroprotection or compensation? *Brain* 133(Pt 8):2210-2216.

Erickson, K. I., C. A. Raji, O. L. Lopez, J. T. Becker, C. Rosano, A. B. Newman, H. M. Gach, P. M. Thompson, A. J. Ho, and L. H. Kuller. 2010. Physical activity predicts gray matter volume in late adulthood: The Cardiovascular Health Study. *Neurology* 75(16):1415-1422.

Eussen, S. J., L. C. de Groot, L. W. Joosten, R. J. Bloo, R. Clarke, P. M. Ueland, J. Schneede, H. J. Blom, W. H. Hoefnagels, and W. A. van Staveren. 2006. Effect of oral vitamin B-12 with or without folic acid on cognitive function in older people with mild vitamin B-12 deficiency: A randomized, placebo-controlled trial. *American Journal of Clinical Nutrition* 84(2):361-370.

Feart, C., C. Samieri, V. Rondeau, H. Amieva, F. Portet, J. F. Dartigues, N. Scarmeas, and P. Barberger-Gateau. 2009. Adherence to a Mediterranean diet, cognitive decline, and risk of dementia. *JAMA* 302(6):638-648.

Federman, A. D., M. Sano, M. S. Wolf, A. L. Siu, and E. A. Halm. 2009. Health literacy and cognitive performance in older adults. *Journal of the American Geriatrics Society* 57(8):1475-1480.

Finkel, D., R. Andel, M. Gatz, and N. L. Pedersen. 2009. The role of occupational complexity in trajectories of cognitive aging before and after retirement. *Psychology and Aging* 24(3):563-573.

Fonken, L. K., X. Xu, Z. M. Weil, G. Chen, Q. Sun, S. Rajagopalan, and R. J. Nelson. 2011. Air pollution impairs cognition, provokes depressive-like behaviors and alters hippocampal cytokine expression and morphology. *Molecular Psychiatry* 16(10):987-995.

Friedman, E. M., A. S. Karlamangla, D. M. Almeida, and T. E. Seeman. 2012. Social strain and cortisol regulation in midlife in the U.S. *Social Science and Medicine* 74(4):607-615.

Gard, T., B. K. Hölzel, and S. W. Lazar. 2014. The potential effects of meditation on age-related cognitive decline: A systematic review. *Annals of the New York Academy of Sciences* 1307(1):89-103.

Gatto, N. M., V. W. Henderson, H. N. Hodis, J. A. St John, F. Lurmann, J. C. Chen, and W. J. Mack. 2014. Components of air pollution and cognitive function in middle-aged and older adults in Los Angeles. *Neurotoxicology* 40:1-7.

Geda, Y.E., H. M. Topazian, L. A. Roberts, R. O. Roberts, D. S. Knopman, V. S. Pankratz, T. J. Christianson, B. F. Boeve, E. G. Tangalos, R. J. Ivnik, and R. C. Petersen. 2011. Engaging in cognitive activities, aging, and mild cognitive impairment: A population-based study. *Journal of Neuropsychiatry and Clinical Neurosciences* 23(2):149-154.

Genuis, S. J., and K. L. Kelln. 2015. Toxicant exposure and bioaccumulation: A common and potentially reversible cause of cognitive dysfunction and dementia. *Behavioural Neurology* 620143.

Gold, D. R., and M. A. Mittleman. 2013. New insights into pollution and the cardiovascular system: 2010 to 2012. *Circulation* 127(18):1903-1913.

Gourevitch, B., J. M. Edeline, F. Occelli, and J. J. Eggermont. 2014. Is the din really harmless? Long-term effects of non-traumatic noise on the adult auditory system. *Nature Reviews Neuroscience* 15(7):483-491.

Gow, A. J., A. A. Bielak, and D. Gerstorf. 2012. Lifestyle factors and cognitive ageing: Variation across ability and lifestyle domains. *Journal of Aging Research* 143595.

Gow, A. J., K. Avlund, and E. L. Mortensen. 2014. Occupational characteristics and cognitive aging in the Glostrup 1914 Cohort. *The Journals of Gerontology, Series B: Psychological Sciences and Social Sciences* 69(2):228-236.

Granic, A., T. R. Hill, T. B. Kirkwood, K. Davies, J. Collerton, C. Martin-Ruiz, T. von Zglinicki, B. K. Saxby, K. A. Wesnes, D. Collerton, J. C. Mathers, and C. Jagger. 2014. Serum 25-hydroxyvitamin D and cognitive decline in the very old: The Newcastle 85+ Study. *European Journal of Neurology* 22(1):106-115.

Greene, D., J. T. Tschanz, K. R. Smith, T. Ostbye, C. Corcoran, K. A. Welsh-Bohmer, and M. C. Norton. 2014. Impact of offspring death on cognitive health in late life: The Cache County study. *American Journal of Geriatric Psychiatry* 22(11):1307-1315.

Haag, M. 2003. Essential fatty acids and the brain. *Canadian Journal of Psychiatry* 48(3):195-203.

Haskell, W. L., I. M. Lee, R. R. Pate, K. E. Powell, S. N. Blair, B. A. Franklin, C. A. Macera, G. W. Heath, P. D. Thompson, and A. Bauman. 2007. Physical activity and public health: Updated recommendation for adults from the American College of Sports Medicine and the American Heart Association. *Medicine and Science in Sports and Exercise* 39(8):1423-1434.

He, Y., Y. Li, Y. Chen, L. Feng, and Z. Nie. 2014. Homocysteine level and risk of different stroke types: A meta-analysis of prospective observational studies. *Nutrition, Metabolism, and Cardiovascular Diseases* 24(11):1158-1165.

Hendrie, H. C., M. S. Albert, M. A. Butters, S. Gao, D. S. Knopman, L. J. Launer, K. Yaffe, B. N. Cuthbert, E. Edwards, and M. V. Wagster. 2006. The NIH Cognitive and Emotional Health Project. Report of the Critical Evaluation Study Committee. *Alzheimer's & Dementia* 2(1):12-32.

Herbeck, D. M., and M. L. Brecht. 2013. Substance use and mental health characteristics associated with cognitive functioning among adults who use methamphetamine. *Journal of Addictive Diseases* 32(1):11-25.

HHS (U.S. Department of Health and Human Services). 2014a. *Healthy people.* http://www.healthypeople.gov (accessed October 27, 2014).

———. 2014b. *Healthy people 2020 leading health indicators: Nutrition, physical activity, and obesity.* http://www.healthypeople.gov/sites/default/files/HP2020_LHI_Nut_Phys Activ.pdf (accessed January 21, 2015).

Holwerda, T. J., D. J. Deeg, A. T. Beekman, T. G. van Tilburg, M. L. Stek, C. Jonker, and R. A. Schoevers. 2014. Feelings of loneliness, but not social isolation, predict dementia onset: Results from the Amsterdam Study of the Elderly (AMSTEL). *Journal of Neurology, Neurosurgery, and Psychiatry* 85(2):135-142.

Hooper, S. R., D. Woolley, and M. D. De Bellis. 2014. Intellectual, neurocognitive, and academic achievement in abstinent adolescents with cannabis use disorder. *Psychopharmacology* 231(8):1467-1477.

Humphrey, L. L., R. Fu, K. Rogers, M. Freeman, and M. Helfand. 2008. Homocysteine level and coronary heart disease incidence: A systematic review and meta-analysis. *Mayo Clinic Proceedings* 83(11):1203-1212.

Jacobus, J., and S. F. Tapert. 2014. Effects of cannabis on the adolescent brain. *Current Pharmaceutical Design* 20(13):2186-2193.

Jahncke, H. 2012. Open-plan office noise: The susceptibility and suitability of different cognitive tasks for work in the presence of irrelevant speech. *Noise and Health* 14(61):315-320.

Jayasekara, H., D. R. English, R. Room, and R. J. MacInnis. 2014. Alcohol consumption over time and risk of death: A systematic review and meta-analysis. *American Journal of Epidemiology* 179(9):1049-1059.

Jefferson, A. L., L. E. Gibbons, D. M. Rentz, J. O. Carvalho, J. Manly, D. A. Bennett, and R. N. Jones. 2011. A life course model of cognitive activities, socioeconomic status, education, reading ability, and cognition. *Journal of the American Geriatrics Society* 59(8):1403-1411.

Jha, P., C. Ramasundarahettige, V. Landsman, B. Rostron, M. Thun, R. N. Anderson, T. McAfee, and R. Peto. 2013. 21st-century hazards of smoking and benefits of cessation in the United States. *New England Journal of Medicine* 368(4):341-350.

Jorm, A. F., B. Rodgers, A. S. Henderson, A. E. Korten, P. A. Jacomb, H. Christensen, and A. Mackinnon. 1998. Occupation type as a predictor of cognitive decline and dementia in old age. *Age and Ageing* 27(4):477-483.

Kamegaya, T., Y. Araki, H. Kigure, and H. Yamaguchi. 2014. Twelve-week physical and leisure activity programme improved cognitive function in community-dwelling elderly subjects: A randomized controlled trial. *Psychogeriatrics* 14(1):47-54.

Kang, J. H., N. Cook, J. Manson, J. E. Buring, and F. Grodstein. 2006. A randomized trial of vitamin E supplementation and cognitive function in women. *Archives of Internal Medicine* 166(22):2462-2468.

Khalil, N., L. A. Morrow, H. Needleman, E. O. Talbott, J. W. Wilson, and J. A. Cauley. 2009. Association of cumulative lead and neurocognitive function in an occupational cohort. *Neuropsychology* 23(1):10-19.

Koyama, A., D. K. Houston, E. M. Simonsick, J. S. Lee, H. N. Ayonayon, D. R. Shahar, C. Rosano, S. Satterfield, and K. Yaffe. 2014. Association between the Mediterranean diet and cognitive decline in a biracial population. *The Journals of Gerontology, Series A: Biological Sciences and Medical Sciences* 70(3):352-357.

Krahn, D., J. Freese, R. Hauser, K. Barry, and B. Goodman. 2003. Alcohol use and cognition at mid-life: The importance of adjusting for baseline cognitive ability and educational attainment. *Alcoholism, Clinical and Experimental Research* 27(7):1162-1166.

Kramer, A. F., S. Hahn, N. J. Cohen, M. T. Banich, E. McAuley, C. R. Harrison, J. Chason, E. Vakil, L. Bardell, R. A. Boileau, and A. Colcombe. 1999. Ageing, fitness and neurocognitive function. *Nature* 400(6743):418-419.

Kremen, W. S., M. E. Lachman, J. C. Pruessner, M. Sliwinski, and R. S. Wilson. 2012. Mechanisms of age-related cognitive change and targets for intervention: Social interactions and stress. *The Journals of Gerontology, Series A: Biological Sciences and Medical Sciences* 67(7):760-765.

Kuh, D., S. Karunananthan, H. Bergman, and R. Cooper. 2014. A life-course approach to healthy ageing: Maintaining physical capability. *Proceedings of the Nutrition Society* 73(2):237-248.

Lautenschlager, N. T., K. Cox, and E. V. Cyarto. 2012. The influence of exercise on brain aging and dementia. *Biochimica et Biophysica Acta* 1822(3):474-481.

Lee, I. M., E. J. Shiroma, F. Lobelo, P. Puska, S. N. Blair, and P. T. Katzmarzyk. 2012. Effect of physical inactivity on major non-communicable diseases worldwide: An analysis of burden of disease and life expectancy. *Lancet* 380(9838):219-229.

Levin, E. D., O. A. Timofeeva, L. Yang, A. Petro, I. T. Ryde, N. Wrench, F. J. Seidler, and T. A. Slotkin. 2010. Early postnatal parathion exposure in rats causes sex-selective cognitive impairment and neurotransmitter defects which emerge in aging. *Behavioural Brain Research* 208(2):319-327.

Liu, Y., V. Julkunen, T. Paajanen, E. Westman, L. O. Wahlund, A. Aitken, T. Sobow, P. Mecocci, M. Tsolaki, B. Vellas, S. Muehlboeck, C. Spenger, S. Lovestone, A. Simmons, and H. Soininen. 2012. Education increases reserve against Alzheimer's disease—Evidence from structural MRI analysis. *Neuroradiology* 54(9):929-938.

Lourida, I., M. Soni, J. Thompson-Coon, N. Purandare, I. A. Lang, O. C. Ukoumunne, and D. J. Llewellyn. 2013. Mediterranean diet, cognitive function, and dementia: A systematic review. *Epidemiology* 24(4):479-489.

Luanaigh, C. O., and B. A. Lawlor. 2008. Loneliness and the health of older people. *International Journal of Geriatric Psychiatry* 23(12):1213-1221.

Madden, D. J., J. A. Blumenthal, P. A. Allen, and C. F. Emery. 1989. Improving aerobic capacity in healthy older adults does not necessarily lead to improved cognitive performance. *Psychology and Aging* 4(3):307-320.

Malouf, R., and J. Grimley Evans. 2008. Folic acid with or without vitamin B12 for the prevention and treatment of healthy elderly and demented people. *The Cochrane Database of Systematic Reviews* (4):Cd004514.

Manly, J. J., P. Touradji, M. X. Tang, and Y. Stern. 2003. Literacy and memory decline among ethnically diverse elders. *Journal of Clinical and Experimental Neuropsychology* 25(5):680-690.

Manly, J. J., N. Schupf, M. X. Tang, and Y. Stern. 2005. Cognitive decline and literacy among ethnically diverse elders. *Journal of Geriatric Psychiatry and Neurology* 18(4):213-217.

Martinez-Lapiscina, E. H., P. Clavero, E. Toledo, R. Estruch, J. Salas-Salvado, B. San Julian, A. Sanchez-Tainta, E. Ros, C. Valls-Pedret, and M. A. Martinez-Gonzalez. 2013. Mediterranean diet improves cognition: The PREDIMED-NAVARRA randomised trial. *Journal of Neurology, Neurosurgery, and Psychiatry* 84(12):1318-1325.

McEwen, B. S., and J. H. Morrison. 2013. The brain on stress: Vulnerability and plasticity of the prefrontal cortex over the life course. *Neuron* 79(1):16-29.

Mehta, K. M., E. M. Simonsick, R. Rooks, A. B. Newman, S. K. Pope, S. M. Rubin, and K. Yaffe. 2004. Black and white differences in cognitive function test scores: What explains the difference? *Journal of the American Geriatrics Society* 52(12):2120-2127.

Meng, X., and C. D'Arcy. 2012. Education and dementia in the context of the cognitive reserve hypothesis: A systematic review with meta-anaylses and qualitative analyses. *PLoS ONE* 7(6):e38268.

Middleton, L. E., D. E. Barnes, L. Y. Lui, and K. Yaffe. 2010. Physical activity over the life course and its association with cognitive performance and impairment in old age. *Journal of the American Geriatric Society* 58(7):1322-1326.

Miller, E. R., 3rd, R. Pastor-Barriuso, D. Dalal, R. A. Riemersma, L. J. Appel, and E. Guallar. 2005. Meta-analysis: High-dosage vitamin E supplementation may increase all-cause mortality. *Annals of Internal Medicine* 142(1):37-46.

Mortimer, J. A., D. Ding, A. R. Borenstein, C. DeCarli, Q. Guo, Y. Wu, Q. Zhao, and S. Chu. 2012. Changes in brain volume and cognition in a randomized trial of exercise and social interaction in a community-based sample of non-demented Chinese elders. *Journal of Alzheimer's Disease* 30(4):757-766.

Muzet, A. 2007. Environmental noise, sleep and health. *Sleep Medicine Reviews* 11(2):135-142.

NIH (National Institutes of Health). 2013. *Multivitamin/mineral supplements.* http://ods.od.nih.gov/factsheets/MVMS-HealthProfessional (accessed January 8, 2015).

———. 2014a. *What is the DASH eating plan?* http://www.nhlbi.nih.gov/health/health-topics/topics/dash (accessed October 28, 2014).

———. 2014b. *Exercise: Benefits of exercise.* www.nihseniorhealth.gov/exerciseforolderadults/healthbenefits/01.html (accessed December 5, 2014).

Nordling Nilson, L., L. Barregard, G. Sallsten, and S. Hagberg. 2007. Self-reported symptoms and their effects on cognitive functioning in workers with past exposure to solvent-based glues: An 18-year follow-up. *International Archives of Occupational and Environmental Health* 81(1):69-79.

North, A., J. Swant, M. F. Salvatore, J. Gamble-George, P. Prins, B. Butler, M. K. Mittal, R. Heltsley, J. T. Clark, and H. Khoshbouei. 2013. Chronic methamphetamine exposure produces a delayed, long-lasting memory deficit. *Synapse* 67(5):245-257.

Nunomura, A., R. J. Castellani, X. Zhu, P. I. Moreira, G. Perry, and M. A. Smith. 2006. Involvement of oxidative stress in Alzheimer disease. *Journal of Neuropathology and Experimental Neurology* 65(7):631-641.

OHTAC (Ontario Health Technology Advisory Committee). 2013. Vitamin B12 and cognitive function: OHTAC recommendation. Toronto: Queen's Printer for Ontario.

O'Luanaigh, C., H. O'Connell, A. V. Chin, F. Hamilton, R. Coen, C. Walsh, J. B. Walsh, D. Caokley, C. Cunningham, and B. A. Lawlor. 2012. Loneliness and cognition in older people: The Dublin Healthy Ageing Study. *Aging and Mental Health* 16(3):347-352

Pesonen, A. K., K. Raikkonen, K. Heinonen, E. Kajantie, T. Forsen, and J. G. Eriksson. 2007. Depressive symptoms in adults separated from their parents as children: A natural experiment during World War II. *American Journal of Epidemiology* 166(10):1126-1133.

Peters, R., J. Peters, J. Warner, N. Beckett, and C. Bulpitt. 2008a. Alcohol, dementia and cognitive decline in the elderly: A systematic review. *Age and Ageing* 37(5):505-512.

Peters, R., R. Poulter, J. Warner, N. Beckett, L. Burch, and C. Bulpitt. 2008b. Smoking, dementia and cognitive decline in the elderly, a systematic review. *BMC Geriatrics* 8:36.

Plassman, B. L., J. W. Williams, Jr., J. R. Burke, T. Holsinger, and S. Benjamin. 2010. Systematic review: Factors associated with risk for and possible prevention of cognitive decline in later life. *Annals of Internal Medicine* 153(3):182-193.

Querbes, O., F. Aubry, J. Pariente, J. A. Lotterie, J. F. Demonet, V. Duret, M. Puel, I. Berry, J. C. Fort, and P. Celsis. 2009. Early diagnosis of Alzheimer's disease using cortical thickness: Impact of cognitive reserve. *Brain* 132(Pt 8):2036-2047.

Rafnsson, S. B., V. Dilis, and A. Trichopoulou. 2013. Antioxidant nutrients and age-related cognitive decline: A systematic review of population-based cohort studies. *European Journal of Nutrition* 52(6):1553-1567.

Rebok, G. W., M. C. Carlson, T. A. Glass, S. McGill, J. Hill, B. A. Wasik, N. Ialongo, K. D. Frick, L. P. Fried, and M. D. Rasmussen. 2004. Short-term impact of Experience Corps participation on children and schools: results from a pilot randomized trial. *Journal of Urban Health* 81(1):79-93.

Reed, B. R., D. Mungas, S. T. Farias, D. Harvey, L. Beckett, K. Widaman, L. Hinton, and C. DeCarli. 2010. Measuring cognitive reserve based on the decomposition of episodic memory variance. *Brain* 133(Pt 8):2196-2209.

Rickenbach, E. H., D. M. Almeida, T. E. Seeman, and M. E. Lachman. 2014. Daily stress magnifies the association between cognitive decline and everyday memory problems: An integration of longitudinal and diary methods. *Psychology and Aging* 29(4):852-862.

Rikli, R. E., and D. J. Edwards. 1991. Effects of a three-year exercise program on motor function and cognitive processing speed in older women. *Research Quarterly for Exercise and Sport* 62(1):61-67.

Roerecke, M., and J. Rehm. 2012. The cardioprotective association of average alcohol consumption and ischaemic heart disease: A systematic review and meta-analysis. *Addiction* 107(7):1246-1260.

Rosano, C., V. K. Venkatraman, J. Guralnik, A. B. Newman, N. W. Glynn, L. Launer, C. A. Taylor, J. Williamson, S. Studenski, M. Pahor, and H. Aizenstein. 2010. Psychomotor speed and functional brain MRI 2 years after completing a physical activity treatment. *Journal of Gerontology* 65(6):639-647.

Rossom, R. C., M. A. Espeland, J. E. Manson, M. W. Dysken, K. C. Johnson, D. S. Lane, E. S. LeBlanc, F. A. Lederle, K. H. Masaki, and K. L. Margolis. 2012. Calcium and vitamin D supplementation and cognitive impairment in the Women's Health Initiative. *Journal of the American Geriatrics Society* 60(12):2197-2205.

Ruscheweyh, R., C. Willemer, K. Kruger, T. Duning, T. Warnecke, J. Sommer, K. Volker, H. V. Ho, F. Mooren, S. Knecht, and A. Floel. 2011. Physical activity and memory functions: An interventional study. *Neurobiology of Aging* 32(7):1304-1319.

Sabbath, E. L., M. M. Glymour, C. Berr, A. Singh-Manoux, M. Zins, M. Goldberg, and L. F. Berkman. 2012. Occupational solvent exposure and cognition: Does the association vary by level of education? *Neurology* 78(22):1754-1760.

Sachs-Ericsson, N., and D. G. Blazer. 2005. Racial differences in cognitive decline in a sample of community-dwelling older adults: the mediating role of education and literacy. *American Journal of Geriatric Psychiatry* 13(11):968-975.

Salanova, M., S. Llorens, and E. Cifre. 2013. The dark side of technologies: Technostress among users of information and communication technologies. *International Journal of Psychology* 48(3):422-436.

Samieri, C., F. Grodstein, B. A. Rosner, J. H. Kang, N. R. Cook, J. E. Manson, J. E. Buring, W. C. Willett, and O. I. Okereke. 2013. Mediterranean diet and cognitive function in older age: Results from the Women's Health Study. *Epidemiology* 24(4):490-499.

Scarmeas, N., J. A. Luchsinger, N. Schupf, A. M. Brickman, S. Cosentino, M. X. Tang, and Y. Stern. 2009. Physical activity, diet, and risk of Alzheimer disease. *JAMA* 302(6):627-637.

Schaie, K. W. 1996. *Intellectual development in adulthood: The Seattle Longitudinal Study.* New York: Cambridge University Press.

Schneider, A. L., P. L. Lutsey, A. Alonso, R. F. Gottesman, A. R. Sharrett, K. A. Carson, M. Gross, W. S. Post, D. S. Knopman, T. H. Mosley, and E. D. Michos. 2014. Vitamin D and cognitive function and dementia risk in a biracial cohort: The ARIC Brain MRI Study. *European Journal of Neurology* 21(9):1211-1218, e1269-e1270.

Seeman, T. E., D. M. Miller-Martinez, S. Stein Merkin, M. E. Lachman, P. A. Tun, and A. S. Karlamangla. 2011. Histories of social engagement and adult cognition: Midlife in the U.S. Study. *The Journals of Gerontology, Series B: Psychological Sciences and Social Sciences* 66(Suppl 1):i141-i152.

Shah, A. S., J. P. Langrish, H. Nair, D. A. McAllister, A. L. Hunter, K. Donaldson, D. E. Newby, and N. L. Mills. 2013. Global association of air pollution and heart failure: A systematic review and meta-analysis. *Lancet* 382(9897):1039-1048.

Shankar, A., M. Hamer, A. McMunn, and A. Steptoe. 2013. Social isolation and loneliness: Relationships with cognitive function during 4 years of follow-up in the English Longitudinal Study of Ageing. *Psychosomatic Medicine* 75(2):161-170.

Singh-Manoux, A., M. G. Marmot, M. Glymour, S. Sabia, M. Kivimaki, and A. Dugravot. 2011. Does cognitive reserve shape cognitive decline? *Annals of Neurology* 70(2):296-304.

Slinin, Y., M. Paudel, B. C. Taylor, A. Ishani, R. Rossom, K. Yaffe, T. Blackwell, L. Y. Lui, M. Hochberg, and K. E. Ensrud. 2012. Association between serum 25(OH) vitamin D and the risk of cognitive decline in older women. *The Journals of Gerontology, Series A: Biological Sciences and Medical Sciences* 67(10):1092-1098.

Small, B. J., R. A. Dixon, J. J. McArdle, and K. J. Grimm. 2012. Do changes in lifestyle engagement moderate cognitive decline in normal aging? Evidence from the Victoria Longitudinal Study. *Neuropsychology* 26(2):144-155.

Smith, P. J., J. A. Blumenthal, M. A. Babyak, L. Craighead, K. A. Welsh-Bohmer, J. N. Browndyke, T. A. Strauman, and A. Sherwood. 2010a. Effects of the dietary approaches to stop hypertension diet, exercise, and caloric restriction on neurocognition in overweight adults with high blood pressure. *Hypertension* 55(6):1331-1338.

Smith, P. J., J. A. Blumenthal, B. M. Hoffman, H. Cooper, T. A. Strauman, K. Welsh-Bohmer, J. N. Browndyke, and A. Sherwood. 2010b. Aerobic exercise and neurocognitive performance: A meta-analytic review of randomized controlled trials. *Psychosomatic Medicine* 72(3):239-252.

Sole-Padulles, C., D. Bartres-Faz, C. Junque, P. Vendrell, L. Rami, I. C. Clemente, B. Bosch, A. Villar, N. Bargallo, M. A. Jurado, M. Barrios, and J. L. Molinuevo. 2009. Brain structure and function related to cognitive reserve variables in normal aging, mild cognitive impairment and Alzheimer's disease. *Neurobiology of Aging* 30(7):1114-1124.

Spirduso, W. W. 1975. Reaction and movement time as a function of age and physical activity level. *Journal of Gerontology* 30(4):435-440.

Spirduso, W. W., and P. Clifford. 1978. Replication of age and physical activity effects on reaction and movement time. *Journal of Gerontology* 33(1):26-30.

Steptoe, A., A. Shankar, P. Demakakos, and J. Wardle. 2013. Social isolation, loneliness, and all-cause mortality in older men and women. *Proceedings of the National Academy of Sciences of the United States of America* 110(15):5797-5801.

Stern, Y. 2009. Cognitive reserve. *Neuropsychologia* 47(10):2015-2028.

———. 2012. Cognitive reserve in ageing and Alzheimer's disease. *Lancet Neurology* 11(11):1006-1012.

Stine-Morrow, E. A., J. M. Parisi, D. G. Morrow, and D. C. Park. 2008. The effects of an engaged lifestyle on cognitive vitality: A field experiment. *Psychology and Aging* 23(4):778-786.

Stine-Morrow, E. A., B. R. Payne, B. W. Roberts, A. F. Kramer, D. G. Morrow, L. Payne, P. I. Hill, J. J. Jackson, X. Gao, S. R. Noh, and M. C. Janke. 2014. Training versus engagement as paths to cognitive enrichment with aging. *Psychology and Aging* 29(4):891-906.

Szabo, S., Y. Tache, and A. Somogyi. 2012. The legacy of Hans Selye and the origins of stress research: A retrospective 75 years after his landmark brief "letter" to the editor of Nature. *Stress* 15(5):472-478.

Terrett, G., S. N. McLennan, J. D. Henry, K. Biernacki, K. Mercuri, H. V. Curran, and P. G. Rendell. 2014. Prospective memory impairment in long-term opiate users. *Psychopharmacology* 231(13):2623-2632.

Thames, A. D., N. Arbid, and P. Sayegh. 2014. Cannabis use and neurocognitive functioning in a non-clinical sample of users. *Addictive Behaviors* 39(5):994-999.

Thomas, P. A. 2011. Gender, social engagement, and limitations in late life. *Social Science and Medicine* 73(9):1428-1435.

Thomee, S., L. Dellve, A. Harenstam, and M. Hagberg. 2010. Perceived connections between information and communication technology use and mental symptoms among young adults: A qualitative study. *BMC Public Health* 10:66.

Tilvis, R. S., M. H. Kahonen-Vare, J. Jolkkonen, J. Valvanne, K. H. Pitkala, and T. E. Strandberg. 2004. Predictors of cognitive decline and mortality of aged people over a 10-year period. *The Journals of Gerontology, Series A: Biological Sciences and Medical Sciences* 59(3):268-274.

Titova, O. E., E. Ax, S. J. Brooks, P. Sjogren, T. Cederholm, L. Kilander, J. Kullberg, E. M. Larsson, L. Johansson, H. Ahlstrom, L. Lind, H. B. Schioth, and C. Benedict. 2013. Mediterranean diet habits in older individuals: Associations with cognitive functioning and brain volumes. *Experimental Gerontology* 48(12):1443-1448.

Tschanz, J. T., R. Pfister, J. Wanzek, C. Corcoran, K. Smith, B. T. Tschanz, D. C. Steffens, T. Ostbye, K. A. Welsh-Bohmer, and M. C. Norton. 2013. Stressful life events and cognitive decline in late life: Moderation by education and age. The Cache County Study. *International Journal of Geriatric Psychiatry* 28(8):821-830.

Tun, P. A., D. Miller-Martinez, M. E. Lachman, and T. Seeman. 2013. Social strain and executive function across the lifespan: The dark (and light) sides of social engagement. *Neuropsychology, Development, and Cognition. Section B, Aging, Neuropsychology and Cognition* 20(3):320-338.

USDA (U.S. Department of Agriculture). 2014. *Dietary guidelines for Americans*. http://www.cnpp.usda.gov/DietaryGuidelines.htm (accessed October 28, 2014).

van Holst, R. J., and T. Schilt. 2011. Drug-related decrease in neuropsychological functions of abstinent drug users. *Current Drug Abuse Reviews* 4(1):42-56.

Vaynman, S., and F. Gomez-Pinilla. 2005. License to run: Exercise impacts functional plasticity in the intact and injured central nervous system by using neurotrophins. *Neurorehabilitation and Neural Repair* 19(4):283-295.

Vemuri, P., T. G. Lesnick, S. A. Przybelski, M. Machulda, D. S. Knopman, M. M. Mielke, R. O. Roberts, Y. E. Geda, W. A. Rocca, R. C. Petersen, and C. R. Jack. 2014. Association of lifetime intellectual enrichment with cognitive decline in the older population. *JAMA Neurology* 71(8):1017-1024.

Voss, M. W., R. S. Prakash, K. I. Erickson, C. Basak, L. Chaddock, J. S. Kim, H. Alves, S. Heo, A. N. Szabo, S. M. White, T. R. Wojcicki, E. L. Mailey, N. Gothe, E. A. Olson, E. McAuley, and A. F. Kramer. 2010. Plasticity of brain networks in a randomized intervention trial of exercise training in older adults. *Frontiers in Aging Neuroscience* 2.

Voss, M. W., K. I. Erickson, R. S. Prakash, L. Chaddock, J. S. Kim, H. Alves, A. Szabo, S. M. Phillips, T. R. Wojcicki, E. L. Mailey, E. A. Olson, N. Gothe, V. J. Vieira-Potter, S. A. Martin, B. D. Pence, M. D. Cook, J. A. Woods, E. McAuley, and A. F. Kramer. 2013a. Neurobiological markers of exercise-related brain plasticity in older adults. *Brain, Behavior, and Immunity* 28:90-99.

Voss, M. W., C. Vivar, A. F. Kramer, and H. van Praag. 2013b. Bridging animal and human models of exercise-induced brain plasticity. *Trends in Cognitive Science* 17(10):525-544.

Wald, D. S., A. Kasturiratne, and M. Simmonds. 2010. Effect of folic acid, with or without other B vitamins, on cognitive decline: Meta-analysis of randomized trials. *The American Journal of Medicine* 123(6):522-527.

Wang, G. Y., T. A. Wouldes, and B. R. Russell. 2013. Methadone maintenance treatment and cognitive function: A systematic review. *Current Drug Abuse Reviews* 6(3):220-230.

Wengreen, H., R. G. Munger, A. Cutler, A. Quach, A. Bowles, C. Corcoran, J. T. Tschanz, M. C. Norton, and K. A. Welsh-Bohmer. 2013. Prospective study of dietary approaches to stop hypertension- and Mediterranean-style dietary patterns and age-related cognitive change: The Cache County Study on Memory, Health and Aging. *American Journal of Clinical Nutrition* 98(5):1263-1271.

Wilson, R. S., P. A. Scherr, J. A. Schneider, Y. Tang, and D. A. Bennett. 2007. Relation of cognitive activity to risk of developing Alzheimer disease. *Neurology* 69(20):1911-1920.

Wilson, R. S., P. A. Boyle, L. Yu, L. L. Barnes, J. A. Schneider, and D. A. Bennett. 2013. Life-span cognitive activity, neuropathologic burden, and cognitive aging. *Neurology* 81(4):314-321.

Wilson, V. K., D. K. Houston, L. Kilpatrick, J. Lovato, K. Yaffe, J. A. Cauley, T. B. Harris, E. M. Simonsick, H. N. Ayonayon, S. B. Kritchevsky, and K. M. Sink. 2014. Relationship between 25-hydroxyvitamin D and cognitive function in older adults: The Health, Aging and Body Composition Study. *Journal of the American Geriatrics Society* 62(4):636-641.

Wong, H. S., and P. Edwards. 2013. Nature or nurture: A systematic review of the effect of socio-economic status on the developmental and cognitive outcomes of children born preterm. *Maternal and Child Health Journal* 17(9):1689-1700.

Wu, L. T., and D. G. Blazer. 2011. Illicit and nonmedical drug use among older adults: A review. *Journal of Aging and Health* 23(3):481-504.

Wu, L. T., K. R. Gersing, M. S. Swartz, B. Burchett, T. K. Li, and D. G. Blazer. 2013. Using electronic health records data to assess comorbidities of substance use and psychiatric diagnoses and treatment settings among adults. *Journal of Psychiatric Research* 47(4):555-563.

Zahodne, L. B., M. M. Glymour, C. Sparks, D. Bontempo, R. A. Dixon, S. W. MacDonald, and J. J. Manly. 2011. Education does not slow cognitive decline with aging: 12-year evidence from the Victoria Longitudinal Study. *Journal of the International Neuropsychological Society* 17(6):1039-1046.

Zhu, N., D. R. Jacobs, Jr., P. J. Schreiner, K. Yaffe, N. Bryan, L. J. Launer, R. A. Whitmer, S. Sidney, E. Demerath, W. Thomas, C. Bouchard, K. He, J. Reis, and B. Sternfeld. 2014. Cardiorespiratory fitness and cognitive function in middle age: The CARDIA study. *Neurology* 82(15):1339-1346.

4B

Risk and Protective Factors and Interventions: Health and Medical Factors

This is the second of three chapters exploring risk and protective factors and interventions relevant to cognitive aging. Chapter 4A discusses lifestyle factors and the physical environment, and Chapter 4C discusses general approaches to remediation and provides concluding remarks and recommendations on opportunities for next steps in promoting healthy cognitive aging.

This chapter addresses many of the external factors and comorbidities that may affect cognition. The basic overall challenge is that much more needs to be learned about how these factors affect cognitive aging—in particular, whether they have long-term effects on cognitive function. Some of these factors (e.g., certain medications, delirium) may result in easily identifiable short-term risks of cognitive declines, which in some cases it may be possible to completely reverse; in addition, these factors may mediate more long-term changes in cognitive trajectory. For other factors, such as comorbidities and exposures that occur over a period of years, research questions generally focus on the extent to which treating or reducing a comorbidity (e.g., diabetes or uncontrolled hypertension) or reducing or eliminating an exposure will affect long-term cognitive function. Further research is also needed on the biological mechanisms underlying the impact of these factors on cognitive change and the extent to which each is a cause or a mediator of change. As with all aspects of cognitive aging, cognitive function may vary widely both within an individual over time and among individuals.

Each section of this chapter focuses on a specific risk or protective factor and summarizes evidence from available observational studies and intervention studies, then concludes with a summary comment on the strength of the evidence.

MEDICATIONS

Increasingly, certain classes of medicines have been recognized as causing cognitive decline and impairment; these potentially preventable adverse events have risks that are a function of dose, duration, and individual susceptibility (such as preexisting cognitive impairment or dementia or genetic makeup). The impact of these medications on long-term cognitive function is an area of ongoing research.

The role of health care professionals who are interested in preventing adverse effects from medication is made more difficult by a steady influx of new knowledge about the effects and interactions of these medications, by the complex medication regimens that are required to treat many diseases, and by the multiple health care providers that are involved in the care of many older people. Not only is it challenging for health care professionals to stay up to date on the medications they prescribe and to manage medications for individual patients; it is also difficult for them to determine whether the medications they prescribed may have negative or positive cognitive effects when administered in conjunction with other medications. In the United States, older adults represent about 13 percent of the population but are prescribed more than 40 percent of drugs that are prescribed. On average, individuals from ages 65 to 69 years old are prescribed 14 different drugs per year (ASCP, 2015). The high rate of prescription drug use is associated with substantial rates of serious adverse drug events, which are considered preventable in 27 percent of ambulatory, 28 percent of hospitalized, and 42 percent of long-term care patients (Bates et al., 1995; Fick and Semla, 2012). Additionally, some medications with the potential for negative effects on cognition are available over the counter.

Evidence from Observational Studies

Although a number of studies have indicated that there may be an association between these drug classes and dementia, the potential for unrecognized dementia or other confounding conditions in many of these studies prevents the establishment of any causal relationship.

Beers Criteria Medications

Based on a comprehensive and systematic review and a guideline panel process which included the grading of evidence and a public comment period, the 2012 American Geriatrics Society's (AGS's) Beers Criteria for Potentially Inappropriate Medication Use in Older Adults recommended that a number of drugs and classes of drugs be avoided in older adults because of their potential for causing cognitive decline or delirium (AGS, 2012; see Table 4B-1). While a detailed review of all of these drugs is beyond the scope of this report, the usage of anticholinergic and benzodiazepine drugs will be specifically addressed because they remain in common use and are especially at risk for inappropriate use by older individuals.

Anticholinergic Drugs (Including Antihistamines)

Depending on the population studied, about 20 to 50 percent of older persons in the United States are prescribed at least one anticholinergic drug at any given time (Campbell et al., 2009). While definite indications exist for these classes of drugs, such as for the treatment of allergies, nausea, depression, muscle spasm, and many other medical conditions, some of the usage may be inappropriate. Instead, effective less-toxic alternatives should be considered.

Several systematic reviews have documented the association of anticholinergic drugs with both short-term and long-term adverse cognitive effects in older adults (Campbell et al., 2009; Kalisch Ellett et al., 2014; Tannenbaum et al., 2012). Kalisch Ellet and colleagues (2014) analyzed Australian veterans' administrative claims data from 2010 to 2012 and found that using two or more anticholinergic medications increased the risk of hospitalization for confusion or dementia. A listing of drugs with strong anticholinergic properties is provided in Table 4B-2.

A clinical review of 27 studies that included anticholinergic assays and measurement of cognitive performance found that 25 showed associations between the anticholinergic activity of medications and delirium, cognitive impairment, or dementia (Campbell et al., 2009). In a large three-city population study of more than 6,900 older persons (Carriere et al., 2009), continuous anticholinergic drug use was found to be associated with a 1.4- to 2.0-fold higher risk of cognitive decline. In addition, the risk of incident dementia was also increased in continuous users over the 4-year follow-up period (hazard ratio 1.65, 95% confidence interval [CI] 1.0–2.7). The risk increased with the duration of continuous use and was also higher among those with baseline cognitive impairment and dementia (Tannenbaum et al., 2012).

Many antihistamines are available in over-the-counter preparations, including those used for cold, influenza, allergy relief, and sleep ("PM" formulations). Because these antihistamines, such as diphenhydramine, are potent anticholinergic agents, it is important to educate the general public about the potential risks, including the risk of cognitive decline.

TABLE 4B-1 American Geriatrics Society Beers Criteria for Potentially Inappropriate Medication Use in Older Adults Due to Drug–Disease or Drug–Syndrome Interaction That May Exacerbate the Disease or Syndrome

Disease or Syndrome	Drug	Rationale	Recommendation, Quality of Evidence, and Strength of Recommendation
Delirium	All tricyclic antidepressants Anticholinergics (see Table 4B-2) Benzodiazepines Chlorpromazine Corticosteroids H$_2$-receptor antagonists Meperidine Sedative hypnotics Thioridazine	Avoid in older adults with or at high risk of delirium because of inducing or worsening delirium in older adults; if discontinuing drugs used chronically, taper to avoid withdrawal symptoms	**Recommendation:** Avoid **Quality of Evidence:** Moderate **Strength of Recommendation:** Strong
Dementia and Cognitive Impairment	Anticholinergics (see Table 4B-2) Benzodiazepines H$_2$-receptor antagonists Zolpidem Antipsychotics, chronic and as-needed use	Avoid because of adverse central nervous system effects. Avoid antipsychotics for behavioral problems of dementia unless nonpharmacological options have failed, and patient is a threat to themselves or others. Antipsychotics are associated with an increased risk of cerebrovascular accident (stroke) and mortality in persons with dementia	**Recommendation:** Avoid **Quality of Evidence:** High **Strength of Recommendation:** Strong

SOURCE: AGS, 2012. Reprinted with permission of John Wiley & Sons, Inc.

Benzodiazepines

Commonly used to treat anxiety, sleeplessness, and agitation in older persons, benzodiazepines (e.g., alprazolam, lorazepam, chlorazepate, and clonazepam) are associated with a markedly increased risk for delirium, cognitive impairment, falls, fractures, and motor vehicle accidents (Billioti de Gage et al., 2012; de Vries et al., 2013). In a recent systematic review of 68 clinical trials (Tannenbaum et al., 2012), benzodiazepines were consistently associated with both amnestic (involving loss of memory) and non-amnestic cognitive impairment by neuropsychological testing. Given the risks, the use of this class of drugs needs to be carefully assessed for use

TABLE 4B-2 Drugs with Strong Anticholinergic Properties

Antihistamines	Antidepressants	Antimuscarinics (urinary incontinence)	Antiparkinson Agents	Antipsychotics	Antispasmodics	Skeletal Muscle Relaxants
Brompheniramine	Amitriptyline	Darifenacin	Benztropine	Chlorpromazine	Atropine products	Carisoprodol
Carbinoxamine	Amoxapine	Fesoterodine	Trihexyphenidyl	Clozapine	Belladonna alkaloids	Cyclobenzaprine
Chlorpheniramine	Clomipramine	Flavoxate		Fluphenazine	Dicyclomine	Orphenadrine
Clemastine	Desipramine	Oxybutynin		Loxapine	Homatropine	Tizanidine
Cyproheptadine	Doxepin	Solifenacin		Olanzapine	Hyoscyamine products	
Dimenhydrinate	Imipramine	Tolterodine		Perphenazine	Propantheline	
Diphenhydramine	Nortriptyline	Trospium		Pimozide	Scopolamine	
Hydroxyzine	Trimipramine			Prochlorperazine		
Loratadine				Promethazine		
Meclizine				Thioridazine		
				Thiothixene		
				Trifluoperazine		

SOURCE: AGS, 2012. Reprinted with permission of John Wiley & Sons, Inc.

by older persons, with their use reserved for such indications as seizures or other neurological conditions, alcohol withdrawal, severe generalized anxiety disorder, anesthesia, and end-of-life care.

Evidence from Intervention Studies

Several studies conducted in the past decade have tested interventions aimed at reducing the number of high-risk or harmful medications—as well as the total number of medications—that older adults take with the goal of reducing unnecessary side effects, including cognitive decline. A few studies have focused on reducing intake of medications listed on the Beers Criteria (AGS, 2012; Fick and Semla, 2012; Fick et al., 2003; Ray et al., 1986). A 10-year longitudinal study of older women found that they had a high prevalence of inappropriate medication use and high anticholinergic load; this was especially true in women who developed dementia later in life (Koyama et al., 2013).

A study by Gurwitz and colleagues (2000) found that 68 percent of preventable adverse drug events occurred at the ordering (prescribing) stage of care. Such findings have helped encourage the development of computerized decision support and education as a strategy to help decrease adverse drug events in various settings of care (Alldred et al., 2013). A number of studies have found a statistically significant drop in inappropriate prescribing after the implementation of a computerized decision support system[1] that used the electronic health record to alert providers to the use of inappropriate medications (Agostini et al., 2007; Mattison et al., 2010; Raebel et al., 2007; Smith et al., 2006; Tamblyn et al., 2003), but none of these studies measured the impact on cognitive outcomes in older adults. Another intervention that has proved successful in discontinuing some medications in older adults is the use of a consultant pharmacist[2] alone or in combination with other components (Lukazewski et al., 2014).

A systematic review of the impact of anticholinergic discontinuation on cognitive outcomes in older adults by Salahudeen and colleagues (2014) found positive results from empowerment strategies, such as helping older

---

[1] Computerized decision support (CDS) interventions can encompass a variety of levels of support, but most CDS interventions for medication use will alert the provider before the medication is prescribed (when the provider attempts to enter or prescribe the medication) and will offer a suggested drug alternative, a behavioral or non-drug approach, or both a drug and a non-drug alternative.

[2] Consultant pharmacists consult with other health care professionals, patients, and caregivers about high-risk drugs, dosage issues, side effects, cumulative drug burden and drug–drug interactions to ensure appropriate use of medication. Consultant pharmacists practice in a wide variety of settings, including subacute care and assisted living facilities, psychiatric hospitals, hospice programs, and in home- and community-based care (ASCP, 2014).

adults learn about their medications and health status and helping them take the initiative for shared health care decisions to discontinue benzodiazepines. Past efforts at direct-to-consumer advertising by the pharmaceutical industry have been shown to be effective in influencing the public's demand for certain medications (Rosenthal et al., 2002). In another study, the researchers employed a cluster randomized design that assigned community pharmacies to either a treatment group or the control group, with the treatment group being provided with an empowerment process focused on reducing inappropriate benzodiazepine use by the patients. At 6 months, 27 percent of the treatment group had discontinued benzodiazepine use compared with 5 percent of the control group. The empowerment process, which helped older adults gain control and take the initiative to solve the problem, included a detailed patient interview, self-assessment, education, suggestions for non-drug safer substitutions, and the use of peer champions (Tannenbaum et al., 2014).

One over-the-counter antihistamine medication that is commonly used by older adults in the community setting and that worsens cognition is diphenhydramine. Interventions to reduce the use of this medication have been conducted primarily in hospitals. A study by Agostini and colleagues (2007) used a computer-based alert that reminded providers of the side effects of the medication and the dangers of diphenhydramine in older adults and suggested non-drug approaches (such as warm milk and relaxation techniques). This study observed an 18 percent risk reduction in the orders for sedative–hypnotic drugs. A second hospital-based intervention used a computer alert and direct communication between the physician and the pharmacist to achieve a 52 percent reduction in prescribing diphenhydramine (Fosnight et al., 2004). Both of these studies were limited by their prospective, pre–post intervention designs. To date, no research on interventions to limit over-the-counter purchase of diphenhydramine or other related antihistamines by older adults has been published.

Summary

Research has demonstrated that the use of high-risk or potentially inappropriate medications that negatively affect cognition can be effectively reduced or curtailed using techniques such as computerized decision support, consultant pharmacists, and more recently, a direct-to-consumer education approach. However, because of various methodological, clinical, and ethical issues, there has as yet been no research establishing the impact of these initiatives on sustaining or improving cognition. Determining the impact of these medications on cognitive aging will require carefully conducted longitudinal studies. Medication discontinuation interventions need to carefully consider the effects on individuals as well as the various personal preferences of individuals and differing responses to medications and aging. The range of non-drug alternatives is limited by the paucity of strong and individualized evidence for non-drug alternatives in older adults and by the lack of reimbursement for the use of alternatives. Several intervention studies have had moderate methodological limitations, and they have varied widely in how they have measured cognitive function. In the future, studies should use sensitive and validated measures of cognition and should consider issues of dosing, cumulative drug burden effects, effective ways to deliver tailored alternatives, and the impact of medication withdrawal.

MEDICAL CONDITIONS

The evidence on whether treating medical conditions can prevent or reverse cognitive decline and on the impact of medical treatments on long-term cognitive function is complicated. Certain conditions, such as stroke, may result in acute and severe cognitive decline, with the possibility in some cases of regaining some of that cognitive function over time. For stroke and these other conditions, an individual's cognitive trajectory may be determined in large part by the acute event. For other types of conditions, particularly those where prevention and early treatment is the focus (such as diabetes or uncontrolled hypertension), there are many unknowns concerning the extent to which prevention and treatment efforts lead to improvements in cognitive health and how these efforts affect cognitive aging over the life span. For example, reducing the occurrence of strokes will be beneficial to cognitive health; however, much remains to be learned about the effects on cognitive function of treating the individual risk factors for stroke such as hyperlipidemia. Moreover, for some conditions (e.g., hypothyroidism), the benefits of treatment are so compelling—independent of the question of the treatment's effects on cognition—that trials to demonstrate effectiveness on cognition are not needed or ethically justifiable. For these conditions, only observational data are presented, with the assumption that patients with these conditions would be treated and accrue any potential cognitive benefit. For other conditions (e.g., diabetes, obesity) cognitive outcomes are important because they may influence the decisions about the mode or aggressiveness of the treatment. For example, the degree of glycemic or blood pressure control sought for older people with diabetes may need to take into account the adverse consequences of hypoglycemia or hypotension.

Cerebrovascular and Cardiovascular Disease

In the United States, stroke or cerebrovascular accident, which occurs in approximately 2.4 out of every 1,000 persons in the United States (Leys et al., 2005), is a major cause of disability in older adults and the third-leading cause of death in that group (Gorina et al., 2006). There may be considerable overlap between the clinical manifestations of cognitive decline associated with aging and those associated with diagnosed or undiagnosed cardiovascular and cerebrovascular disease (e.g., conditions that may show up as white matter hyperintensities [leukoaraiosis] with magnetic resonance imaging [MRI]). Treatment of cerebrovascular and cardiovascular risk factors might be expected to prevent some of these events and, consequently, the related cognitive declines.

Cognitive decline and dementia are well-recognized sequelae of stroke. For example, one study found dementia in 26 percent of older persons evaluated 3 months after a stroke (Tatemichi et al., 1994). Large strokes can lead to stepwise declines in cognitive functioning, while multiple small strokes may result in only a modestly accelerated course of cognitive decline. While milder degrees of cerebrovascular disease (such as microvascular disease or transient ischemia) have been associated with cognitive decline, the consistency and degree of association has not been clear. In a systematic review of 16 population-based studies (Savva and Stephan, 2010), the occurrence of stroke was found to be associated with a doubling in the risk of incident dementia in the older population. In a systematic review of 30 studies (involving a total of 7,565 patients), the incidence of new dementia following a first-ever stroke was 7.4 percent (95% CI 4.8–10.0) in the first year and 1.7 percent per year (95% CI 1.4–2.0) thereafter (Pendlebury, 2009). Two studies reviewed by Savva and Stephan (2010) suggested that the impact of stroke on the future risk of dementia may be stronger in people with a specific genetic risk factor for Alzheimer's disease (those who are APOE ε4 negative), but the association in three other studies was inconsistent.

The committee supports efforts to improve cardiovascular health in older adults, including through the management of blood pressure, the control of cholesterol, and the maintenance of a healthy body weight (see Chapter 6). Hypoglycemia and hypotension should be avoided because their well-documented harms likely outweigh any potential benefits. The long-term impacts on cognitive aging are largely unknown.

Hypertension

Hypertension is present in approximately 65 percent of people age 60 years and older (Hajjar and Kotchen, 2003) and has been identified in systematic reviews as an important potentially preventable risk factor for cognitive decline and dementia with an increased hazard ratio of between 1.24 and 1.59, depending on the study (Etgen et al., 2011). While the studies vary somewhat in their definition of hypertension, in general, most studies considered a participant to be hypertensive if the average systolic blood pressure was 140 mmHg or higher, the average diastolic blood pressure was 90 mmHg or higher, or the participant was currently receiving antihypertensive medications.

Evidence from Observational Studies

There is robust longitudinal data to support a relationship between blood pressure and cognitive decline (Elias et al., 2012; Etgen et al., 2011) with more consistent associations observed for midlife hypertension; by contrast, late-life hypertension might not be a critical risk factor for cognitive aging (Qiu et al., 2005) More recent studies have also suggested an important role for modification by APOE status (Andrews et al., 2015; Bangen et al., 2013). The impact of hypertension on cognition is likely mediated by a number of mechanisms, including small and large vessel disease, microinfarcts, leukoaraiosis, and changes in cerebral metabolism (Gasecki et al., 2013). Observational studies also indicate that the cognitive function of older adults may possibly benefit from antihypertensive medications (Rouch et al., 2015). Thus, blood pressure control will likely remain an important prevention target in any multifactorial approach to preventing age-related cognitive decline (see Chapter 4C).

Evidence from Intervention Studies

Evidence from blood pressure treatment trials, such as ADVANCE, HYVET-COG, and SCOPE, varies, with some demonstrating a benefit and others reporting no effect on cognition. A recent meta-analysis found that antihypertensive medication had no significant impact on the incidence of Alzheimer's disease, cognitive impairment, or cognitive decline (Chang-Quan et al., 2011). This may reflect differences in the classes of drugs used for hypertension therapy as well as in the timing and duration of treatment (Rouch et al., 2015; Staessen et al., 2011). To gain a better understanding of the effects of blood pressure treatment, the ongoing Systolic Blood Pressure Intervention Trial (SPRINT) will monitor the course of cognitive decline in people undergoing intensive blood pressure control.

Summary

Although the evidence from clinical trials does not demonstrate a clear cognitive benefit from hypertension treatment and the long-term impact on cognitive aging is not known, the benefits for preventing heart attack and stroke, both of which are linked to cognitive decline, are evident. However, in older persons it is particularly important to maintain prudent therapy, with an avoidance of overtreatment, which is associated with adverse cognitive effects as well as falls.

Hyperlipidemia

Hyperlipidemia, or high levels of blood lipids (including triglycerides and cholesterol), is present in approximately 50.8 percent of the older U.S. population (Crawford et al., 2010).

Evidence from Observational Studies

Multiple large population-based observational studies have found that hyperlipidemia, especially hypercholesterolemia, is associated with cognitive decline, with hazard ratio ranging from 1.4 to 1.9 (Etgen et al., 2011). Lipid regulation plays a critical role in neuronal plasticity and survival (Ledesma et al., 2012), and like hypertension, hyperlipidemia may be a stronger risk factor in midlife cognitive decline than in late life (Reynolds et al., 2010; van Vliet, 2012). In addition, some observational studies have found the use of statins (drugs that reduce cholesterol levels) to protect against cognitive impairment (Etgen et al., 2011).

A longitudinal study by Steenland and colleagues (2013) assembled a group—1,244 statin users and 2,363 non-users—and gave them a battery of cognitive tests several times over 3.4 years. They controlled for several potentially confounding conditions, including diabetes, hypertension, and heart disease, and looked for differences in changes in cognitive functioning between the users and non-users of statins. They found that people who had normal cognition at baseline and who used statins had better scores on tests of sustained attention and executive functioning than non-users. Similar benefits for cognition have been observed in large, observational cohorts of older adults without dementia (Bettermann et al., 2012; Solomon et al., 2009).

Evidence from Intervention Studies

In contrast to the above findings, several large randomized controlled trials (RCTs), including the Heart Protection Study and the PROSPER trial (Prospective Study of Pravastatin in the Elderly at Risk), have failed to demonstrate a protective effect of statin treatment on cognitive functioning (McGuinness et al., 2009). A 2009 Cochrane review identified two large RCTs that indicated no benefit of statins on cognitive measures despite their having achieved reductions in serum cholesterol (McGuinness et al., 2009). Similarly, a recent meta-analysis found inconsistent evidence for the effect of statins on cognition among people who were cognitively intact

(Richardson et al., 2013). Some drug post-marketing safety reports have suggested that statins might actually impair cognition, which prompted the Food and Drug Administration (FDA) to issue an alert about potential memory loss associated with this class of drugs (FDA, 2012), although a more recent meta-analysis reported no increased risk of adverse cognitive effects related to statin use (Richardson et al., 2013).

Consistent with these studies, a 2010 systematic review of clinical trials of the treatment of cardiovascular risk factors to prevent cognitive decline concluded that there is no apparent cognitive benefit from treating hyperlipidemia and that the treatment of hypertension has only a suggestive effect on cognitive decline (Ligthart et al., 2010).

Summary

Although studies of the benefits of treating hyperlipidemia on cognitive health have had inconsistent results (Plassman et al., 2010), clinical practice guidelines still recommend that high lipid levels be treated because of the beneficial effect on cardiovascular and cerebrovascular diseases (Etgen et al., 2011). Further research will be necessary to identify any specific impact that lipid-lowering drugs have on long-term cognitive functioning.

Diabetes Mellitus and Metabolic Syndrome

Diabetes occurs in about 27 percent of the older U.S. population (CDC, 2011). In addition, metabolic syndrome is estimated to be present in about 42 percent of the population age 70 years and older (Ford et al., 2002). Metabolic syndrome is defined as participants having three or more of the following: abdominal obesity, hypertriglyceridemia, high blood pressure, high fasting glucose, and low high-density lipoproteins. Metabolic syndrome is often unrecognized, and thus its prevalence is underreported (Giannini and Testa, 2003).

Evidence from Observational Studies

Both diabetes and metabolic syndrome have been found to be associated with long-term cognitive decline and an increased risk of dementia in both cross-sectional and long-term observational studies (Plassman et al., 2010; Spauwen et al., 2013; Yaffe et al., 2004). Diabetes is associated with approximately a 1.2-fold increase in risk of cognitive decline, mild cognitive impairment, and dementia (McCrimmon et al., 2012; Plassman et al., 2010). Glycemic control may be a critical factor in this association (Yaffe et al., 2012) and could contribute to both neurodegenerative and vascular damage (Biessels et al., 2014). Because the metabolic syndrome includes both cardiovascular and metabolic components, it may be an especially crucial risk factor for accelerated cognitive aging (Yaffe, 2007).

Evidence from Intervention Studies

People with type 2 diabetes have a higher risk for developing cardiovascular and cerebrovascular disease and may stand to gain more from an aggressive treatment of hypertension and hyperlipidemia. Currently, results from clinical trials are inconsistent as to whether tight glucose control improves cognitive outcomes in type 2 diabetes, and this must be weighed against evidence that too-aggressive efforts to reduce blood sugar levels may increase mortality among high-risk individuals (ACCORD et al., 2008). Moreover, a large RCT conducted in people with type 2 diabetes that examined the effects of an intensive lowering of blood pressure (to systolic target of 120 mmHg) and the treatment of lipids with fenofibrate, found no benefit from either of the two interventions on a wide variety of measures of cognition (including the Mini-Mental State Examination [MMSE], the digit-symbol substitution test, and Stroop, Rey, and auditory verbal learning tests). In preliminary trials, long-acting intranasal insulin has shown promise in improving cognitive function in adults with mild cognitive impairment (MCI) or early Alzheimer's disease (Claxton et al., 2015; Craft et al., 2012). Currently, there is a lack of consistent evidence from clinical trials that tight glucose control improves cognitive outcomes in type 2 diabetes, but there is important evidence that tight control may increase mortality (NHLBI, 2014); furthermore, hypoglycemia may harm cognition (NHLBI, 2014; Yaffe et al., 2012).

Summary

The early recognition and prudent management of diabetes and metabolic syndrome has potential benefit for cognitive health by reducing the risk for cardiovascular and cerebrovascular disease, but much remains to be learned about the direct impact of these factors on cognitive aging. There are specific issues concerning the effects that treatment of these conditions might have on cognitive function that warrant attention. The committee believes that any goals for glycemic control should be consistent with those goals issued by the American Diabetes Association (ADA, 2014).

Obesity

Almost one-third of Americans age 60 years and older are severely overweight or obese, defined as having a body mass index (BMI) of 30 kg/m2 or greater (Wang and Beydoun, 2007).

Evidence from Observational Studies

Although more longitudinal studies are needed (Plassman et al., 2010), evidence is emerging to support the existence of obesity-related brain changes and dysfunction in cognition (Sellbom and Gunstad, 2012). While the effects of obesity may be mediated through other pathways, such as through the well-described effects of diabetes or metabolic syndrome (i.e., inflammation, insulin resistance, endothelial dysfunction, and microvascular disease) and through the complications of obesity, such as obstructive sleep apnea, obesity may also increase risk of cognitive aging directly through the presence of excess adipose tissue and the secretion of inflammatory proteins such as leptin, which have been linked to cognitive impairment and decline (Gustafson, 2012; Holden et al., 2009; Zeki Al Hazzouri et al., 2013). A meta-analysis also suggests that the effects of BMI on cognition may differ between midlife and late life (Anstey et al., 2011).

Evidence from Intervention Studies

A randomized trial among middle-aged overweight or obese individuals that compared an energy-restricted low-calorie diet with a conventional low-fat diet with no change in calorie intake found a time-effect improvement on working memory in both groups at 1 year but no differences between groups; these diets had no effect on speed of mental processing (Brinkworth et al., 2009).

A recent RCT among obese older individuals compared the effects of four regimens—a diet aimed at reducing caloric intake by 500–750 kcal/day below requirements, exercise using a multicomponent progressive training program, both diet and exercise, and neither—and found that those assigned to diet alone performed better than the control group on the modified-MMSE but not as well as those assigned to exercise alone; the combination of diet and exercise was no more effective than exercise alone. The effects of diet alone on other measures, including word-list fluency and the Trail Making Test, Parts A and B, were not significant (Napoli et al., 2014). A 2011 meta-analysis concluded that weight loss had inconsistent effects on memory and modest beneficial effects on attention/executive function, generally in obese subjects (Siervo et al., 2011). Among obese middle-aged persons, bariatric surgery resulted in improvement on a verbal list learning test compared to obese controls when assessed 24 months after surgery (Alosco et al., 2014).

Summary

While the exact mechanism by which obesity contributes to cognitive decline remains unclear, given its prevalence and serious associated complications, morbid obesity may act on mediating pathways (e.g., through diabetes and hypertension) to produce long-term cognitive impairment (Etgen et al., 2011; Plassman et al., 2010). The studies reviewed here are those focusing on weight loss itself rather than any particular diet; specific diets are addressed in Chapter 4A. Further research is needed on the effect of weight loss and bariatric surgery on cognitive outcomes.

Delirium and Hospitalization

Nearly every individual will experience at least one acute medical illness, surgery, or hospitalization, and nearly one-third of the older U.S. population is hospitalized each year (HHS, 2013). Delirium, an acute disorder of attention and confusion, is the most common complication of acute illness and hospitalization for older people in the United States, occurring in an estimated 2.6 million individuals per year (HHS, 2011). Up to 50 percent of all Americans age 65 years and older will develop delirium during the course of a hospitalization, with the associated increased risks of institutionalization and death leading to health care costs that exceed $160 billion per year (Inouye et al., 2014).

Evidence from Observational Studies

Delirium Although common, delirium is preventable in some 30 to 50 percent of cases (Inouye et al., 2014), and every effort should be made to prevent it, as it significantly increases a person's risk for long-term cognitive decline and dementia. A systematic review and meta-analysis found two studies involving 241 patients demonstrating an increased odds ratio for incident dementia following delirium (Witlox et al., 2010). Another study of 225 cardiac surgery patients age 60 years and older demonstrated that delirium is independently associated with cognitive decline at 1 year post-surgery; the time pattern of cognitive functioning showed an initially steep decline followed by improvement but with residual impairment (Saczynski et al., 2012). A study of 821 intensive care unit (ICU) patients found that a longer duration of delirium was independently associated with worse global cognitive function and executive function at 3 and 12 months follow-up (Pandharipande et al., 2013). The adverse impact of delirium on cognitive trajectory is magnified among patients with underlying dementia (Fong et al., 2009; Gross et al., 2012).

A recent comprehensive review found six prospective studies document delirium's association with long-term cognitive decline after hospitalization, whether a follow-up occurred soon (2 months) or a longer time (12 months) afterward (Mathews et al., 2014). Some of the studies in this review lacked baseline (pre-hospitalization) cognitive testing, however. The disparate reasons for hospitalization (acute illness, surgery, intensive care, palliative care) may have different prognostic implications for cognitive decline.

Hospitalization Regardless of admitting diagnosis, hospitalization is increasingly recognized as a major stressor for older adults and an important independent contributor to cognitive and functional decline (Krumholz, 2013). A study of 1,870 community-dwelling older adults demonstrated an independent 2.4-fold increase in the rate of cognitive decline following a first hospitalization, even after controlling for demographic factors, illness severity, and pre-hospital cognitive trajectory (Wilson et al., 2012). The impact of hospitalization was greatest on short-term memory and executive functioning. Another study of 2,929 patients admitted to a hospital or ICU who were followed afterward for a median of 4 years found an increased rate of cognitive decline following either hospitalization or ICU stay and an increased hazard ratio for incident dementia at follow-up of 1.4 (95% CI 1.1–1.7) and 2.3 (95% CI 0.9–5.7) after the hospitalization and ICU stay, respectively (Ehlenbach et al., 2010).

Mathews and colleagues (2014) found six studies (five prospective and one retrospective) showing that acute hospitalization was associated with long-term cognitive decline, but several of these studies did not include formal preadmission cognitive testing. Despite those studies' limited and heterogeneous nature, a consistent picture is emerging that points to the important contributions of delirium, acute illness, and hospitalization to long-term cognitive decline and possibly dementia.

Evidence from Intervention Studies

Catalyzed by the strong observational evidence summarized above, delirium prevention has emerged as a priority in the prevention of cognitive decline following major illness, hospitalization, or surgery. Authoritative guidelines and systematic reviews recommend multicomponent, non-pharmacologic intervention strategies targeted toward patients with delirium risk factors and implemented by skilled interdisciplinary teams (Greer et al., 2011; O'Mahony et al., 2011). Two recent systematic reviews and meta-analyses (AGS Expert Panel 2014; Hshieh et al., 2014) of 10 and 14 intervention studies, respectively, have documented the effectiveness of these approaches. The interventions were largely based on the Hospital Elder Life Program (the original model of which has been widely disseminated with consistent effectiveness) (Inouye, 2000; Inouye et al., 1999, 2006; Rubin et al., 2011; Zaubler et al., 2013) and included the following approaches: cognitive orientation, sleep enhancement (i.e., non-pharmacologic sleep protocol and sleep hygiene), early mobility and/or physical rehabilitation, adaptations for visual and hearing impairment, nutrition and fluid replenishment, pain management, appropriate medication usage, adequate oxygenation, and prevention of constipation (HELP, 2014). Rounds by an interdisciplinary team and associated strategies to assure adherence to recommended interventions were important to the protocol's effectiveness. At least five of the studies demonstrated a "dose–response" relationship between the level of adherence and the intervention's effectiveness (Holt et al., 2013; Inouye et al., 1999, 2000, 2003; Vidan et al., 2009).

In addition to the prevention of incident delirium, these studies demonstrated consistent beneficial impact for the following outcomes: cognitive decline, functional decline, length of hospital stay, nursing home placement, falls, and health care costs. In a meta-analysis of 14 studies, 11 studies demonstrated significant reductions in delirium duration and incidence (odds ratio: 0.47; 95% CI 0.38–0.58) (Hshieh et al., 2014).

Summary

Because one-third of older Americans will be hospitalized each year for acute illness or surgery, putting them at increased risk of delirium and subsequent cognitive decline in addition to them facing the associated higher morbidity, mortality, and health care costs, the committee believes that the implementation of proven cost-effective multicomponent non-pharmacologic delirium-prevention strategies is vital. These regimens should be implemented by interdisciplinary teams and targeted to patients with demonstrated risk factors, who should have cognitive assessments either before or immediately after hospital admission or surgery (HELP, 2014). More needs to be learned about the long-term impacts of delirium on cognitive aging.

Major Surgery and General Anesthesia

The association of major surgery and general anesthesia with cognitive decline has gained recent widespread attention. Previous epidemiologic studies have documented a persistent cognitive decline following major surgery, yet it has been assumed that this decline may be due more to patients' pre-operative trajectories than to the effects of the surgery or anesthesia (Selnes et al., 2012). Some of the older studies have lacked pre-surgical baseline cognitive trajectories and have inadequately controlled for potential confounding variables. Thus, it has been difficult to determine whether any cognitive impairment arising after surgery is attributable to the surgery or anesthesia (Avidan and Evers, 2011; Rudolph et al., 2010; van Dijk et al., 2000) rather than to associated comorbidity, delirium, or stressors related to the hospitalization. Furthermore, previous studies have failed to demonstrate any difference in cognitive outcomes between patients who received general and regional anesthesia (Newman et al., 2007). This is an important area of research that could assist in the exploration of the long-term impacts on cognitive aging.

OTHER MEDICAL CONDITIONS

A number of other medical conditions may be associated with cognitive changes and decline. Because the prevention and treatment of each of these conditions have been the subjects of extensive research, albeit not focused on cognitive outcomes, this report does not summarize the intervention literature. For each condition, little is known about how the medical condition might or might not affect cognitive aging.

Thyroid Disorders

Both hypo- and hyperthyroidism have been long identified as major reversible causes of cognitive decline and are screened for in many cases of cognitive impairment. However, the contribution to impaired cognition by subclinical thyroid disease, defined as abnormal levels of thyroid-stimulating hormone (TSH) in the face of normal levels of thyroxine (T4) and triiodothyronine (T3), is less clear. The presence of subclinical thyroid disease increases with age, with rates from 7 to 25 percent in persons age 60 years and older (Ceresini et al., 2009; Etgen et al., 2011).

In a recent systematic review of 11 studies, including six population-based prospective studies and five cross-sectional studies, six of the studies supported the association between subclinical hypothyroidism and cognitive impairment (Annerbo and Lokk, 2013). The confounding influence of acute illness, comorbidity, and medications—which can substantially affect TSH, T4, and T3 levels—were not controlled for in many studies (Roberts et al., 2006). Given the inconsistent association and the small number of studies, subclinical thyroid disease is not considered to be a major risk factor for cognitive decline at this time; however, it remains of interest for future investigation and the possible development of preventive interventions.

Chronic Kidney Disease

Chronic kidney disease, defined as having kidney damage or a glomerular filtration rate (GFR) of less than 60 mL/min/1.73 m^2, is a highly prevalent condition, present in more than 45 percent of adults age 70 years and older (Anand et al., 2014). Emerging evidence indicates that chronic kidney disease is an independent contributor to decline in cognitive function. An estimated 70 percent of hemodialysis patients 55 years of age and older will have moderate to severe cognitive impairment (Elias et al.,

2013); however, even milder degrees of renal impairment are associated with cognitive impairment.

A recent systematic review and meta-analysis involving seven cross-sectional and 10 prospective studies with more than 54,000 participants who were pre-dialysis but with mild to severe renal impairment demonstrated an increased relative risk for cognitive decline of 1.65 (95% CI 1.32–2.05) and 1.39 (95% CI 1.15–1.68), respectively, even after adjustment for confounding factors (Etgen et al., 2012). Importantly, the reviewers found a dose–response relationship with the more severe degrees of renal failure (GFR >60) creating a greater risk for cognitive decline than did milder degrees of renal impairment (GFR of 45 to 60 or GFR <45). There are a number of possible mechanisms that could potentially explain the association of chronic kidney disease with cognitive decline, including vascular risk factors (hypertension, diabetes, hyperlipidemia, cardiovascular disease), cerebral ischemia/stroke, elevated homocysteine, hypercoagulability, oxidative stress, inflammation, anemia, metabolic derangements (hyperparathyroidism, malnutrition, hypoalbuminemia), polypharmacy, depression, and sleep disorders (Elias et al., 2013; Etgen et al., 2012). Many of these represent important potential targets for secondary prevention of cognitive decline among people with chronic kidney disease.

Cancer

Approximately 9 million persons, or 3 percent of the U.S. population, are cancer survivors (Anderson-Hanley et al., 2003). Cognitive functioning among cancer patients may be influenced by the malignancy itself as well as by the effects of the associated treatments, including chemotherapy, surgery, radiation, hormonal therapy, and biologics, alone or in combination.

A meta-analysis of 30 studies involving a total of 838 patients examined at 1 month to several years following cancer treatment showed significant decreases in neuropsychological testing scores due to the above causes, with the largest impact on the areas of executive functioning and verbal memory (Anderson-Hanley et al., 2003). A twin study of 702 cancer survivors demonstrated that the twin who had cancer was significantly more likely (relative risk [RR] 2.10, 95% CI 1.36–3.24) to develop cognitive decline than the co-twin (Heflin et al., 2005). In addition, the risk of dementia was doubled, although it did not reach statistical significance.

While these studies are suggestive, the evidence that cancer and its treatment leads to cognitive impairment and dementia remains equivocal, particularly in light of potential confounding by vascular disease, other comorbidities, and their treatment. Moreover, few older people are included in most cancer trials and follow-up studies. In a systematic review of 88 articles (Bial et al., 2006), no conclusions about cognition could be reached because of the small and heterogeneous nature of the studies, along with the shortage of older persons included. This important gap will need to be addressed.

Depression

Depression is a common mental health problem across the life span, with one in five U.S. adults experiencing at least one depressive episode during a lifetime (Byers and Yaffe, 2011). The prevalence of depression ranges from 7 to 36 percent in older adult populations (Crocco et al., 2010).

Midlife depression has been consistently associated with about a twofold increased risk for subsequent cognitive decline or dementia (Byers and Yaffe, 2011). While a similar association has been demonstrated for late-life depression, caution is warranted in interpreting these studies since dementia has a long prodromal phase and can coexist with cognitive decline or dementia; establishing whether depression represents a cause, an effect, a manifestation of a shared mechanism, or a chance co-occurrence can be challenging. Nonetheless, a recent systematic review supported a strong relationship between late-life depression and subsequent dementia, with the strongest risk for vascular dementia.

A meta-analysis of 23 population-based studies examining late-life depression and involving more than 49,000 people demonstrated a significantly increased risk for all-cause dementia (RR 1.85, 95% CI 1.67–2.04), Alzheimer's disease (RR 1.65, 95% CI 1.42–1.92), and vascular dementia (RR 2.52, 95% CI 1.77–3.59) (Diniz et al., 2013). An earlier review of 13 studies involving more than 32,000 people found relative risks of 1.5 to 6.0 for cognitive decline or dementia (Plassman et al., 2010).

Potential mechanisms by which depression may contribute to cognitive decline and dementia include alterations in the glucocorticoid–stress hormone pathway and hippocampal atrophy, inflammatory changes, vascular disease with involvement of the frontal-striatal pathway, and accelerated deposition of beta-amyloid (Byers and Yaffe, 2011; Crocco et al., 2010). While the exact relationship between depression and cognition awaits clarification, given depression's prevalence and potential implications, its prevention and intervention should be an important goal in enhancing functioning and quality of life for older adults.

TRAUMATIC BRAIN INJURY

Brain trauma can occur at any age, and it varies dramatically in its severity, comorbid effects, and clinical outcomes. It may occur multiple times to the same individual, such as from repeated falls, from recurring concussions in sports participation, from military service, or from multiple injuries associated with chronic substance abuse. Falls are the leading cause of brain trauma among older adults. Traumatic brain injury (TBI) is often divided into mild and severe categories; while criteria for these categories have been promulgated and are useful, they require additional research and validation (Arciniegas and Silver, 2001).

Severe TBI usually is associated with some period of coma, hospitalization, and prolonged rehabilitation. There is usually gross anatomic brain damage (e.g., a penetrating wound, hemorrhage, or displaced or destroyed brain tissue). Persistent pathological problems may emerge, including hydrocephalus, vascular compromise, and fibrosis. These sequelae of brain injury may lead to long-term cognitive impairments, which cause substantial functional disability (Vincent et al., 2014). The trajectories after severe TBI need to be better understood, including determining risk factors for improvement and adverse effects on later life cognitive function.

Mild TBI may be associated with concussion, but unconsciousness is likely to be brief, and mild TBI less often requires hospitalization or long-term rehabilitation. Remaining TBI symptoms, the so-called post-concussion syndrome—irritability, headache, fatigue, and dizziness—may persist for days or weeks (Eisenberg et al., 2014) and can be frustrating to patients and clinicians and may impede conventional cognitive evaluation. Concerning single or multiple mild TBI episodes that appear to resolve to clinical "normalcy," the central questions are whether they lead to later increases in the risk of cognitive decrements, and if so, what the range of severity is and how those at greater risk can be identified.

Many but not all studies find TBI to be associated with cognitive decrements in later life compared to control groups, as determined both by cognitive testing and by brain anatomic and physiological characteristics (Ashman et al., 2008; Broglio et al., 2012; Konrad et al., 2011; Moretti et al., 2012). In addition, an older age at the time of the TBI and a greater interval between the injury and the evaluation have been independently associated with worse cognitive outcomes (Ponsford and Schonberger, 2010; Ponsford et al., 2008; Senathi-Raja et al., 2010). Some follow-up studies of 30 years or more (Isoniemi et al., 2006) have detected differences in some elements of cognitive performance between people with past TBI and control groups (Barnes et al., 2014). However, one systematic review found chronic cognitive impairment in mild TBI patients to have occurred only among those who had complications in their clinical course (Godbolt et al., 2014). TBI in general has been associated with increased risk of dementia among U.S. military veterans (Barnes et al., 2014).

The evidence for the long-term role of mild TBI in chronic cognitive impairment is mixed and far from definitive. This is a challenging area to study because of differences in the types and severity of injury, the selection of appropriate control groups, the need for lengthy follow-up, the presence of comorbidities, and the existence of many alternative potential causes of cognitive change. Definitions of cognitive impairment also vary. Although long-term studies are difficult to perform, they are critical to evaluating this exposure and are particularly important because they have the potential to strengthen public health efforts aimed at TBI prevention.

Summary for Medical Conditions

The evidence for the contributions of the medical conditions examined in this section on the cognitive aging process is mounting, yet the impact and mechanisms often remain unclear. In addition, targeted intervention strategies to prevent cognitive decline associated with these conditions have not been well examined. This is a priority for future research.

HEARING AND VISION LOSS

Alterations in sensation and perception with aging can have substantial effects on daily function, and ongoing research is investigating the role of hearing and vision loss in cognitive performance. Vision loss and low visual acuity, both of which are common among older adults, have been associated with decreased cognitive function (Clemons et al., 2006), but the precise effect depends on the type of eye disease (Keller et al., 1999; Tay et al., 2006). Age-related changes in vision include: declines in visual acuity and in the range of visual accommodation, loss of contrast sensitivity, decreases in abilities to visually adapt to darkness, declines in color sensitivity, and heightened sensitivity to glare (Czaja and Lee, 2003).

Some causes of visual impairment, such as cataracts or retinitis, are related to pathology in eye structures; others may be related to brain diseases, such as neurodegenerative conditions, where there are underlying problems in visual-spatial perception. The mechanisms by which declining visual acuity relates to cognitive aging are not always clear, but they may include decreased social activity and increased risk of falls, possibly leading to head injury (Wood et al., 2011). Some types of visual impairment, such as decreased near vision, may be risk factors for cognitive impairment (Reyes-Ortiz et al., 2005). Also, because both cognitive changes and visual loss emerge slowly, it can be difficult to determine which came first. Nonetheless, there is reasonably strong evidence that visual impairment is a risk factor for cognitive change, even after controlling for mental status and comorbidity (Clemons et al., 2006; Lin et al., 2004; Reyes-Ortiz et al., 2005).

Age-related losses in hearing include a loss of sensitivity for pure tones, especially high-frequency tones; difficulty understanding speech, especially if the speech is distorted or embedded in noise; problems related to localizing sounds and binaural hearing; and increased sensitivity to loudness

(Schieber and Baldwin, 1996). While severe hearing loss can make it difficult to assess cognitive function, this sensory impairment has been identified in several studies as a risk factor for cognitive decline, incident dementia, and severity of cognitive dysfunction (Lin et al., 2011, 2013; Uhlmann et al., 1989). Studies of combined hearing and visual impairment have also found an association with cognitive aging (Lin et al., 2004). Preexisting neurodegenerative diseases may preclude accurate auditory testing.

Irrespective of the relationship between vision or auditory impairment and cognitive function, improving and maximizing sensory function is important to quality of life and general function and mobility for older adults, and it should be addressed (Genther et al., 2013; Lin et al., 2004). These changes can affect interactions with the health care system as well. For example, age-related changes in vision might make it difficult for an older person to read labels on a medication bottle, which may in turn affect the proper use of prescription drugs. Similarly, age-related changes in hearing might make it difficult for an older adult to engage in a conversation or to understand oral instructions, particularly when speech is rapid.

SLEEP

Evidence from Observational Studies

Epidemiological studies of self-reported sleep quality have generally shown an association among poorer cognitive function, insomnia symptoms, and poor sleep quality (Fortier-Brochu et al., 2012; Schmutte et al., 2007), although the results of studies evaluating cognitive impairment and sleep patterns have been mixed. Some studies have shown a roughly two- to four-fold increase in the risk of cognitive decline or impairment among those who reported sleep disturbances (Elwood et al., 2011; Jelicic et al., 2002; Potvin et al., 2012; Sterniczuk et al., 2013), while others have found no association (Foley et al., 2001; Jaussent et al., 2012; Merlino et al., 2010; Tworoger et al., 2006). Differing results across studies using self-reports about sleep patterns may be due in part to the heterogeneity of the study methods and design. The majority of studies using objective measures to determine sleep quality have supported a greater risk of cognitive decline, impairment, and Alzheimer's disease being associated with disturbed sleep, as measured by non-invasive actigraphy, including associated longer time needed to fall asleep, increased sleep fragmentation, and waking after sleep onset (Blackwell et al., 2006, 2011; Lim et al., 2013a). Furthermore, better sleep consolidation has been shown to reduce the incidence of cognitive decline (Lim et al., 2013b). Observational studies have suggested that there may be a U-shaped association between sleep duration and cognition, with worse cognitive outcomes associated with both long and short sleep durations compared to more intermediate sleep lengths of 7 to 8 hours (Yaffe et al., 2014).

Disordered breathing during sleep, typically involving apneas (the cessation of breathing) and hypopneas (reduced or shallow breathing), also has been associated with impairments in cognitive function. In some cross-sectional studies, indicators of sleep disordered breathing have been associated with worse cognition (Beebe et al., 2003; Spira et al., 2008), but not all studies have found this (Blackwell et al., 2011; Foley et al., 2003). Prospective studies have shown older adults with sleep disordered breathing have greater cognitive decline (Cohen-Zion et al., 2004) and an increased risk of MCI or dementia than those without disordered breathing during sleep (Yaffe et al., 2011). Taken together, these results suggest that improving sleep may prove beneficial for cognitive outcomes among older adults.

Evidence from Intervention Studies

A number of treatments have been shown to be effective in improving sleep among older adults, but few trials have evaluated the cognitive benefits of these treatments. A small study among older adults with insomnia showed improvements in both sleep quality (falling asleep sooner and staying asleep) and cognitive performance after 8 weeks of a computerized cognitive training program (Haimov and Shatil, 2013). Exercise, primarily aerobic, has also shown potential for benefiting sleep and well-being among older adults with and without insomnia (Benloucif et al., 2004; Montgomery and Dennis, 2002; Reid et al., 2010), but further study is needed to evaluate effects on cognitive aging.

Promising results have also been demonstrated for the use of light therapy to ameliorate sleep and circadian rhythm disturbances in people with Alzheimer's disease and other dementias, although the cognitive benefits have not yet been determined (Hanford and Figueiro, 2013; McCurry et al., 2011; Salami et al., 2011). Several small trials have shown that acetylcholinesterase inhibitors may improve sleep and cognitive outcomes among both healthy adults and those with Alzheimer's disease (Ancoli-Israel et al., 2005; Cooke et al., 2006; Hornung et al., 2009; Mizuno et al., 2004; Moraes Wdos et al., 2006; Schliebs and Arendt, 2006); however, the benefits must be weighed against the potential side effects (Inglis, 2002), and larger prospective trials are needed to determine long-term outcomes.

Sleep disordered breathing is a promising modifiable risk factor for improving cognitive outcomes; however, the timing and duration of its treatment as well as the optimal treatment population are still unclear. A meta-analysis of 13 treatment studies found improvements in attention, but most trials were short-term and underpowered (a mean sample size of 54) (Kylstra et al., 2013). In one small 3-month study of sleep apnea patients, continuous positive airway pressure (CPAP) treatment resulted in improved cognitive function in several domains that corresponded to gray matter volume increases in hippocampal and frontal regions (Canessa et al., 2011). Another small study found that compliant use of CPAP for 3 months was associated with broad improvements in cognitive functioning, such as in attention, psychomotor speed, executive functioning, and nonverbal delayed recall (Aloia et al., 2003). Results from the recent Apnea Positive Pressure Long-term Efficacy Study (APPLES) trial showed improvements in executive function among patients with severe obstructive sleep apnea following CPAP therapy over 2 and 6 months, but no improvement on tests of attention, psychomotor function, or memory (Kushida et al., 2012). Another study evaluating functional MRI changes in 17 participants undergoing 2 months of CPAP treatment suggested that treatment improves cognitive function but that the potential to reverse neuronal damage may be limited (Prilipko et al., 2012).

Some promise has been shown for certain drugs, such as donepezil and fluticasone, in treating obstructive sleep apnea and improving cognitive outcomes; however, the evidence is currently insufficient to recommend the use of drug therapy in treating obstructive sleep apnea, and additional studies among larger populations with long durations of follow-up are needed (Mason et al., 2013).

Summary

In aggregate, observational and intervention studies suggest that insomnia and sleep disorders may impair cognitive function in older adults and that their treatment has the potential to ameliorate this effect. The long-term effects on cognitive aging are unknown. Most intervention trials have been small and short-term, and additional studies among larger populations and longer follow-up are needed (Mason et al., 2013). The treatment of sleep disordered breathing has particular promise for improving cognitive outcomes. The mainstay of current treatment for obstructive sleep apnea consists of non-pharmacologic approaches, including CPAP and weight reduction.

GENETIC FACTORS: APOE STATUS

Advances in genetics and molecular biology have prompted substantial exploration of a possible genetic basis for age-related cognitive impairment. Most of these "risk factor" investigations have attempted to identify genetic predictors and correlates of Alzheimer's disease and other neurodegenerative dementias. Currently, interest in possible genetic impacts on other late-life cognitive changes, both negative and positive, is increasing. To date, the gene (and surrounding genetic regions) found to be most closely related to decreased cognitive function in later life secondary to Alzheimer's disease is the APOE ε4 allele (Davies et al., 2014). This has been established in many studies and summarized in a meta-analysis by Small and colleagues (2004). However, while this finding is important for use in clinical prediction or in evaluating early or familial cognitive syndromes, the committee is not aware of any U.S. national expert group that has recommended routine APOE ε4 screening in asymptomatic adults. Furthermore, evidence suggests that the APOE ε4 allele has different cognitive effects at different ages (Qiu et al., 2004).

It is difficult to assess the significance of other genes and related genetic markers that have been identified in diverse studies related to cognitive maintenance (Payton, 2009). The studies have several methodological features that impede comparison, including varied study populations, the strength of the association is usually small, findings vary in different study populations, studies often fail to consider relevant comorbid conditions, different studies find associations with different cognitive outcomes, and biological interactions exist among implicated genes (Adamczuk et al., 2012).

A recent meta-analysis reported on more than 20 genetic loci that have demonstrated modest but significant effects on dementia risk (Bertram and Tanzi, 2008). In at least one recent genome-wide association study, yet another genetic location (on chromosome 11) appeared to be associated with cognitive maintenance in older adults (Yokoyama et al., 2014). Other such genetic factors may exist. Thus, new and potentially important genetic variants continue to be identified that may turn out to be relevant to maintaining late-life cognitive performance (Sweet et al., 2012; Yokoyama et al., 2014), and other genetic factors, such as epigenetic determinants, may also be operative (Akbarian et al., 2013).

Summary

Overall, it appears that while genetic forces must be ultimately important in cognitive aging, the research is at an early stage, the particular genes and related mechanisms have not been identified, and the research quest continues. At present, the exact role of genetic factors in cognitive maintenance and decline remains unclear, with little reason at this time to perform genetic testing among older persons in the general population either to predict cognitive risk or to guide treatment decisions. Further research in this area is clearly needed.

REFERENCES

ACCORD (Action to Control Cardiovascular Risk in Diabetes) Study Group, H. C. Gerstein, M. E. Miller, R. P. Byington, D. C. Goff, Jr., J. T. Bigger, J. B. Buse, W. C. Cushman, S. Genuth, F. Ismail-Beigi, R. H. Grimm, Jr., J. L. Probstfield, D. G. Simons-Morton, and W. T. Friedewald. 2008. Effects of intensive glucose lowering in type 2 diabetes. *New England Journal of Medicine* 358(24):2545-2559.

ADA (American Diabetes Association). 2014. *Checking your blood glucose.* http://www.diabetes.org/living-with-diabetes/treatment-and-care/blood-glucose-control/checking-your-blood-glucose.html (accessed November 4, 2014).

Adamczuk, K., A.-S. De Weer, K. Sleegers, N. Nelissen, G. Farrar, L. Thurfjell, C. Van Broeckhoven, K. Van Laere, and R. Vandenberghe. 2012. Gene-gene interaction and subclinical amyloid levels in cognitively intact elderly individuals. *Alzheimer's & Dementia* 8(4):P619.

Agostini, J. V., Y. Zhang, and S. K. Inouye. 2007. Use of a computer-based reminder to improve sedative-hypnotic prescribing in older hospitalized patients. *Journal of the American Geriatrics Society* 55(1):43-48.

AGS (American Geriatrics Society). 2012. Beers Criteria Update Expert Panel. American Geriatrics Society updated Beers Criteria for potentially inappropriate medication use in older adults. *Journal of the American Geriatrics Society* 60(4):616-631.

———. 2014. American Geriatrics Society Expert Panel on Postoperative Delirium in Older Adults. Postoperative delirium in older adults: Best practice statement from the American Geriatrics Society. *Journal of the American College of Surgeons* 220(2):136-148.

Akbarian, S., M. S. Beeri, and V. Haroutunian. 2013. Epigenetic determinants of healthy and diseased brain aging and cognition. *JAMA Neurology* 70(6):711-718.

Alldred, D. P., D. K. Raynor, C. Hughes, N. Barber, T. F. Chen, and P. Spoor. 2013. Interventions to optimise prescribing for older people in care homes. *The Cochrane Database of Systematic Reviews* 2:Cd009095.

Aloia, M. S., N. Ilniczky, P. Di Dio, M. L. Perlis, D. W. Greenblatt, and D. E. Giles. 2003. Neuropsychological changes and treatment compliance in older adults with sleep apnea. *Journal of Psychosomatic Research* 54(1):71-76.

Alosco, M. L., M. B. Spitznagel, G. Strain, M. Devlin, R. Cohen, R. D. Crosby, J. E. Mitchell, and J. Gunstad. 2014. The effects of cystatin C and alkaline phosphatase changes on cognitive function 12-months after bariatric surgery. *Journal of the Neurological Sciences* 345(1-2):176-180.

Anand, S., K. L. Johansen, and M. Kurella Tamura. 2014. Aging and chronic kidney disease: The impact on physical function and cognition. *The Journals of Gerontology, Series A: Biological Sciences and Medical Sciences* 69(3):315-322.

Ancoli-Israel, S., J. Amatniek, S. Ascher, K. Sadik, and K. Ramaswamy. 2005. Effects of galantamine versus donepezil on sleep in patients with mild to moderate Alzheimer disease and their caregivers: A double-blind, head-to-head, randomized pilot study. *Alzheimer Disease and Associated Disorders* 19(4):240-245.

Anderson-Hanley, C., M. L. Sherman, R. Riggs, V. B. Agocha, and B. E. Compas. 2003. Neuropsychological effects of treatments for adults with cancer: A meta-analysis and review of the literature. *Journal of the International Neuropsychological Society* 9(7):967-982.

Andrews, S., D. Das, K. J. Anstey, and S. Easteal. 2015. Interactive effect of APOE genotype and blood pressure on cognitive decline: The path through life study. *Journal of Alzheimer's Disease* 44(4):1087-1098.

Annerbo, S., and J. Lokk. 2013. A clinical review of the association of thyroid stimulating hormone and cognitive impairment. *ISRN Endocrinology* 856017.

Anstey, K. J., N. Cherbuin, M. Budge, and J. Young. 2011. Body mass index in midlife and late-life as a risk factor for dementia: A meta-analysis of prospective studies. *Obesity Reviews* 12(5):e426-e437.

Arciniegas, D. B., and J. M. Silver. 2001. Regarding the search for a unified definition of mild traumatic brain injury. *Brain Injury* 15(7):649-652.

ASCP (American Society of Consultant Pharmacists). 2014. *What is a consultant pharmacist?* https://www.ascp.com/articles/what-consultant-pharmacist (accessed October 11, 2014).

———. 2015. *ASCP fact sheet.* https://www.ascp.com/articles/about-ascp/ascp-fact-sheet (accessed on February 27, 2015).

Ashman, T. A., J. B. Cantor, W. A. Gordon, A. Sacks, L. Spielman, M. Egan, and M. R. Hibbard. 2008. A comparison of cognitive functioning in older adults with and without traumatic brain injury. *Journal of Head Trauma Rehabilitation* 23(3):139-148.

Avidan, M. S., and A. S. Evers. 2011. Review of clinical evidence for persistent cognitive decline or incident dementia attributable to surgery or general anesthesia. *Journal of Alzheimer's Disease* 24(2):201-216.

Bangen, K. J., A. Beiser, L. Delano-Wood, D. A. Nation, M. Lamar, D. J. Libon, M. W. Bondi, S. Seshadri, P. A. Wolf, and R. Au. 2013. APOE genotype modifies the relationship between midlife vascular risk factors and later cognitive decline. *Journal of Stroke and Cerebrovascular Disease* 22(8):1361-1369.

Barnes, D. E., A. Kaup, K. A. Kirby, A. L. Byers, R. Diaz-Arrastia, and K. Yaffe. 2014. Traumatic brain injury and risk of dementia in older veterans. *Neurology* 83(4):312-319.

Bates, D. W., D. J. Cullen, N. Laird, L. A. Petersen, S. D. Small, D. Servi, G. Laffel, B. J. Sweitzer, B. F. Shea, R. Hallisey, M. V. Vliet, R. Nemeskal, L. L. Leape, for the ADE Prevention Study Group. 1995. Incidence of adverse drug events and potential adverse drug events. Implications for prevention. *JAMA* 274(1):29-34.

Beebe, D. W., L. Groesz, C. Wells, A. Nichols, and K. McGee. 2003. The neuropsychological effects of obstructive sleep apnea: A meta-analysis of norm-referenced and case-controlled data. *Sleep* 26(3):298-307.

Benloucif, S., L. Orbeta, R. Ortiz, I. Janssen, S. I. Finkel, J. Bleiberg, and P. C. Zee. 2004. Morning or evening activity improves neuropsychological performance and subjective sleep quality in older adults. *Sleep* 27(8):1542-1551.

Bertram, L., and R. E. Tanzi. 2008. Thirty years of Alzheimer's disease genetics: The implications of systematic meta-analyses. *Nature Reviews Neuroscience* 9(10):768-778.

Bettermann, K., A. M. Arnold, J. Williamson, S. Rapp, K. Sink, J. F. Toole, M. C. Carlson, S. Yasar, S. Dekosky, and G. L. Burke. 2012. Statins, risk of dementia, and cognitive function: Secondary analysis of the ginkgo evaluation of memory study. *Journal of Stroke and Cerebrovascular Disease* 21(6):436-444.

Bial, A. K., R. L. Schilsky, and G. A. Sachs. 2006. Evaluation of cognition in cancer patients: Special focus on the elderly. *Critical Reviews in Oncology/Hematology* 60(3):242-255.

Biessels, G. J., M. W. Strachan, F. L. Visseren, L. J. Kappelle, and R. A. Whitmer. 2014. Dementia and cognitive decline in type 2 diabetes and prediabetic stages: Towards targeted interventions. *The Lancet Diabetes and Endocrinology* 2(3):246-255.

Billioti de Gage, S., B. Begaud, F. Bazin, H. Verdoux, J. F. Dartigues, K. Peres, T. Kurth, and A. Pariente. 2012. Benzodiazepine use and risk of dementia: Prospective population based study. *BMJ (Clinical Research Edition)* 345:e6231.

Blackwell, T., K. Yaffe, S. Ancoli-Israel, J. L. Schneider, J. A. Cauley, T. A. Hillier, H. A. Fink, and K. L. Stone. 2006. Poor sleep is associated with impaired cognitive function in older women: The study of osteoporotic fractures. *The Journals of Gerontology, Series A: Biological Sciences and Medical Sciences* 61(4):405-410.

Blackwell, T., K. Yaffe, S. Ancoli-Israel, S. Redline, K. E. Ensrud, M. L. Stefanick, A. Laffan, and K. L. Stone. 2011. Associations between sleep architecture and sleep-disordered breathing and cognition in older community-dwelling men: The osteoporotic fractures in men sleep study. *Journal of the American Geriatrics Society* 59(12):2217-2225.

Brinkworth, G. D., J. D. Buckley, M. Noakes, P. M. Clifton, and C. J. Wilson. 2009. Long-term effects of a very low-carbohydrate diet and a low-fat diet on mood and cognitive function. *Archives of Internal Medicine* 169(20):1873-1880.

Broglio, S. P., J. T. Eckner, H. L. Paulson, and J. S. Kutcher. 2012. Cognitive decline and aging: The role of concussive and subconcussive impacts. *Exercise and Sport Sciences Reviews* 40(3):138-144.

Byers, A. L., and K. Yaffe. 2011. Depression and risk of developing dementia. *Nature Reviews Neurology* 7(6):323-331.

Campbell, N., M. Boustani, T. Limbil, C. Ott, C. Fox, I. Maidment, C. C. Schubert, S. Munger, D. Fick, D. Miller, and R. Gulati. 2009. The cognitive impact of anticholinergics: A clinical review. *Clinical Interventions of Aging* 4:225-233.

Canessa, N., V. Castronovo, S. F. Cappa, M. S. Aloia, S. Marelli, A. Falini, F. Alemanno, and L. Ferini-Strambi. 2011. Obstructive sleep apnea: Brain structural changes and neurocognitive function before and after treatment. *American Journal of Respiratory and Critical Care Medicine* 183(10):1419-1426.

Carriere, I., A. Fourrier-Reglat, J. F. Dartigues, O. Rouaud, F. Pasquier, K. Ritchie, and M. L. Ancelin. 2009. Drugs with anticholinergic properties, cognitive decline, and dementia in an elderly general population: The 3-city study. *Archives of Internal Medicine* 169(14):1317-1324.

CDC (Centers for Disease Control and Prevention). 2011. *National diabetes fact sheet: National estimates and general information on diabetes and prediabetes in the United States, 2011.* http://www.cdc.gov/diabetes/pubs/pdf/ndfs_2011.pdf (accessed March 2, 2015).

Ceresini, G., F. Lauretani, M. Maggio, G. P. Ceda, S. Morganti, E. Usberti, C. Chezzi, R. Valcavi, S. Bandinelli, J. M. Guralnik, A. R. Cappola, G. Valenti, and L. Ferrucci. 2009. Thyroid function abnormalities and cognitive impairment in elderly people: Results of the Invecchiare in Chianti study. *Journal of the American Geriatrics Society* 57(1):89-93.

Chang-Quan, H., W. Hui, W. Chao-Min, W. Zheng-Rong, G. Jun-Wen, L. Yong-Hong, L. Yan-You, and L. Qing-Xiu. 2011. The association of antihypertensive medication use with risk of cognitive decline and dementia: A meta-analysis of longitudinal studies. *International Journal of Clinical Practice* 65(12):1295-1305.

Claxton, A., L. D. Baker, A. Hanson, E. H. Trittschuh, B. Cholerton, A. Morgan, M. Callaghan, M. Arbuckle, C. Behl, and S. Craft. 2015. Long-acting intranasal insulin detemir improves cognition for adults with mild cognitive impairment or early-stage Alzheimer's disease dementia. *Journal of Alzheimer's Disease* 44(3):897-906.

Clemons, T. E., M. W. Rankin, and W. L. McBee. 2006. Cognitive impairment in the age-related eye disease study: AREDS report no. 16. *Archives of Ophthalmology* 124(4):537-543.

Cohen-Zion, M., C. Stepnowsky, S. Johnson, M. Marler, J. E. Dimsdale, and S. Ancoli-Israel. 2004. Cognitive changes and sleep disordered breathing in elderly: Differences in race. *Journal of Psychosomatic Research* 56(5):549-553.

Cooke, J. R., J. S. Loredo, L. Liu, M. Marler, J. Corey-Bloom, L. Fiorentino, T. Harrison, and S. Ancoli-Israel. 2006. Acetylcholinesterase inhibitors and sleep architecture in patients with Alzheimer's disease. *Drugs and Aging* 23(6):503-511.

Craft, S., L. D. Baker, T. J. Montine, S. Minoshima, G. S. Watson, A. Claxton, M. Arbuckle, M. Callaghan, E. Tsai, S. R. Plymate, P. S. Green, J. Leverenz, D. Cross, and B. Gerton. 2012. Intranasal insulin therapy for Alzheimer disease and amnestic mild cognitive impairment: A pilot clinical trial. *Archives of Neurology* 69(1):29-38.

Crawford, A. G., C. Cote, J. Couto, M. Daskiran, C. Gunnarsson, K. Haas, S. Haas, S. C. Nigam, and R. Schuette. 2010. Prevalence of obesity, Type II diabetes mellitus, hyperlipidemia, and hypertension in the United States: Findings from the GE Centricity electronic medical record database. *Population Health Management* 13(3):151-161.

Crocco, E. A., K. Castro, and D. A. Loewenstein. 2010. How late-life depression affects cognition: Neural mechanisms. *Current Psychiatry Reports* 12(1):34-38.

Czaja, S. J., and C. C. Lee. 2003. Designing computer systems for older adults. In *The human-computer interaction handbook: Fundamentals, evolving technologies, and emerging applications.* Edited by A. Sears and J. A. Jacko. Mahwah, NJ: Lawrence Erlbaum Associates. Pp. 413-427.

Davies, G., S. E. Harris, C. A. Reynolds, A. Payton, H. M. Knight, D. C. Liewald, L. M. Lopez, M. Luciano, A. J. Gow, J. Corley, R. Henderson, C. Murray, A. Pattie, H. C. Fox, P. Redmond, M. W. Lutz, O. Chiba-Falek, C. Linnertz, S. Saith, P. Haggarty, G. McNeill, X. Ke, W. Ollier, M. Horan, A. D. Roses, C. P. Ponting, D. J. Porteous, A. Tenesa, A. Pickles, J. M. Starr, L. J. Whalley, N. L. Pedersen, N. Pendleton, P. M. Visscher, and I. J. Deary. 2014. A genome-wide association study implicates the APOE locus in nonpathological cognitive ageing. *Molecular Psychiatry* 19(1):76-87.

de Vries, O. J., G. Peeters, P. Elders, C. Sonnenberg, M. Muller, D. J. Deeg, and P. Lips. 2013. The elimination half-life of benzodiazepines and fall risk: Two prospective observational studies. *Age and Ageing* 42(6):764-770.

Diniz, B. S., M. A. Butters, S. M. Albert, M. A. Dew, and C. F. Reynolds, 3rd. 2013. Late-life depression and risk of vascular dementia and Alzheimer's disease: Systematic review and meta-analysis of community-based cohort studies. *The British Journal of Psychiatry: The Journal of Mental Science* 202(5):329-335.

Ehlenbach, W. J., C. L. Hough, P. K. Crane, S. J. Haneuse, S. S. Carson, J. R. Curtis, and E. B. Larson. 2010. Association between acute care and critical illness hospitalization and cognitive function in older adults. *JAMA* 303(8):763-770.

Eisenberg, M. A., W. P. Meehan, 3rd, and R. Mannix. 2014. Duration and course of post-concussive symptoms. *Pediatrics* 133(6):999-1006.

Elias, M. F., A. L. Goodell, and G. A. Dore. 2012. Hypertension and cognitive functioning: A perspective in historical context. *Hypertension* 60(2):260-268.

Elias, M. F., G. A. Dore, and A. Davey. 2013. Kidney disease and cognitive function. *Contributions to Nephrology* 179:42-57.

Elwood, P. C., A. J. Bayer, M. Fish, J. Pickering, C. Mitchell, and J. E. Gallacher. 2011. Sleep disturbance and daytime sleepiness predict vascular dementia. *Journal of Epidemiology and Community Health* 65(9):820-824.

Etgen, T., D. Sander, H. Bickel, and H. Forstl. 2011. Mild cognitive impairment and dementia: The importance of modifiable risk factors. *Deutsches Arzteblatt International* 108(44):743-750.

Etgen, T., M. Chonchol, H. Forstl, and D. Sander. 2012. Chronic kidney disease and cognitive impairment: A systematic review and meta-analysis. *American Journal of Nephrology* 35(5):474-482.

FDA (Food and Drug Administration). 2012. *FDA safety communication: Important safety label changes to cholesterol-lowering statin drugs.* February 28, 2012. http://www.fda.gov/Drugs/DrugSafety/ucm293101.htm#sa (accessed January 9, 2105).

Fick, D. M., and T. P. Semla. 2012. 2012 American Geriatrics Society Beers Criteria: New year, new criteria, new perspective. *Journal of the American Geriatrics Society* 60(4):614-615.

Fick, D. M., J. W. Cooper, W. E. Wade, J. L. Waller, J. R. Maclean, and M. H. Beers. 2003. Updating the Beers Criteria for potentially inappropriate medication use in older adults: Results of a U.S. consensus panel of experts. *Archives of Internal Medicine* 163(22):2716-2724.

Foley, D., A. Monjan, K. Masaki, W. Ross, R. Havlik, L. White, and L. Launer. 2001. Daytime sleepiness is associated with 3-year incident dementia and cognitive decline in older Japanese-American men. *Journal of the American Geriatrics Society* 49(12):1628-1632.
Foley, D. J., K. Masaki, L. White, E. K. Larkin, A. Monjan, and S. Redline. 2003. Sleep-disordered breathing and cognitive impairment in elderly Japanese-American men. *Sleep* 26(5):596-599.
Fong, T. G., R. N. Jones, P. Shi, E. R. Marcantonio, L. Yap, J. L. Rudolph, F. M. Yang, D. K. Kiely, and S. K. Inouye. 2009. Delirium accelerates cognitive decline in Alzheimer disease. *Neurology* 72(18):1570-1575.
Ford, E. S., W. H. Giles, and W. H. Dietz. 2002. Prevalence of the metabolic syndrome among U.S. adults: Findings from the third National Health and Nutrition Examination Survey. *JAMA* 287(3):356-359.
Fortier-Brochu, E., S. Beaulieu-Bonneau, H. Ivers, and C. M. Morin. 2012. Insomnia and daytime cognitive performance: A meta-analysis. *Sleep Medicine Reviews* 16(1):83-94.
Fosnight, S. M., C. M. Holder, K. R. Allen, and S. Hazelett. 2004. A strategy to decrease the use of risky drugs in the elderly. *Cleveland Clinic Journal of Medicine* 71(7):561-568.
Gasecki, D., M. Kwarciany, W. Nyka, and K. Narkiewicz. 2013. Hypertension, brain damage and cognitive decline. *Current Hypertension Reports* 15(6):547-558.
Genther, D. J., K. D. Frick, D. Chen, J. Betz, and F. R. Lin. 2013. Association of hearing loss with hospitalization and burden of disease in older adults. *JAMA* 309(22):2322-2324.
Giannini, E., and R. Testa. 2003. The metabolic syndrome: All criteria are equal, but some criteria are more equal than others. *Archives of Internal Medicine* 163(22):2787-2788; author reply 2788.
Godbolt, A. K., C. Cancelliere, C. A. Hincapie, C. Marras, E. Boyle, V. L. Kristman, V. G. Coronado, and J. D. Cassidy. 2014. Systematic review of the risk of dementia and chronic cognitive impairment after mild traumatic brain injury: Results of the International Collaboration on Mild Traumatic Brain Injury Prognosis. *Archives of Physical Medicine and Rehabilitation* 95(3 Suppl):S245-S256.
Gorina, Y., D. Hoyert, H. Lentzner, and M. Goulding. 2006. *Trends in causes of death among older persons in the United States.* Aging Trends, No 6. Hyattsville, MD: National Center for Health Statistics.
Greer, N., R. Rossom, P. Anderson, R. MacDonald, J. Tacklind, I. Rutks, and T. J. Wilt. 2011. VA evidence-based synthesis program reports. In *Delirium: Screening, prevention, and diagnosis—A systematic review of the evidence.* Washington, DC: Department of Veterans Affairs. http://www.hsrd.research.va.gov/publications/esp/delirium-REPORT.pdf (accessed January 9, 2015).
Gross, A. L., R. N. Jones, D. A. Habtemariam, T. G. Fong, D. Tommet, L. Quach, E. Schmitt, L. Yap, and S. K. Inouye. 2012. Delirium and long-term cognitive trajectory among persons with dementia. *Archives of Internal Medicine* 172(17):1324-1331.
Gurwitz, J. H., T. S. Field, J. Avorn, D. McCormick, S. Jain, M. Eckler, M. Benser, A. C. Edmondson, and D. W. Bates. 2000. Incidence and preventability of adverse drug events in nursing homes. *American Journal of Medicine* 109(2):87-94.
Gustafson, D. R. 2012. Adiposity and cognitive decline: Underlying mechanisms. *Journal of Alzheimer's Disease* 30(Suppl 2):S97-S112.
Haimov, I., and E. Shatil. 2013. Cognitive training improves sleep quality and cognitive function among older adults with insomnia. *PLoS ONE* 8(4):e61390.
Hajjar, I., and T. A. Kotchen. 2003. Trends in prevalence, awareness, treatment, and control of hypertension in the United States, 1988–2000. *JAMA* 290(2):199-206.
Hanford, N., and M. Figueiro. 2013. Light therapy and Alzheimer's disease and related dementia: Past, present, and future. *Journal of Alzheimer's Disease* 33(4):913-922.

Heflin, L. H., B. E. Meyerowitz, P. Hall, P. Lichtenstein, B. Johansson, N. L. Pedersen, and M. Gatz. 2005. Cancer as a risk factor for long-term cognitive deficits and dementia. *Journal of the National Cancer Institute* 97(11):854-856.

HELP (Hospital Elder Life Program). 2014. *What we do*. http://www.hospitalelderlifeprogram.org/about/what-we-do (accessed November 4, 2014).

HHS (U.S. Department of Health and Human Services). 2011. *A profile of older Americans: 2011*. http://www.aoa.gov/Aging_Statistics/Profile/2011/docs/2011profile.pdf (accessed March 24, 2015).

———. 2013. *A profile of older Americans: 2013*. http://www.aoa.acl.gov/Aging_Statistics/Profile/2013/docs/2013_Profile.pdf (accessed February 20, 2015).

Holden, K. F., K. Lindquist, F. A. Tylavsky, C. Rosano, T. B. Harris, and K. Yaffe. 2009. Serum leptin level and cognition in the elderly: Findings from the Health ABC study. *Neurobiology of Aging* 30(9):1483-1489.

Holt, R., J. Young, and D. Heseltine. 2013. Effectiveness of a multi-component intervention to reduce delirium incidence in elderly care wards. *Age and Ageing* 42(6):721-727.

Hornung, O. P., F. Regen, H. Dorn, I. Anghelescu, N. Kathmann, M. Schredl, H. Danker-Hopfe, and I. Heuser. 2009. The effects of donepezil on postlearning sleep EEG of healthy older adults. *Pharmacopsychiatry* 42(1):9-13.

Hshieh, T. T., J. Yue, E. Oh, M. Puelle, S. Dowal, T. Travison, and S. K. Inouye. 2014. Effectiveness of multi-component non-pharmacologic delirium interventions: A systematic review and meta-analysis. *JAMA Internal Medicine* [Epub] 7779.

Inglis, F. 2002. The tolerability and safety of cholinesterase inhibitors in the treatment of dementia. *International Journal of Clinical Practice Supplement* (127):45-63.

Inouye, S. K. 2000. Prevention of delirium in hospitalized older patients: Risk factors and targeted intervention strategies. *Annals of Medicine* 32(4):257-263.

Inouye, S. K., S. T. Bogardus, Jr., P. A. Charpentier, L. Leo-Summers, D. Acampora, T. R. Holford, and L. M. Cooney, Jr. 1999. A multicomponent intervention to prevent delirium in hospitalized older patients. *New England Journal of Medicine* 340(9):669-676.

Inouye, S. K., S. T. Bogardus, Jr., D. I. Baker, L. Leo-Summers, and L. M. Cooney, Jr. 2000. The Hospital Elder Life Program: A model of care to prevent cognitive and functional decline in older hospitalized patients. *Journal of the American Geriatrics Society* 48(12):1697-1706.

Inouye, S. K., S. T. Bogardus, Jr., C. S. Williams, L. Leo-Summers, and J. V. Agostini. 2003. The role of adherence on the effectiveness of nonpharmacologic interventions: Evidence from the delirium prevention trial. *Archives of Internal Medicine* 163(8):958-964.

Inouye, S. K., D. I. Baker, P. Fugal, and E. H. Bradley. 2006. Dissemination of the Hospital Elder Life Program: Implementation, adaptation, and successes. *Journal of the American Geriatrics Society* 54(10):1492-1499.

Inouye, S. K., R. G. Westendorp, and J. S. Saczynski. 2014. Delirium in elderly people. *Lancet* 383(9920):911-922.

Isoniemi, H., O. Tenovuo, R. Portin, L. Himanen, and V. Kairisto. 2006. Outcome of traumatic brain injury after three decades—relationship to APOE genotype. *Journal of Neurotrauma* 23(11):1600-1608.

Jaussent, I., J. Bouyer, M. L. Ancelin, C. Berr, A. Foubert-Samier, K. Ritchie, M. M. Ohayon, A. Besset, and Y. Dauvilliers. 2012. Excessive sleepiness is predictive of cognitive decline in the elderly. *Sleep* 35(9):1201-1207.

Jelicic, M., H. Bosma, R. W. Ponds, M. P. Van Boxtel, P. J. Houx, and J. Jolles. 2002. Subjective sleep problems in later life as predictors of cognitive decline. Report from the Maastricht Ageing Study (MAAS). *International Journal of Geriatric Psychiatry* 17(1):73-77.

Kalisch Ellett, L. M., N. L. Pratt, E. N. Ramsay, J. D. Barratt, and E. E. Roughead. 2014. Multiple anticholinergic medication use and risk of hospital admission for confusion or dementia. *Journal of the American Geriatrics Society* 62(10):1916-1922.

Keller, B. K., J. L. Morton, V. S. Thomas, and J. F. Potter. 1999. The effect of visual and hearing impairments on functional status. *Journal of the American Geriatrics Society* 47(11):1319-1325.

Konrad, C., A. J. Geburek, F. Rist, H. Blumenroth, B. Fischer, I. Husstedt, V. Arolt, H. Schiffbauer, and H. Lohmann. 2011. Long-term cognitive and emotional consequences of mild traumatic brain injury. *Psychological Medicine* 41(6):1197-1211.

Koyama, A., M. Steinman, K. Ensrud, T. A. Hillier, and K. Yaffe. 2013. Ten-year trajectory of potentially inappropriate medications in very old women: Importance of cognitive status. *Journal of the American Geriatrics Society* 61(2):258-263.

Krumholz, H. M. 2013. Post-hospital syndrome—an acquired, transient condition of generalized risk. *New England Journal of Medicine* 368(2):100-102.

Kushida, C. A., D. A. Nichols, T. H. Holmes, S. F. Quan, J. K. Walsh, D. J. Gottlieb, R. D. Simon, Jr., C. Guilleminault, D. P. White, J. L. Goodwin, P. K. Schweitzer, E. B. Leary, P. R. Hyde, M. Hirshkowitz, S. Green, L. K. McEvoy, C. Chan, A. Gevins, G. G. Kay, D. A. Bloch, T. Crabtree, and W. C. Dement. 2012. Effects of continuous positive airway pressure on neurocognitive function in obstructive sleep apnea patients: The Apnea Positive Pressure Long-term Efficacy Study (APPLES). *Sleep* 35(12):1593-1602.

Kylstra, W. A., J. A. Aaronson, W. F. Hofman, and B. A. Schmand. 2013. Neuropsychological functioning after CPAP treatment in obstructive sleep apnea: A meta-analysis. *Sleep Medicine Reviews* 17(5):341-347.

Ledesma, M. D., M. G. Martin, and C. G. Dotti. 2012. Lipid changes in the aged brain: Effect on synaptic function and neuronal survival. *Progress in Lipid Research* 51(1):23-35.

Leys, D., H. Henon, M. A. Mackowiak-Cordoliani, and F. Pasquier. 2005. Poststroke dementia. *Lancet Neurology* 4(11):752-759.

Ligthart, S. A., E. P. Moll van Charante, W. A. Van Gool, and E. Richard. 2010. Treatment of cardiovascular risk factors to prevent cognitive decline and dementia: A systematic review. *Vascular Health and Risk Management* 6:775-785.

Lim, A. S., M. Kowgier, L. Yu, A. S. Buchman, and D. A. Bennett. 2013a. Sleep fragmentation and the risk of incident Alzheimer's disease and cognitive decline in older persons. *Sleep* 36(7):1027-1032.

Lim, A. S., L. Yu, M. Kowgier, J. A. Schneider, A. S. Buchman, and D. A. Bennett. 2013b. Modification of the relationship of the apolipoprotein e epsilon4 allele to the risk of Alzheimer disease and neurofibrillary tangle density by sleep. *JAMA Neurology* 70(12):1544-1551.

Lin, F. R., E. J. Metter, R. J. O'Brien, S. M. Resnick, A. B. Zonderman, and L. Ferrucci. 2011. Hearing loss and incident dementia. *Archives of Neurology* 68(2):214-220.

Lin, F. R., K. Yaffe, J. Xia, Q. L. Xue, T. B. Harris, E. Purchase-Helzner, S. Satterfield, H. N. Ayonayon, L. Ferrucci, and E. M. Simonsick. 2013. Hearing loss and cognitive decline in older adults. *JAMA Internal Medicine* 173(4):293-299.

Lin, M. Y., P. R. Gutierrez, K. L. Stone, K. Yaffe, K. E. Ensrud, H. A. Fink, C. A. Sarkisian, A. L. Coleman, and C. M. Mangione. 2004. Vision impairment and combined vision and hearing impairment predict cognitive and functional decline in older women. *Journal of the American Geriatrics Society* 52(12):1996-2002.

Lukazewski, A., B. Martin, D. Sokhal, K. Hornemann, and A. Schwartzwald. 2014. Screening for adverse drug events in older adults: The impact of interventions. *The Consultant Pharmacist* 29(10):689-697.

Mason, M., E. J. Welsh, and I. Smith. 2013. Drug therapy for obstructive sleep apnoea in adults. *The Cochrane Database of Systematic Reviews* 5:Cd003002.

Mathews, S. B., S. E. Arnold, and C. N. Epperson. 2014. Hospitalization and cognitive decline: Can the nature of the relationship be deciphered? *American Journal of Geriatric Psychiatry* 22(5):465-480.

Mattison, M. L., K. A. Afonso, L. H. Ngo, and K. J. Mukamal. 2010. Preventing potentially inappropriate medication use in hospitalized older patients with a computerized provider order entry warning system. *Archives of Internal Medicine* 170(15):1331-1336.

McCrimmon, R. J., C. M. Ryan, and B. M. Frier. 2012. Diabetes and cognitive dysfunction. *Lancet* 379(9833):2291-2299.

McCurry, S. M., K. C. Pike, M. V. Vitiello, R. G. Logsdon, E. B. Larson, and L. Teri. 2011. Increasing walking and bright light exposure to improve sleep in community-dwelling persons with Alzheimer's disease: Results of a randomized, controlled trial. *Journal of the American Geriatrics Society* 59(8):1393-1402.

McGuinness, B., S. Todd, P. Passmore, and R. Bullock. 2009. Blood pressure lowering in patients without prior cerebrovascular disease for prevention of cognitive impairment and dementia. *The Cochrane Database of Systematic Reviews* (4):Cd004034.

Merlino, G., A. Piani, G. L. Gigli, I. Cancelli, A. Rinaldi, A. Baroselli, A. Serafini, B. Zanchettin, and M. Valente. 2010. Daytime sleepiness is associated with dementia and cognitive decline in older Italian adults: A population-based study. *Sleep Medicine* 11(4):372-377.

Mizuno, S., A. Kameda, T. Inagaki, and J. Horiguchi. 2004. Effects of donepezil on Alzheimer's disease: The relationship between cognitive function and rapid eye movement sleep. *Psychiatry and Clinical Neurosciences* 58(6):660-665.

Montgomery, P., and J. Dennis. 2002. Physical exercise for sleep problems in adults aged 60+. *The Cochrane Database of Systematic Reviews* (4):Cd003404.

Moraes Wdos, S., D. R. Poyares, C. Guilleminault, L. R. Ramos, P. H. Bertolucci, and S. Tufik. 2006. The effect of donepezil on sleep and REM sleep EEG in patients with Alzheimer disease: A double-blind placebo-controlled study. *Sleep* 29(2):199-205.

Moretti, L., I. Cristofori, S. M. Weaver, A. Chau, J. N. Portelli, and J. Grafman. 2012. Cognitive decline in older adults with a history of traumatic brain injury. *Lancet Neurology* 11(12):1103-1112.

Napoli, N., K. Shah, D. L. Waters, D. R. Sinacore, C. Qualls, and D. T. Villareal. 2014. Effect of weight loss, exercise, or both on cognition and quality of life in obese older adults. *American Journal of Clinical Nutrition* 100(1):189-198.

Newman, S., J. Stygall, S. Hirani, S. Shaefi, and M. Maze. 2007. Postoperative cognitive dysfunction after noncardiac surgery: A systematic review. *Anesthesiology* 106(3):572-590.

NHLBI (National Health, Lung, and Blood Institute). 2014. *Action to Control Cardiovascular Risk in Diabetes* (ACCORD). https://clinicaltrials.gov/ ct2/show/NCT00000620 (accessed January 7, 2015).

O'Mahony, R., L. Murthy, A. Akunne, and J. Young. 2011. Synopsis of the National Institute for Health and Clinical Excellence guideline for prevention of delirium. *Annals of Internal Medicine* 154(11):746-751.

Pandharipande, P. P., T. D. Girard, J. C. Jackson, A. Morandi, J. L. Thompson, B. T. Pun, N. E. Brummel, C. G. Hughes, E. E. Vasilevskis, A. K. Shintani, K. G. Moons, S. K. Geevarghese, A. Canonico, R. O. Hopkins, G. R. Bernard, R. S. Dittus, and E. W. Ely. 2013. Long-term cognitive impairment after critical illness. *New England Journal of Medicine* 369(14):1306-1316.

Payton, A. 2009. The impact of genetic research on our understanding of normal cognitive ageing: 1995 to 2009. *Neuropsychology Review* 19(4):451-477.

Pendlebury, S. T. 2009. Stroke-related dementia: Rates, risk factors and implications for future research. *Maturitas* 64(3):165-171.

Plassman, B. L., J. W. Williams, Jr., J. R. Burke, T. Holsinger, and S. Benjamin. 2010. Systematic review: Factors associated with risk for and possible prevention of cognitive decline in later life. *Annals of Internal Medicine* 153(3):182-193.

Ponsford, J., and M. Schonberger. 2010. Family functioning and emotional state two and five years after traumatic brain injury. *Journal of the International Neuropsychological Society* 16(2):306-317.

Ponsford, J., K. Draper, and M. Schonberger. 2008. Functional outcome 10 years after traumatic brain injury: Its relationship with demographic, injury severity, and cognitive and emotional status. *Journal of the International Neuropsychological Society* 14(2):233-242.

Potvin, O., D. Lorrain, H. Forget, M. Dube, S. Grenier, M. Preville, and C. Hudon. 2012. Sleep quality and 1-year incident cognitive impairment in community-dwelling older adults. *Sleep* 35(4):491-499.

Prilipko, O., N. Huynh, S. Schwartz, V. Tantrakul, C. Kushida, T. Paiva, and C. Guilleminault. 2012. The effects of CPAP treatment on task positive and default mode networks in obstructive sleep apnea patients: An fMRI study. *PLoS ONE* 7(12):e47433.

Qiu, C., M. Kivipelto, H. Agüero-Torres, B. Winblad, and L. Fratiglioni. 2004. Risk and protective effects of APOE gene towards Alzheimer's disease in the Kungsholmen project: variation by age and sex. *Journal of Neurology, Neurosurgery & Psychiatry* 75(6):828-833.

Qiu, C., B. Winblad, and L. Fratiglioni. 2005. The age-dependent relation of blood pressure to cognitive function and dementia. *Lancet Neurology* 4(8):487-499.

Raebel, M. A., J. Charles, J. Dugan, N. M. Carroll, E. J. Korner, D. W. Brand, and D. J. Magid. 2007. Randomized trial to improve prescribing safety in ambulatory elderly patients. *Journal of the American Geriatrics Society* 55(7):977-985.

Ray, W. A., D. G. Blazer, 2nd, W. Schaffner, C. F. Federspiel, and R. Fink. 1986. Reducing long-term diazepam prescribing in office practice. A controlled trial of educational visits. *JAMA* 256(18):2536-2539.

Reid, K. J., K. G. Baron, B. Lu, E. Naylor, L. Wolfe, and P. C. Zee. 2010. Aerobic exercise improves self-reported sleep and quality of life in older adults with insomnia. *Sleep Medicine* 11(9):934-940.

Reyes-Ortiz, C. A., Y. F. Kuo, A. R. DiNuzzo, L. A. Ray, M. A. Raji, and K. S. Markides. 2005. Near vision impairment predicts cognitive decline: Data from the Hispanic Established Populations for Epidemiologic Studies of the Elderly. *Journal of the American Geriatrics Society* 53(4):681-686.

Reynolds, C. A., M. Gatz, J. A. Prince, S. Berg, and N. L. Pedersen. 2010. Serum lipid levels and cognitive change in late life. *Journal of the American Geriatrics Society* 58(3):501-509.

Richardson, K., M. Schoen, B. French, C. A. Umscheid, M. D. Mitchell, S. E. Arnold, P. A. Heidenreich, D. J. Rader, and E. M. deGoma. 2013. Statins and cognitive function: A systematic review. *Annals of Internal Medicine* 159(10):688-697.

Roberts, L. M., H. Pattison, A. Roalfe, J. Franklyn, S. Wilson, F. D. Hobbs, and J. V. Parle. 2006. Is subclinical thyroid dysfunction in the elderly associated with depression or cognitive dysfunction? *Annals of Internal Medicine* 145(8):573-581.

Rosenthal, M. B., E. R. Berndt, J. M. Donohue, R. G. Frank, and A. M. Epstein. 2002. Promotion of prescription drugs to consumers. *New England Journal of Medicine* 346(7):498-505.

Rouch, L., P. Cestac, O. Hanon, C. Cool, C. Helmer, B. Bouhanick, B. Chamontin, J. F. Dartigues, B. Vellas, and S. Andrieu. 2015. Antihypertensive drugs, prevention of cognitive decline and dementia: A systematic review of observational studies, randomized controlled trials and meta-analyses, with discussion of potential mechanisms. *CNS Drugs* 29(2):113-130.

Rubin, F. H., K. Neal, K. Fenlon, S. Hassan, and S. K. Inouye. 2011. Sustainability and scalability of the Hospital Elder Life Program at a community hospital. *Journal of the American Geriatrics Society* 59(2):359-365.

Rudolph, J. L., K. A. Schreiber, D. J. Culley, R. E. McGlinchey, G. Crosby, S. Levitsky, and E. R. Marcantonio. 2010. Measurement of post-operative cognitive dysfunction after cardiac surgery: A systematic review. *Acta Anaesthesiologica Scandinavica* 54(6):663-677.

Saczynski, J. S., E. R. Marcantonio, L. Quach, T. G. Fong, A. Gross, S. K. Inouye, and R. N. Jones. 2012. Cognitive trajectories after postoperative delirium. *New England Journal of Medicine* 367(1):30-39.

Salahudeen, M. S., S. B. Duffull, and P. S. Nishtala. 2014. Impact of anticholinergic discontinuation on cognitive outcomes in older people: A systematic review. *Drugs & Aging* 31(3):185-192.

Salami, O., C. Lyketsos, and V. Rao. 2011. Treatment of sleep disturbance in Alzheimer's dementia. *International Journal of Geriatric Psychiatry* 26(8):771-782.

Savva, G. M., and B. C. Stephan. 2010. Epidemiological studies of the effect of stroke on incident dementia: A systematic review. *Stroke* 41(1):e41-e46.

Schieber, F., and C. L. Baldwin. 1996. Vision, audition, and aging research. In *Perspectives on cognitive change in adulthood and aging*. Edited by F. Blanchard-Fields and T. H. Hess. New York: McGraw-Hill. Pp. 122-162.

Schliebs, R., and T. Arendt. 2006. The significance of the cholinergic system in the brain during aging and in Alzheimer's disease. *Journal of Neural Transmission* 113(11):1625-1644.

Schmutte, T., S. Harris, R. Levin, R. Zweig, M. Katz, and R. Lipton. 2007. The relation between cognitive functioning and self-reported sleep complaints in nondemented older adults: Results from the Bronx Aging Study. *Behavioral Sleep Medicine* 5(1):39-56.

Sellbom, K. S., and J. Gunstad. 2012. Cognitive function and decline in obesity. *Journal of Alzheimer's Disease* 30(Suppl 2):S89-S95.

Selnes, O. A., R. F. Gottesman, M. A. Grega, W. A. Baumgartner, S. L. Zeger, and G. M. McKhann. 2012. Cognitive and neurologic outcomes after coronary-artery bypass surgery. *New England Journal of Medicine* 366(3):250-257.

Senathi-Raja, D., J. Ponsford, and M. Schonberger. 2010. The association of age and time postinjury with long-term emotional outcome following traumatic brain injury. *Journal of Head Trauma Rehabilitation* 25(5):330-338.

Siervo, M., R. Arnold, J. C. Wells, A. Tagliabue, A. Colantuoni, E. Albanese, C. Brayne, and B. C. Stephan. 2011. Intentional weight loss in overweight and obese individuals and cognitive function: A systematic review and meta-analysis. *Obesity Reviews* 12(11):968-983.

Small, B. J., C. B. Rosnick, L. Fratiglioni, and L. Backman. 2004. Apolipoprotein e and cognitive performance: A meta-analysis. *Psychology and Aging* 19(4):592-600.

Smith, D. H., N. Perrin, A. Feldstein, X. Yang, D. Kuang, S. R. Simon, D. F. Sittig, R. Platt, and S. B. Soumerai. 2006. The impact of prescribing safety alerts for elderly persons in an electronic medical record: An interrupted time series evaluation. *Archives of Internal Medicine* 166(10):1098-1104.

Solomon, A., I. Kareholt, T. Ngandu, B. Wolozin, S. W. Macdonald, B. Winblad, A. Nissinen, J. Tuomilehto, H. Soininen, and M. Kivipelto. 2009. Serum total cholesterol, statins and cognition in non-demented elderly. *Neurobiology of Aging* 30(6):1006-1009.

Spauwen, P. J., S. Kohler, F. R. Verhey, C. D. Stehouwer, and M. P. van Boxtel. 2013. Effects of type 2 diabetes on 12-year cognitive change: Results from the Maastricht Aging Study. *Diabetes Care* 36(6):1554-1561.

Spira, A. P., T. Blackwell, K. L. Stone, S. Redline, J. A. Cauley, S. Ancoli-Israel, and K. Yaffe. 2008. Sleep-disordered breathing and cognition in older women. *Journal of the American Geriatrics Society* 56(1):45-50.

Staessen, J. A., L. Thijs, T. Richart, A. N. Odili, and W. H. Birkenhager. 2011. Placebo-controlled trials of blood pressure-lowering therapies for primary prevention of dementia. *Hypertension* 57(2):e6-e7.

Steenland, K., L. Zhao, F. C. Goldstein, and A. I. Levey. 2013. Statins and cognitive decline in older adults with normal cognition or mild cognitive impairment. *Journal of the American Geriatrics Society* 61(9):1449-1455.

Sterniczuk, R., O. Theou, B. Rusak, and K. Rockwood. 2013. Sleep disturbance is associated with incident dementia and mortality. *Current Alzheimer Research* 10(7):767-775.

Sweet, R. A., H. Seltman, J. E. Emanuel, O. L. Lopez, J. T. Becker, J. C. Bis, E. A. Weamer, M. A. DeMichele-Sweet, and L. H. Kuller. 2012. Effect of Alzheimer's disease risk genes on trajectories of cognitive function in the cardiovascular health study. *American Journal of Psychiatry* 169(9):954-962.

Tamblyn, R., A. Huang, R. Perreault, A. Jacques, D. Roy, J. Hanley, P. McLeod, and R. Laprise. 2003. The medical office of the 21st century (MOXXI): Effectiveness of computerized decision-making support in reducing inappropriate prescribing in primary care. *Canadian Medical Association Journal* 169(6):549-556.

Tannenbaum, C., A. Paquette, S. Hilmer, J. Holroyd-Leduc, and R. Carnahan. 2012. A systematic review of amnestic and non-amnestic mild cognitive impairment induced by anticholinergic, antihistamine, gabaergic and opioid drugs. *Drugs & Aging* 29(8):639-658.

Tannenbaum, C., P. Martin, R. Tamblyn, A. Benedetti, and S. Ahmed. 2014. Reduction of inappropriate benzodiazepine prescriptions among older adults through direct patient education: The EMPOWER cluster randomized trial. *JAMA Internal Medicine* 174(6):890-898.

Tatemichi, T. K., M. Paik, E. Bagiella, D. W. Desmond, M. Pirro, and L. K. Hanzawa. 1994. Dementia after stroke is a predictor of long-term survival. *Stroke* 25(10):1915-1919.

Tay, T., J. J. Wang, A. Kifley, R. Lindley, P. Newall, and P. Mitchell. 2006. Sensory and cognitive association in older persons: Findings from an older Australian population. *Gerontology* 52(6):386-394.

Tworoger, S. S., S. Lee, E. S. Schernhammer, and F. Grodstein. 2006. The association of self-reported sleep duration, difficulty sleeping, and snoring with cognitive function in older women. *Alzheimer Disease and Associated Disorders* 20(1):41-48.

Uhlmann, R. F., E. B. Larson, T. S. Rees, T. D. Koepsell, and L. G. Duckert. 1989. Relationship of hearing impairment to dementia and cognitive dysfunction in older adults. *JAMA* 261(13):1916-1919.

van Dijk, D., A. M. Keizer, J. C. Diephuis, C. Durand, L. J. Vos, and R. Hijman. 2000. Neurocognitive dysfunction after coronary artery bypass surgery: A systematic review. *Journal of Thoracic and Cardiovascular Surgery* 120(4):632-639.

van Vliet, P. 2012. Cholesterol and late-life cognitive decline. *Journal of Alzheimer's Disease* 30(Suppl 2):S147-S162.

Vidan, M. T., E. Sanchez, M. Alonso, B. Montero, J. Ortiz, and J. A. Serra. 2009. An intervention integrated into daily clinical practice reduces the incidence of delirium during hospitalization in elderly patients. *Journal of the American Geriatrics Society* 57(11):2029-2036.

Vincent, A. S., T. M. Roebuck-Spencer, and A. Cernich. 2014. Cognitive changes and dementia risk after traumatic brain injury: Implications for aging military personnel. *Alzheimer's & Dementia* 10(3 Suppl):S174-S187.

Wang, Y., and M. A. Beydoun. 2007. The obesity epidemic in the United States—gender, age, socioeconomic, racial/ethnic, and geographic characteristics: A systematic review and meta-regression analysis. *Epidemiologic Reviews* 29:6-28.

Wilson, R. S., L. E. Hebert, P. A. Scherr, X. Dong, S. E. Leurgens, and D. A. Evans. 2012. Cognitive decline after hospitalization in a community population of older persons. *Neurology* 78(13):950-956.

Witlox, J., L. S. Eurelings, J. F. de Jonghe, K. J. Kalisvaart, P. Eikelenboom, and W. A. van Gool. 2010. Delirium in elderly patients and the risk of postdischarge mortality, institutionalization, and dementia: A meta-analysis. *JAMA* 304(4):443-451.

Wood, J. M., P. Lacherez, A. A. Black, M. H. Cole, M. Y. Boon, and G. K. Kerr. 2011. Risk of falls, injurious falls, and other injuries resulting from visual impairment among older adults with age-related macular degeneration. *Investigative Ophthalmology and Visual Science* 52(8):5088-5092.

Yaffe, K. 2007. Metabolic syndrome and cognitive disorders: Is the sum greater than its parts? *Alzheimer's Disease and Associated Disorders* 21(2):167-171.

Yaffe, K., T. Blackwell, A. M. Kanaya, N. Davidowitz, E. Barrett-Connor, and K. Krueger. 2004. Diabetes, impaired fasting glucose, and development of cognitive impairment in older women. *Neurology* 63(4):658-663.

Yaffe, K., A. M. Laffan, S. L. Harrison, S. Redline, A. P. Spira, K. E. Ensrud, S. Ancoli-Israel, and K. L. Stone. 2011. Sleep-disordered breathing, hypoxia, and risk of mild cognitive impairment and dementia in older women. *JAMA* 306(6):613-619.

Yaffe, K., C. Falvey, N. Hamilton, A. V. Schwartz, E. M. Simonsick, S. Satterfield, J. A. Cauley, C. Rosano, L. J. Launer, E. S. Strotmeyer, and T. B. Harris. 2012. Diabetes, glucose control, and 9-year cognitive decline among older adults without dementia. *Archives of Neurology* 69(9):1170-1175.

Yaffe, K., C. M. Falvey, and T. Hoang. 2014. Connections between sleep and cognition in older adults. *Lancet Neurology* 13(10):1017-1028.

Yokoyama, J. S., D. S. Evans, G. Coppola, J. H. Kramer, G. J. Tranah, and K. Yaffe. 2014. Genetic modifiers of cognitive maintenance among older adults. *Human Brain Mapping* 35(9):4556-4565.

Zaubler, T. S., K. Murphy, L. Rizzuto, R. Santos, C. Skotzko, J. Giordano, R. Bustami, and S. K. Inouye. 2013. Quality improvement and cost savings with multicomponent delirium interventions: Replication of the Hospital Elder Life Program in a community hospital. *Psychosomatics* 54(3):219-226.

Zeki Al Hazzouri, A., K. L. Stone, M. N. Haan, and K. Yaffe. 2013. Leptin, mild cognitive impairment, and dementia among elderly women. *The Journals of Gerontology, Series A: Biological Sciences and Medical Sciences* 68(2):175-180.

4C

Risk and Protective Factors and Interventions: General Cognitive Aging Interventions and Next Steps

This chapter explores interventions that are aimed at improving cognition or slowing cognitive decline but that are not aimed at specific risk factors. Among the many approaches that fall into this category are cognitive stimulation through memory and other cognitive skills training, participation in the arts, technology-based cognitive stimulation, electrical stimulation, medications, and chemical stimulation such as the use of nootropic drugs or supplements. The chapter reviews studies that examine the effects on cognition of combining several interventions (e.g., physical activity, diet, cognitive stimulation) in multimodal interventions and concludes with the committee's recommendations on next steps.

COGNITIVE STIMULATION AND TRAINING

There has been considerable scholarly and commercial interest over the past several years in the question of whether cognitive stimulation, either through such everyday activities as completing crossword puzzles, participating in a book club, playing card games, learning to play a musical instrument, and learning a new language (see Chapter 4A) or through more formal training, can assist in the maintenance or enhancement of cognitive function as people age. A second, equally important question is whether cognitive stimulation and training will transfer to real-world activities and tasks (i.e., transfer effects). For example, can a computer-based memory training program help people better remember their shopping list, medical and other appointments, and the names and faces of new acquaintances?

Or can computer-based, cognitive training improve driving performance and safety?

Fortunately, an increasing number of randomized controlled trials (RCTs) are assessing whether cognitive training, such as adaptive computer-based programs, can create improvements in trained performance and whether the benefits of such training will transfer to untrained tasks and skills. In general, these studies reveal that older adults can indeed benefit from training, albeit often at a slower rate than younger adults do (Baltes et al., 1989; Willis et al., 2006; Winocur et al., 2007). Transfer effects (benefits for untrained-for tasks) are often quite limited, as a study by Ball and colleagues (2002) illustrates. In this study, the largest RCT of cognitive training to date, 2,800 older adults were randomized among three training groups (training for memory, reasoning, and speed of processing) and a no-contact control group. Participants did improve on the trained tasks and other measures of these processes. However, no significant transfer occurred between the trained and untrained cognitive processes (e.g., those individuals receiving memory training did not improve on speed of processing and vice versa). Interestingly, the benefits of training were still observed for the reasoning and speed-of-processing groups, as compared with the control group, after 10 years. Participants in each of the three training groups also reported less difficulty with instrumental activities of daily living (IADLs), although no differences were observed for the performance-based everyday activities (Rebok et al., 2014). The IADL results should be interpreted with caution, since they might be partly attributable to expectancy differences between the training groups and the no-contact controls (Boot et al., 2013b).

Another major focus of the cognitive training literature has been on improving working memory (also see Chapter 2), on which many other cognitive processes depend (Bopp and Verhaeghen, 2005; Hale et al., 2011), which makes working memory an important target for training. It is now relatively well established that young adults show near-transfer effects with working memory. However, the transfer results for older adults have been mixed, with some studies failing to observe any transfer, even to similar memory tasks (Dahlin et al., 2008; Zinke et al., 2012), while other studies have reported transfer to similar memory tasks (Li et al., 2008; Zinke et al., 2014). A number of factors that might mediate transfer have been suggested, including age, health, general cognitive ability, baseline performance, motivation, and expectancies (Boot et al., 2011; Brehmer et al., 2011; Fairchild et al., 2013).

Another approach to strengthening cognitive skills for older adults has been the use of video games, which employ a somewhat different set of training strategies than the computer-based training. For example, Anguera and colleagues (2013) worked with video games incorporating cognitive training tasks that have shown some promise in training and transfer in the scientific literature. These video games are believed to be more entertaining (and motivating) than most of the cognitive tasks designed by cognitive scientists, and they can adaptively increase their difficulty level as the user's skill increases, just as "off-the-shelf" video games designed for entertainment do.

A study by Smith and colleagues (2009) used a commercially available adaptive cognitive training program focused on auditory detection, discrimination, and comprehension. The researchers compared an experimental group to an active control group that watched educational videos (1 hour daily for 40 sessions). Older adults in the active group improved, relative to the control group, on auditory measures from the Repeatable Battery for the Assessment of Neuropsychological Status as well as on other measures of attention and memory. Effect sizes were generally small to modest, and a subset of these effects was maintained over a 3-month period (Nouchi et al., 2012; Zelinski et al., 2011). Not all video game-based cognitive training programs have been as successful, with some failing to find any transfer of training effects (Ackerman et al., 2010; Owen et al., 2010) and others observing very limited transfer of training (van Muijden et al., 2012). Research on the use of video games designed for enjoyment (rather than specifically for cognitive training) has produced a mixed pattern of effects in older adults, with some showing transfer effects (Basak et al., 2008; Belchior et al., 2013) and others failing to observe them (Boot et al., 2013a).

In this report the committee does not attempt to compare one approach to cognitive training with another; rather, it considers the overall literature on this topic. The committee recognizes that future studies will better inform the research community and the general public about the effectiveness of these approaches to training, especially in whether the skills they support transfer to everyday tasks and challenges.

Ongoing debate by experts in the field about the utility of commercial cognitive training games (Cognitive Training Data, 2015; Stanford Center on Longevity, 2014) points to the need for careful evaluation of these efforts. Given the early stage of research in this field and the need to demonstrate and validate transfer effects from cognitive training products to real-life situations, consumers need information from independent evaluations of commercial cognitive training products. Questions to be examined by consumer organizations and evaluation researchers include

- Has the product demonstrated transfer of training to other laboratory tasks that measure the same cognitive construct as the training task (e.g., if some aspect of memory is being targeted in the product, is transfer demonstrated to other memory tasks)?

- Has the product demonstrated transfer of training to relevant real-world tasks?
- Has the product performance been evaluated using an active control group whose members have the same expectations of cognitive benefits as do members of the experimental group?
- How long are the trained skills retained?
- Have the purported benefits of the training product been replicated by research groups other than those selling the product?

Furthermore, the committee recommends a review of regulatory policies and guidelines (see Recommendations section) and the development of consumer product evaluation criteria for cognition-related products (see Chapter 6).

In summary, the literature on cognitive stimulation and cognitive training is promising, in that studies have shown that older adults can improve on trained abilities, albeit often at a slower pace than that of younger adults (for an exception, see Kramer et al., 1999), and that improvements on the tasks can be maintained over time (Rebok et al., 2014; Zelinski et al., 2011). Studies of the transfer of training effects to other tasks have had mixed results, with few showing transfer effects extending to tasks that are dissimilar to the training tasks (including transfer to real-world tasks and skills). As the developers of cognitive training products strive to demonstrate the benefits of these products in real-life situations, claims regarding the effectiveness of their products will require careful evaluation by consumers and in regulatory review.

ARTS

Engagement in the arts has been gaining increasing interest as a potential intervention to maintain or improve a variety of aspects of health, including cognition. In general, these approaches have focused on "participatory" arts, in which the older adult is actually creating art or doing the activity rather than observing performances or discussing art. The state of the science regarding the impact of participation in writing, theater, music, dance, and visual arts has been reviewed (Noice et al., 2014). Much of the published literature reports the results of studies employing quasi-experimental and intervention designs. Moreover, many of the studies have substantial limitations in design and implementation (e.g., small sample sizes and unrepresentative samples, short follow-up, use of composite measures that may not have clinical relevance, or incomplete reporting of results). Methodological rigor might be improved by creating teams of researchers who have content and research expertise.

To date, some RCT evidence supports the use of theatrical acting, dance, and piano playing to improve specific aspects of cognition (e.g., executive function and working memory [piano playing]; selective attention/concentration and a composite cognition measure [dance]; recall, problem solving, and verbal fluency [acting]) (Bugos et al., 2007; Kattenstroth et al., 2013; Noice and Noice, 2009, 2013; Noice et al., 2014). However, many of the studies have inconsistent results or do not show persistent benefits. A 6-month, once-weekly dance intervention was found to improve many aspects of cognitive and physical function along with subjective well-being, without causing any improvement in physical fitness (Kattenstroth et al., 2013). Furthermore, virtually no studies directly compare different arts interventions.

In summary, despite the limitations of existing research, the results are promising. Additional studies on the influence of the arts on cognitive health are needed that have the methodological rigor that teams of researchers with expertise in the arts, cognition, and methodology can bring.

PHARMACOLOGICS, NOOTROPICS, AND SUPPLEMENTS

Pharmacologics and Nootropics

Continued controversy exists on the usefulness of medications and pharmacologics for preventing cognitive decline and for enhancing or improving cognitive function in older adults. Several medications evaluated over the past decade are thought to have cognitive-enhancing properties either directly or through disease modification. Although a few have been found to slow cognitive decline in older people with dementia, the few controlled studies in people without dementia have had mostly mixed or no results. The majority of these studies are observational, have some methodological shortcomings in design, and vary widely in how they measured cognitive function. This section highlights a few specific pharmacologics and introduces the category of nootropic medications. (As noted in Chapter 4B, there also are a number of medications that can cause cognitive decline.)

Cognitive outcomes have been examined as secondary outcomes in some studies, but few studies have focused specifically on cognitive outcomes. A 2012 prospective cohort study looked at the effects of low doses of acetylsalicylic acid on women who had high cardiovascular disease risk and were free of dementia; the women given the acetylsalicylic acid showed smaller declines in Mini-Mental State Examination (MMSE) scores than a comparison group, but the differences in scores were small. There were no differences between the groups for risk of dementia (Kern et al., 2012). A 2010 observational study of non-steroidal anti-inflammatory drug users without dementia (N = 2,300) from the Baltimore Longitudinal Study of Aging showed less decline in cognitive performance over time among users of non-steroidal anti-inflammatory drugs when assessed on the Blessed I-M-C test (memory and attention) and Trail Making Part B. Study participants taking acetylsalicylic acid declined on several measures (Waldstein et al., 2010).

Studies of the effects of hormone therapy on cognitive function have found very small or adverse effects. A 4-year RCT of hormone treatment in postmenopausal women with cardiovascular disease did not find improvements in cognitive function compared to the use of a placebo (Grady et al., 2002). A 2008 Cochrane review of 16 double-blind RCTs showed no effects of hormone replacement therapy (either estrogen alone or in combination with progestagen) in preventing cognitive impairment (Lethaby et al., 2008). Participants in the meta-analysis were followed for an average of 4 to 5 years, and some negative effects were found after 1 year of estrogen replacement therapy and 3 and 4 years of the combined form.

Continued controversy exists regarding the hypothesis that hormone replacement therapy may confer cognitive and other benefits depending on the timing, formulation, dosage, and duration of treatment, and additional research is needed (Maki, 2013). Some have argued that cognition and verbal memory, in particular, may benefit from early hormone therapy, although this may apply only to specific combinations of hormones (Maki, 2013; Sherwin et al., 2011). Several trials are under way to attempt to address some of the questions regarding hormone therapy safety and to ascertain its impact on cognitive outcomes. The KEEPS Cognitive and Affective Study is a multicenter clinical trial investigating the benefits of hormone replacement therapies administered to perimenopausal women. This study includes women 42 to 58 years of age. The study's primary cognitive outcome measures will include performance on tests of verbal memory and attention/executive function. Final results have not yet been published (NIH, 2014).

Nootropics are a broad range of medications, supplements, and nutriceuticals that aim to stimulate cognitive performance or facilitate learning. Most have not been evaluated in clinical trials of older people without dementia and are not focused on preventing or remediating decline. Nootropics have been classified by their mechanism of action into 19 separate categories (Froestl et al., 2014a,b,c). Some are intended to enhance cognition directly, whereas others are reputed to enhance neuronal health. Accordingly, many studies of presumed nootropics have focused on specific situations (e.g., during sleep deprivation) rather than examining the effects of long-term use on cognition. Classes of nootropics for which some evidence exists about their efficacy in people who do not have dementia include

- Racetams (e.g., piracetam): A meta-analysis of studies involving patients undergoing coronary bypass surgery suggested that racetams have short-term benefits on several dimensions of cognitive function, such as pictured object recall, delayed pictured object recall, delayed picture recognition, immediate word recall, and letter interference (Fang et al., 2014).
- Cholinesterase inhibitors (e.g., donepezil): In small, short-term (14- to 42-day) trials, donepezil improved the retention of training on complex aviation tasks and verbal memory. Studies on episodic memory show mixed results. In one study, donepezil reduced the memory and attention deficits resulting from 24 hours of sleep deprivation (Repantis et al., 2010a).
- Phenylethylamines (e.g., methylphenidate): Methylphenidate had short-term benefit on memory, especially spatial working memory, but not on attention or other dimensions of cognition (Repantis et al., 2010b).
- Eugeroics (e.g., modafinil): Modafinil improved attention for well-rested individuals, and in sleep-deprived individuals it showed beneficial effects on wakefulness, memory, and executive functions (Repantis et al., 2010b).
- Other putative nootropics (e.g., selegiline, phosphadiylserine, atomoxetine, bupropion) have not been shown to have positive benefits on cognition in humans.

The potential harms of medications and pharmacologics also need to be considered, including bleeding and effects on the central nervous and gastrointestinal systems.

Summary

The committee did not identify evidence that nootropic compounds lead to long-term improvement or the preservation of cognition. Studies that have looked for any cognition-enhancing properties of these substances have been limited by various methodological shortcomings and the risk of bias, including the lack of a consistent and standard definition for improved cognition, a paucity of RCTs, variability in the measurement of cognitive change or improvement, the short-term scale of the follow-up, and variations in drug formulations, dosages, and duration of treatment. Some of the studies cited above were designed to evaluate other questions or conditions such as cardiovascular disease or dementia.

The studies that showed minor improvements in cognitive measures did not demonstrate clinically important changes, and their impact on cognitive functioning and daily life was less clear. In conclusion, although the situation may become clearer over time with further RCTs and larger studies, no consistent associations have yet been found. No currently available medication, either prescribed or over-the-counter, has been shown to effectively delay cognitive decline or enhance or promote cognition in healthy older adults.

Supplements

Ginko Biloba

Gingko biloba, an herbal extract used as a part of traditional Chinese medicine, is sold as a nutritional supplement (Birks and Grimley Evans, 2009). Numerous mechanisms have been proposed for its possible benefits, including antioxidant effects, mitochondrial protection, the promotion of hippocampal neurogenesis, decreasing blood viscosity, and the enhancing of microperfusion in the brain (Amieva et al., 2013).

In a prospective study of 3,612 cognitively healthy French men and women who were age 65 years and older at baseline and who were followed for 20 years, the scores of gingko users declined less than did those of non-supplement users on the MMSE (Amieva et al., 2013). By contrast, in a large RCT conducted in 3,069 Americans age 72 to 96 years, twice-daily supplementation with 120 mg of gingko did not affect the rate of change in scores on the MMSE compared with study participants receiving a placebo, over 6 years of follow-up (Snitz et al., 2009). A recent meta-analysis that examined the effects of gingko on cognition did not separately examine the subgroup without dementia or mild cognitive impairment (Tan et al., 2014). Given the current results of RCTs, gingko is not considered effective in preventing cognitive decline.

Caffeine

Coffee and tea, purportedly because of their caffeine content, are central nervous system stimulants, which increase alertness and arousal. The literature on caffeine's effects on cognition is inconsistent but has some support in both animal and human studies. In laboratory studies of older rats, 8 weeks of coffee-supplemented diets resulted in enhanced performance on psychomotor testing and on a working memory task; the most beneficial dose was equivalent to 10 cups of coffee per day (Shukitt-Hale et al., 2013). Based on further tests in which caffeine alone did not appear to explain all of the enhanced cognitive effects, the authors concluded that other bioactive compounds in coffee may play a role (Shukitt-Hale et al., 2013).

In humans, short-term studies of caffeine have demonstrated improved perceptual speed and vigilance (Childs and de Wit, 2006). In a recent laboratory study of 24 healthy older adults who were asked to perform a demanding working memory task and undergo functional magnetic resonance imaging (fMRI), the activity in the part of the brain where working memory takes places was enhanced with acute caffeine administration compared to a placebo (Haller et al., 2013).

Reviews of prospective studies have found considerable variation in their results (Arab et al., 2013; Carman et al., 2014; Vercambre et al., 2013). In a 2014 comprehensive review, 3 of 11 prospective studies and 4 of 7 cross-sectional studies found associations between caffeine intake and cognitive outcomes, with these associations being more consistent among women and for coffee consumption (Beydoun et al., 2014). Some studies found modestly reduced levels of cognitive decline associated with caffeine intake, especially coffee, while other studies showed non-significant or no associations or evidence only for coffee intake, or benefit only for women or specific exposures. For example, in the Cardiovascular Health Study (2,722 women, 2,077 men), tea and coffee intake were associated with less cognitive decline in women but not in men (Arab et al., 2011). Among 2,475 women age 65 years and older who were at high vascular risk and participated in the Women's Antioxidant Cardiovascular Study, consumption of caffeinated coffee, but not tea, cola, or chocolate intake, was associated with a slower cognitive decline, including slower declines in global cognition, verbal memory, and category fluency (Vercambre et al., 2013).

Both animal and human short-term interventional studies support the beneficial effect of caffeine on some aspects of cognition. However, the published studies do not permit conclusions about dose or duration or about whether the effects are enduring or only short term. Data on long-term benefits are only observational and inconsistent. The dose and source (e.g., coffee versus other beverages or supplements) and whether only specific populations (e.g., women) benefit are all issues that will require further research.

TRANSCRANIAL DIRECT CURRENT STIMULATION (tDCS)

Recent studies have suggested that transcranial direct current stimulation (tDCS) may improve learning and cognitive performance by modulating the excitability of cortical brain networks (Coffmann et al., 2012; Utz et al., 2010), which are assumed to be prime brain regions that support different cognitive processes. However, much remains to be learned about the process's safety and efficacy. tDCS uses a weak electric current (1–2 mA) administered through an electrode for 20 to 40 minutes (Brunoni et al., 2012).

Surface-anodal tDCS increases excitability in the cortex near the positive electrode through weak but coherent polarization of the membrane potential of radially oriented axons (Reato et al., 2010). Long-term potentiation has been proposed as a possible mechanism for the longer-term and behavior-enhancing effects of tDCS (Nitsche and Paulus, 2000). At a cognitive level, tDCS may engender learning, in part, by enhancing an individual's attention to critical stimuli and events within new tasks (Coffman et al., 2012). For example, a small study with the electrode over the right temporal parietal cortex resulted in improvement in the ability to retain object–location learning at 1 week (Floel et al., 2012). Application over the right dorsolateral prefrontal cortex was associated with increases in the proportion of performance errors that were consciously detected (Harty et al., 2014). Moreover, using a crossover sham-controlled design, tDCS administered to the left inferior frontal gyrus led to improvement in overt semantic word generation and the inducement of a more "youth-like" connectivity pattern during resting-state fMRI (Meinzer et al., 2013).

A number of theoretical and methodological issues require further study. For example, although animal studies have begun to reveal the biophysics of direct current stimulation (Bikson et al., 2004), there is still much to learn about the dependence of tDCS's effects on N-methyl-D-aspartate glutamate receptors and on long-term potentiation and depression and also about the optimal placement and size of the stimulating electrodes and current strength, as well as about alternative stimulation techniques, such as alternating current and random noise stimulation (Fertonani et al., 2011).

In summary, tDCS shows some promise for enhancing learning and selective aspects of cognition, but further testing for both safety (especially for long-term application) and efficacy is needed before tDCS can be recommended for improving cognition and before it is known which situations are appropriate for such stimulation.

MULTI-DOMAIN TRIALS

Given that some of the modifiable risk factors for cognitive decline are interrelated and that an intervention with multiple components might be more beneficial for cognitive health than one involving a single factor, multi-domain interventions are emerging as a new strategy. Of the six completed multi-domain trials described below, four have produced cognitive improvements through a combination of physical and mental activities. Two trials found that combining physical activity and cognitive training among healthy older adults was more effective at improving cognitive test scores than either intervention alone (Fabre et al., 2002; Oswald et al., 2006). Another trial examining physical activity and vitamin E supplementation found improvements in cognitive outcomes associated with physical activity but no added benefit with vitamin E (Cetin et al., 2010). Among participants in the Mental Activity and Exercise (MAX) trial, which evaluated mental and physical activity interventions, global cognitive function improved over time, but there was no difference between intervention and control groups (Barnes et al., 2013). Two other trials, one evaluating a physical and cognitive activity intervention among older adults at risk for cognitive decline (Legault et al., 2011) and the other a diet, social, and physical activity intervention among frail older adults (de Jong et al., 2001), found no effects on cognitive outcomes. Overall, findings from multi-domain trials look promising, although conclusions cannot yet be drawn regarding any additive or synergistic effects from targeting multiple factors or about which domains yield the greatest effect.

At least seven multi-domain trials have been recently completed or are currently under way, and all have included a physical activity component. Two combined cognitive and physical activity (Gates et al., 2011; O'Dwyer et al., 2007), while another is evaluating aerobic versus resistance exercise alone or in combination with a diet intervention (Kouki et al., 2012). Another trial among frail older adults is examining the benefits of omega-3 supplementation alone or in combination with physical activity, cognitive training, and social activities (University Hospital Toulouse, 2014), and two trials involve behavioral interventions targeting mental activity and lifestyle factors related to cognitive health such as nutrition, physical and social activities, and vascular risk factors (HealthPartners Institute for Education and Research, 2009; National Institute for Health and Welfare Finland, 2014; Ngandu et al., 2014). Yet another trial is evaluating whether an intervention targeting medication compliance, blood pressure control, diet changes, and physical activity will help prevent cognitive decline among those who have had an ischemic stroke (Brainin et al., 2013; Danube University Krems, 2012).

In summary, results from multi-domain trials appear promising. Future studies should provide greater clarity regarding which combinations of factors (and which levels, duration, and treatments) yield positive benefits for general or selective aspects of cognition.

NEXT STEPS AND RECOMMENDATIONS

This and the two preceding chapters have described strengths and limitations in the evidence base for preventing and mitigating cognitive decline and promoting cognitive health. The following recommendations offer actions that individuals and their families can take, policy and regulatory efforts that are needed, and priority areas for future research.

Take Action to Support Cognitive Health

In examining the evidence base for actions by individuals and behavior changes that could be recommended, the committee found a paucity of research that focuses on preventing cognitive decline or promoting cognitive health in individuals across the life span and in those who are not diagnosed with mild cognitive impairment or neurodegenerative diseases, such as Alzheimer's disease and other dementias. Although it is not possible to define "normal" cognitive aging because individuals vary so widely in their baseline cognition and in the way their cognitive function changes with aging, strong evidence supports several actions as having a positive impact: engaging in physical activity, monitoring medications, being aware of and preventing delirium-related cognitive changes, and reducing cardiovascular disease risk. Examples of the resources available to individuals and their families to make these changes are provided in Chapter 6. Other actions, such as getting adequate sleep, may have a positive impact on cognition, but further research is needed on non-disease-related cognitive effects and on disentangling confounding factors. At present there is a great deal of research focused on cognitive training and on games aimed at improving cognitive function. Among the issues being explored in this research are the retention of training effects and how best to transfer the gains made in gaming/training into changes in cognitive function in daily life and into related areas of cognition.

Recommendation 3: *Take Actions to Reduce Risks of Cognitive Decline with Aging*
Individuals of all ages and their families should take actions to maintain and sustain their cognitive health, realizing that there is wide variability in cognitive health among individuals.

Specifically, individuals should:
- Be physically active.
- Reduce and manage cardiovascular disease risk factors (including hypertension, diabetes, smoking).
- Regularly discuss and review health conditions and medications that might influence cognitive health with a health care professional.
- Take additional actions that may promote cognitive health, including
  - Be socially and intellectually engaged, and engage in lifelong learning;
  - Get adequate sleep and receive treatment for sleep disorders if needed;

- Take steps to avoid the risk of cognitive changes due to delirium if hospitalized; and
- Carefully evaluate products advertised to consumers to improve cognitive health, such as medications, nutritionals, and cognitive training.

Increase Research on Risk and Protective Factors and Interventions

As noted throughout the chapters, much remains to be learned about the relationship between lifestyle and risk factors and the maintenance of cognitive health throughout the adult life span. While many studies have examined dementia-based outcomes, few have examined non-dementia-related cognitive changes. For some risk factors, there are few high-quality studies examining cognitive aging, including population-based longitudinal studies and RCTs of risk factor modification. Many studies do not include sufficient numbers of older adults for valid inferences. In addition, studies are needed that consider the effects of multiple risk factors and multimorbidity, in order to better understand the cumulative contributions of different risk factors and the impact of risk factor reduction.

The assessment of cognitive function is a particular challenge (see Chapter 2). Measurement procedures (and tasks used to measure cognition) improve over time, as does the conception of various aspects of cognition. Careful measurement of baseline cognitive function, preferably at the latent variable level, is needed, as are various measurements repeated over time. Minimizing cultural, ethnic, racial, and socioeconomic biases in the measurement of risk factors and outcomes is an additional concern.

Recommendation 4: *Increase Research on Risk and Protective Factors and Interventions to Promote Cognitive Health and Prevent or Reduce Cognitive Decline*
The National Institutes of Health, the Centers for Disease Control and Prevention, other relevant government agencies, nonprofit organizations, and research foundations should expand research on risk and protective factors for cognitive aging and on interventions aimed at preventing or reducing cognitive decline and maintaining cognitive health.
Research efforts should:
- Develop collaborative approaches between ongoing longitudinal studies across the life span that focus on cognitive aging outcomes in order to maximize the amount and comparability of data available on risk and protective factors.
- Examine risk factors and interventions in under-studied and vulnerable populations, including people 85 years and older and those with childhood or youth trauma or developmental

delay, mental illness, learning disabilities, or genetic intellectual disabilities and spanning ethnic/cultural and socioeconomic groups.
- Conduct single- and multicomponent clinical trials of promising interventions to promote cognitive health and prevent cognitive decline, testing for both cognitive status and functional outcomes.
- Assess cognitive outcomes in clinical trials that target the reduction of cardiovascular and other risk factors likely related to cognitive health.
- Explore older adults' preferences and values regarding cognitive health and aging and regarding specific cognitive interventions and training modalities.
- Identify effective approaches to sustaining behavior changes that promote healthy cognition across the life span.

Policies and Regulatory Review for Cognition-Related Products

Health-related products and the advertising of those products are subject to the guidelines and regulations of the Food and Drug Administration (FDA) and the Federal Trade Commission (FTC). FDA has the responsibility to assure the safety, effectiveness, quality, and security of drugs and medical devices and the safety and security of dietary supplements (FDA, 2014), and FTC acts to prevent "unfair, deceptive or fraudulent practices in the marketplace" (FTC, 2015). Among its responsibilities, FTC has authority to examine claims of deceptive advertising. Depending on the category of the product, federal agencies have a range of tools for regulation and review. For instance, when manufacturers wish to shift a medication from a prescription drug to an over-the-counter (OTC) medicine, FDA follows a process of evaluating safety data that will result in a product gaining or failing to gain OTC status (FDA, 2011). FDA also has the authority to review new evidence regarding the safety and side effects of medications and can consider a number of remedies in the face of newly documented risks. Depending on the severity of the risk, appropriate regulatory measures could include required changes to product labeling, such as a specific warning of a side effect. More drastic measures might include a shift from OTC status to prescription use only or an outright ban on sales of the product. As discussed in Chapter 4B, antihistamines, sedatives, and other medications that have strong anticholinergic activity, many of which are sold over the counter, have the potential to impair cognition. Although giving OTC status to popular medicines has many advantages for consumers, those advantages disappear if a medication's risks are substantial. The risks for older consumers of the OTC products listed above indicate that additional consumer protections may be warranted. A reexamination of product labels and OTC status could focus on the cognitive effects of these products for older adults and include a comprehensive review of currently available data regarding adverse events.

For products that claim to enhance cognitive function or to maintain current levels of function (including cognitive training products, nutriceuticals, supplements, or medications), a review of policies and regulatory guidance is needed. In 1994 the passage of the Dietary Supplement Health and Education Act[1] required that dietary supplements be regulated like foods, not drugs, which denied FDA the authority to require safety and efficacy data before marketing. Consumers may believe that dietary supplements are safe because they are "natural" products; however, manufacturers of dietary supplements are not required to list risks and side effects on their packaging, and some supplements (for instance, the now-banned ephedra), have substantial risks. FDA can remove clearly dangerous products from the market, but this process is neither fast nor simple. For dietary supplements, FTC and FDA have an agreement outlining the responsibilities of each agency; FDA has primary responsibility for claims on product labeling and point-of-sale materials and FTC has the lead in responsibility for claims made in media advertising (FTC, 2001).

While the regulation of dietary supplements by FDA is difficult, the potential for FDA to regulate cognitive training products is still more uncertain. FDA would have to determine that a cognitive training product meets the definition of a medical device, and that it falls within the category of devices of sufficient risk to require oversight. Devices that may pose a major health risk if they malfunction are a focus of regulatory attention. For instance, FDA plans to oversee mobile apps that perform electrocardiography (Cortez et al., 2014). Cognitive training products seem unlikely to carry the amount of risk that currently triggers FDA scrutiny.

Current FTC and FDA guidelines and regulations allow products that are not medications to make certain general statements about the function of the product but require a substantial evidence base in order to allow specific medical claims that the product is effective in treating a specific disease (FTC, 2001). For example, either a dietary supplement or a cognitive training product would be permitted to make general claims about promoting health or cognition but would not be able to say "treats or prevents dementia." The committee believes that in the area of cognition-related products and related product claims, current FTC and FDA guidelines and regulations need specific reconsideration from a regulatory and policy perspective to ensure that new information regarding adverse events for older

---

[1] Dietary Supplement Health and Education Act of 1994, Public Law 103-417, 103rd Cong., 2nd sess. (October 25, 1994).

adults is appropriately reviewed and that policies reflect the current level of estimated risk. This relates to a wide range of products, including OTC medications, dietary supplements, and cognitive training products.

Recommendation 5: *Ensure Appropriate Review, Policies, and Guidelines for Products That Affect Cognitive Function or Assert Claims Regarding Cognitive Health*
The Food and Drug Administration and the Federal Trade Commission, in conjunction with other relevant federal agencies and consumer organizations, should determine the appropriate regulatory review, policies, and guidelines for

- over-the-counter medications (such as antihistamines, sedatives, and other medications that have strong anticholinergic activity) that may affect cognitive function, and
- interventions (such as cognitive training, nutriceuticals, supplements, or medications) that do not target a disease but may assert claims about cognitive enhancement or maintaining cognitive abilities such as memory or attention.

REFERENCES

Ackerman, P. L., R. Kanfer, and C. Calderwood. 2010. Use it or lose it?: Wii brain exercise practice and reading for domain knowledge. *Psychology and Aging* 25(4):753-766.
Amieva, H., C. Meillon, C. Helmer, P. Barberger-Gateau, and J. F. Dartigues. 2013. Ginkgo biloba extract and long-term cognitive decline: A 20-year follow-up population-based study. *PLoS ONE* 8(1):e52755.
Anguera, J. A., J. Boccanfuso, J. L. Rintoul, O. Al-Hashimi, F. Faraji, J. Janowich, E. Kong, Y. Larraburo, C. Rolle, E. Johnston, and A. Gazzaley. 2013. Video game training enhances cognitive control in older adults. *Nature* 501(7465):97-101.
Arab, L., M. L. Biggs, E. S. O'Meara, W. T. Longstreth, P. K. Crane, and A. L. Fitzpatrick. 2011. Gender differences in tea, coffee, and cognitive decline in the elderly: The Cardiovascular Health Study. *Journal of Alzheimer's Disease* 27(3):553-566.
Arab, L., F. Khan, and H. Lam. 2013. Epidemiologic evidence of a relationship between tea, coffee, or caffeine consumption and cognitive decline. *Advances in Nutrition* 4(1):115-122.
Ball, K., D. B. Berch, K. F. Helmers, J. B. Jobe, M. D. Leveck, M. Marsiske, J. N. Morris, G. W. Rebok, D. M. Smith, S. L. Tennstedt, F. W. Unverzagt, and S. L. Willis. 2002. Effects of cognitive training interventions with older adults: A randomized controlled trial. *JAMA* 288(18):2271-2281.
Baltes, P. B., D. Sowarka, and R. Kliegl. 1989. Cognitive training research on fluid intelligence in old age: What can older adults achieve by themselves? *Psychology and Aging* 4(2):217-221.
Barnes, D. E., W. Santos-Modesitt, G. Poelke, A. F. Kramer, C. Castro, L. E. Middleton, and K. Yaffe. 2013. The Mental Activity and Exercise (MAX) trial: A randomized controlled trial to enhance cognitive function in older adults. *JAMA Internal Medicine* 173(9):797-804.

Basak, C., W. R. Boot, M. W. Voss, and A. F. Kramer. 2008. Can training in a real-time strategy video game attenuate cognitive decline in older adults? *Psychology and Aging* 23(4):765-777.
Belchior, P., M. Marsiske, S. M. Sisco, A. Yam, D. Bavelier, K. Ball, and W. C. Mann. 2013. Video game training to improve selective visual attention in older adults. *Computers in Human Behavior* 29(4):1318-1324.
Beydoun, M. A., H. A. Beydoun, A. A. Gamaldo, A. Teel, A. B. Zonderman, and Y. Wang. 2014. Epidemiologic studies of modifiable factors associated with cognition and dementia: Systematic review and meta-analysis. *BMC Public Health* 14:643.
Bikson, M., M. Inoue, H. Akiyama, J. K. Deans, J. E. Fox, H. Miyakawa, and J. G. Jefferys. 2004. Effects of uniform extracellular DC electric fields on excitability in rat hippocampal slices in vitro. *Journal of Physiology* 557(Pt 1):175-190.
Birks, J., and J. Grimley Evans. 2009. Ginkgo biloba for cognitive impairment and dementia. *Cochrane Database of Systematic Reviews* (1):Cd003120.
Boot, W. R., D. P. Blakely, and D. J. Simons. 2011. Do action video games improve perception and cognition? *Frontiers in Psychology* 2:226.
Boot, W. R., M. Champion, D. P. Blakely, T. Wright, D. J. Souders, and N. Charness. 2013a. Video games as a means to reduce age-related cognitive decline: Attitudes, compliance, and effectiveness. *Frontiers in Psychology* 4:31.
Boot, W. R., D. J. Simons, C. Stothart, and C. Stutts. 2013b. The pervasive problem with placebos in psychology: Why active control groups are not sufficient to rule out placebo effects. *Perspectives on Psychological Science* 8(4):445-454.
Bopp, K. L., and P. Verhaeghen. 2005. Aging and verbal memory span: A meta-analysis. *The Journals of Gerontology: Series B, Psychological Sciences and Social Sciences* 60(5):P223-233.
Brainin, M., K. Matz, M. Nemec, Y. Teuschl, A. Dachenhausen, S. Asenbaum-Nan, C. Bancher, B. Kepplinger, S. Oberndorfer, M. Pinter, P. Schnider, J. Tuomilehto, and ASPIS Study Group. 2013. Prevention of poststroke cognitive decline: ASPIS—A multicenter, randomized, observer-blind, parallel group clinical trial to evaluate multiple lifestyle interventions—Study design and baseline characteristics. *International Journal of Stroke* 10(4):627-635.
Brehmer, Y., A. Rieckmann, M. Bellander, H. Westerberg, H. Fischer, and L. Backman. 2011. Neural correlates of training-related working-memory gains in old age. *Neuroimage* 58(4):1110-1120.
Brunoni, A. R., M. A. Nitsche, N. Bolognini, M. Bikson, T. Wagner, L. Merabet, D. J. Edwards, A. Valero-Cabre, A. Rotenberg, A. Pascual-Leone, R. Ferrucci, A. Priori, P. Boggio, and F. Fregni. 2012. Clinical research with transcranial direct current stimulation (tDCS): Challenges and future directions. *Brain Stimulation* 5(3):175-195.
Bugos, J. A., W. M. Perlstein, C. S. McCrae, T. S. Brophy, and P. H. Bedenbaugh. 2007. Individualized piano instruction enhances executive functioning and working memory in older adults. *Aging and Mental Health* 11(4):464-471.
Carman, A. J., P. A. Dacks, R. F. Lane, D. W. Shineman, and H. M. Fillit. 2014. Current evidence for the use of coffee and caffeine to prevent age-related cognitive decline and Alzheimer's disease. *Journal of Nutrition, Health, and Aging* 18(4):383-392.
Cetin, E., E. C. Top, G. Sahin, Y. G. Ozkaya, H. Aydin, and F. Toraman. 2010. Effect of vitamin E supplementation with exercise on cognitive functions and total antioxidant capacity in older people. *Journal of Nutrition, Health, and Aging* 14(9):763-769.
Childs, E., and H. de Wit. 2006. Subjective, behavioral, and physiological effects of acute caffeine in light, nondependent caffeine users. *Psychopharmacology* 185(4):514-523.

Coffman, B. A., M. C. Trumbo, R. A. Flores, C. M. Garcia, A. J. van der Merwe, E. M. Wassermann, M. P. Weisend, and V. P. Clark. 2012. Impact of tDCS on performance and learning of target detection: Interaction with stimulus characteristics and experimental design. *Neuropsychologia* 50(7):1594-1602.

Cognitive Training Data. 2015. *Cognitive Training Data: An open letter.* http://www.cognitive trainingdata.org (accessed February 27, 2015).

Cortez, N. G., I. G. Cohen, and A. S. Kesselheim. 2014. FDA regulation of mobile health technologies. *New England Journal of Medicine* 371(4):372-379.

Dahlin, E., L. Nyberg, L. Backman, and A. S. Neely. 2008. Plasticity of executive functioning in young and older adults: Immediate training gains, transfer, and long-term maintenance. *Psychology and Aging* 23(4):720-730.

Danube University Krems. 2012. *Austrian Polyintervention Study to Prevent Cognitive Decline After Ischemic Stroke (ASPIS).* https://clinicaltrials.gov/ct2/show/NCT01109836 (accessed January 7, 2015).

de Jong, N., A. P. M. J. Chin, L. C. de Groot, R. A. Rutten, D. W. Swinkels, F. J. Kok, and W. A. van Staveren. 2001. Nutrient-dense foods and exercise in frail elderly: Effects on B vitamins, homocysteine, methylmalonic acid, and neuropsychological functioning. *American Journal of Clinical Nutrition* 73(2):338-346.

Fabre, C., K. Chamari, P. Mucci, J. Masse-Biron, and C. Prefaut. 2002. Improvement of cognitive function by mental and/or individualized aerobic training in healthy elderly subjects. *International Journal of Sports Medicine* 23(6):415-421.

Fairchild, J. K., L. Friedman, A. C. Rosen, and J. A. Yesavage. 2013. Which older adults maintain benefit from cognitive training? Use of signal detection methods to identify long-term treatment gains. *International Psychogeriatrics* 25(4):607-616.

Fang, Y., Z. Qiu, W. Hu, J. Yang, X. Yi, L. Huang, and S. Zhang. 2014. Effect of piracetam on the cognitive performance of patients undergoing coronary bypass surgery: A meta-analysis. *Experimental and Therapeutic Medicine* 7(2):429-434.

FDA (Food and Drug Administration). 2011. *Now available without a prescription.* http://www.fda.gov/Drugs/ResourcesForYou/Consumers/ucm143547.htm (accessed February 26, 2015).

———. 2014. *FDA fundamentals.* http://www.fda.gov/AboutFDA/Transparency/Basics/ucm 192695.htm (accessed February 26, 2015).

Fertonani, A., C. Pirulli, and C. Miniussi. 2011. Random noise stimulation improves neuroplasticity in perceptual learning. *Journal of Neuroscience* 31(43):15416-15423.

Floel, A., W. Suttorp, O. Kohl, J. Kurten, H. Lohmann, C. Breitenstein, and S. Knecht. 2012. Non-invasive brain stimulation improves object-location learning in the elderly. *Neurobiology of Aging* 33(8):1682-1689.

Froestl, W., A. Muhs, and A. Pfeifer. 2014a. Cognitive enhancers (nootropics). Part 1: Drugs interacting with receptors. Update 2014. *Journal of Alzheimer's Disease* 41(4):961-1019.

———. 2014b. Cognitive enhancers (nootropics). Part 2: Drugs interacting with enzymes. Update 2014. *Journal of Alzheimer's Disease* 42(1):1-68.

Froestl, W., A. Pfeifer, and A. Muhs. 2014c. Cognitive enhancers (nootropics). Part 3: Drugs interacting with targets other than receptors or enzymes. Disease-modifying drugs. Update 2014. *Journal of Alzheimer's Disease* 42(4):1079-1149.

FTC (Federal Trade Commission). 2001. *Dietary supplements: An advertising guide for industry.* http://www.ftc.gov/system/files/documents/plain-language/bus09-dietary-supplements-advertising-guide-industry.pdf (accessed February 26, 2015).

———. 2015. *About the FTC.* http://www.ftc.gov/about-ftc/what-we-do (accessed February 26, 2015).

Gates, N. J., M. Valenzuela, P. S. Sachdev, N. A. Singh, B. T. Baune, H. Brodaty, C. Suo, N. Jain, G. C. Wilson, Y. Wang, M. K. Baker, D. Williamson, N. Foroughi, and M. A. Fiatarone Singh. 2011. Study of Mental Activity and Regular Training (SMART) in at risk individuals: A randomised double blind, sham controlled, longitudinal trial. *BMC Geriatrics* 11:19.

Grady, D., K. Yaffe, M. Kristof, F. Lin, C. Richards, and E. Barrett-Connor. 2002. Effect of postmenopausal hormone therapy on cognitive function: The Heart and Estrogen/progestin Replacement Study. *American Journal of Medicine* 113(7):543-548.

Hale, S., N. S. Rose, J. Myerson, M. J. Strube, M. Sommers, N. Tye-Murray, and B. Spehar. 2011. The structure of working memory abilities across the adult life span. *Psychology and Aging* 26(1):92-110.

Haller, S., C. Rodriguez, D. Moser, S. Toma, J. Hofmeister, I. Sinanaj, D. Van De Ville, P. Giannakopoulos, and K. O. Lovblad. 2013. Acute caffeine administration impact on working memory-related brain activation and functional connectivity in the elderly: A BOLD and perfusion MRI study. *Neuroscience* 250:364-371.

Harty, S., I. H. Robertson, C. Miniussi, O. C. Sheehy, C. A. Devine, S. McCreery, and R. G. O'Connell. 2014. Transcranial direct current stimulation over right dorsolateral prefrontal cortex enhances error awareness in older age. *Journal of Neuroscience* 34(10):3646-3652.

HealthPartners Institute for Education and Research. 2009. *Passport to Brain Wellness in Sedentary Adults.* https://clinicaltrials.gov/ct2/show/NCT00979446 (accessed January 7, 2015).

Kattenstroth, J. C., T. Kalisch, S. Holt, M. Tegenthoff, and H. R. Dinse. 2013. Six months of dance intervention enhances postural, sensorimotor, and cognitive performance in elderly without affecting cardio-respiratory functions. *Frontiers in Aging Neuroscience* 5:5.

Kern, S., I. Skoog, S. Ostling, J. Kern, and A. Borjesson-Hanson. 2012. Does low-dose acetylsalicylic acid prevent cognitive decline in women with high cardiovascular risk? A 5-year follow-up of a non-demented population-based cohort of Swedish elderly women. *BMJ Open* 2(5).

Kouki, R., U. Schwab, T. A. Lakka, M. Hassinen, K. Savonen, P. Komulainen, B. Krachler, and R. Rauramaa. 2012. Diet, fitness and metabolic syndrome—The DR's EXTRA Study. *Nutrition, Metabolism, and Cardiovascular Diseases* 22(7):553-560.

Kramer, A. F., J. Larish, T. Weber, and L. Bardell. 1999. Training for executive control: Task coordination strategies and aging. In *Attention and Performance XVII*. Edited by D. Gopher and A. Koriat. Cambridge, MA: MIT Press. Pp. 617-652.

Legault, C., J. M. Jennings, J. A. Katula, D. Dagenbach, S. A. Gaussoin, K. M. Sink, S. R. Rapp, W. J. Rejeski, S. A. Shumaker, and M. A. Espeland. 2011. Designing clinical trials for assessing the effects of cognitive training and physical activity interventions on cognitive outcomes: The Seniors Health and Activity Research Program Pilot (SHARP-P) study, a randomized controlled trial. *BMC Geriatrics* 11:27.

Lethaby, A., E. Hogervorst, M. Richards, A. Yesufu, and K. Yaffe. 2008. Hormone replacement therapy for cognitive function in postmenopausal women. *Cochrane Database of Systematic Reviews* (1):Cd003122.

Li, S. C., F. Schmiedek, O. Huxhold, C. Rocke, J. Smith, and U. Lindenberger. 2008. Working memory plasticity in old age: Practice gain, transfer, and maintenance. *Psychology and Aging* 23(4):731-742.

Maki, P. M. 2013. Critical window hypothesis of hormone therapy and cognition: A scientific update on clinical studies. *Menopause* 20(6):695-709.

Meinzer, M., R. Lindenberg, D. Antonenko, T. Flaisch, and A. Floel. 2013. Anodal transcranial direct current stimulation temporarily reverses age-associated cognitive decline and functional brain activity changes. *Journal of Neuroscience* 33(30):12470-12478.

National Institute for Health and Welfare Finland. 2014. *Finnish Geriatric Intervention Study to Prevent Cognitive Impairment and Disability (FINGER)*. https://clinicaltrials.gov/ct2/show/NCT01041989 (accessed January 7, 2015).

Ngandu, T., J. Lehtisalo, E. Levalahti, T. Laatikainen, J. Lindstrom, M. Peltonen, A. Solomon, S. Ahtiluoto, R. Antikainen, T. Hanninen, A. Jula, F. Mangialasche, T. Paajanen, S. Pajala, R. Rauramaa, T. Strandberg, J. Tuomilehto, H. Soininen, and M. Kivipelto. 2014. Recruitment and baseline characteristics of participants in the Finnish Geriatric Intervention Study to Prevent Cognitive Impairment and Disability (FINGER)—A randomized controlled lifestyle trial. *International Journal of Environmental Research and Public Health* 11(9):9345-9360.

NIH (National Institutes of Health). 2014. *KEEPS cognitive and affective study*. http://clinicaltrials.gov/show/NCT00623311 (accessed December 5, 2014).

Nitsche, M. A., and W. Paulus. 2000. Excitability changes induced in the human motor cortex by weak transcranial direct current stimulation. *Journal of Physiology* 527(Pt 3):633-639.

Noice, H., and T. Noice. 2009. An arts intervention for older adults living in subsidized retirement homes. *Neuropsychology, Development, and Cognition. Section B, Aging, Neuropsychology and Cognition* 16(1):56-79.

———. 2013. Extending the reach of an evidence-based theatrical intervention. *Experimental Aging Research* 39(4):398-418.

Noice, T., H. Noice, and A. F. Kramer. 2014. Participatory arts for older adults: A review of benefits and challenges. *The Gerontologist* 54(5):741-753.

Nouchi, R., Y. Taki, H. Takeuchi, H. Hashizume, Y. Akitsuki, Y. Shigemune, A. Sekiguchi, Y. Kotozaki, T. Tsukiura, Y. Yomogida, and R. Kawashima. 2012. Brain training game improves executive functions and processing speed in the elderly: A randomized controlled trial. *PLoS ONE* 7(1):e29676.

O'Dwyer, S. T., N. W. Burton, N. A. Pachana, and W. J. Brown. 2007. Protocol for fit bodies, fine minds: A randomized controlled trial on the affect of exercise and cognitive training on cognitive functioning in older adults. *BMC Geriatrics* 7:23.

Oswald, W., T. Gunzelmann, R. Rupprecht, and B. Hagen. 2006. Differential effects of single versus combined cognitive and physical training with older adults: The SIMA study in a 5-year perspective. *European Journal of Ageing* 3(4):179-192.

Owen, A. M., A. Hampshire, J. A. Grahn, R. Stenton, S. Dajani, A. S. Burns, R. J. Howard, and C. G. Ballard. 2010. Putting brain training to the test. *Nature* 465(7299):775-778.

Reato, D., A. Rahman, M. Bikson, and L. C. Parra. 2010. Low-intensity electrical stimulation affects network dynamics by modulating population rate and spike timing. *Journal of Neuroscience* 30(45):15067-15079.

Rebok, G. W., K. Ball, L. T. Guey, R. N. Jones, H. Y. Kim, J. W. King, M. Marsiske, J. N. Morris, S. L. Tennstedt, F. W. Unverzagt, and S. L. Willis. 2014. Ten-year effects of the advanced cognitive training for independent and vital elderly cognitive training trial on cognition and everyday functioning in older adults. *Journal of the American Geriatrics Society* 62(1):16-24.

Repantis, D., O. Laisney, and I. Heuser. 2010a. Acetylcholinesterase inhibitors and memantine for neuroenhancement in healthy individuals: A systematic review. *Pharmacological Research* 61(6):473-481.

Repantis, D., P. Schlattmann, O. Laisney, and I. Heuser. 2010b. Modafinil and methylphenidate for neuroenhancement in healthy individuals: A systematic review. *Pharmacological Research* 62(3):187-206.

Sherwin, B. B., H. Chertkow, H. Schipper, and Z. Nasreddine. 2011. A randomized controlled trial of estrogen treatment in men with mild cognitive impairment. *Neurobiology of Aging* 32(10):1808-1817.

Shukitt-Hale, B., M. G. Miller, Y. F. Chu, B. J. Lyle, and J. A. Joseph. 2013. Coffee, but not caffeine, has positive effects on cognition and psychomotor behavior in aging. *Age (Dordrecht, Netherlands)* 35(6):2183-2192.

Smith, G. E., P. Housen, K. Yaffe, R. Ruff, R. F. Kennison, H. W. Mahncke, and E. M. Zelinski. 2009. A cognitive training program based on principles of brain plasticity: Results from the Improvement in Memory with Plasticity-based Adaptive Cognitive Training (IMPACT) study. *Journal of the American Geriatrics Society* 57(4):594-603.

Snitz, B. E., E. S. O'Meara, M. C. Carlson, A. M. Arnold, D. G. Ives, S. R. Rapp, J. Saxton, O. L. Lopez, L. O. Dunn, K. M. Sink, and S. T. DeKosky. 2009. Ginkgo biloba for preventing cognitive decline in older adults: A randomized trial. *JAMA* 302(24):2663-2670.

Stanford Center on Longevity. 2014. *A consensus on the brain training industry from the scientific community.* http://longevity3.stanford.edu/blog/2014/10/15/the-consensus-on-the-brain-training-industry-from-the-scientific-community (accessed November 24, 2014).

Tan, M. S., J. T. Yu, C. C. Tan, H. F. Wang, X. F. Meng, C. Wang, T. Jiang, X. C. Zhu, and L. Tan. 2014. Efficacy and adverse effects of ginkgo biloba for cognitive impairment and dementia: A systematic review and meta-analysis. *Journal of Alzheimer's Disease* 43(2):589-603.

University Hospital Toulouse. 2014. *Omega-3 fatty acids and/or multi-domain intervention in the prevention of age-related cognitive decline (MAPT).* https://clinicaltrials.gov/ct2/show/NCT00672685 (accessed January 7, 2015).

Utz, K. S., V. Dimova, K. Oppenlander, and G. Kerkhoff. 2010. Electrified minds: Transcranial direct current stimulation (TDCS) and galvanic vestibular stimulation (GVS) as methods of non-invasive brain stimulation in neuropsychology—A review of current data and future implications. *Neuropsychologia* 48(10):2789-2810.

van Muijden, J., G. P. Band, and B. Hommel. 2012. Online games training aging brains: Limited transfer to cognitive control functions. *Frontiers in Human Neuroscience* 6:221.

Vercambre, M. N., C. Berr, K. Ritchie, and J. H. Kang. 2013. Caffeine and cognitive decline in elderly women at high vascular risk. *Journal of Alzheimer's Disease* 35(2):413-421.

Waldstein, S. R., C. R. Wendell, S. L. Seliger, L. Ferrucci, E. J. Metter, and A. B. Zonderman. 2010. Nonsteroidal anti-inflammatory drugs, aspirin, and cognitive function in the Baltimore Longitudinal Study of Aging. *Journal of the American Geriatrics Society* 58(1):38-43.

Willis, S. L., S. L. Tennstedt, M. Marsiske, K. Ball, J. Elias, K. M. Koepke, J. N. Morris, G. W. Rebok, F. W. Unverzagt, A. M. Stoddard, and E. Wright. 2006. Long-term effects of cognitive training on everyday functional outcomes in older adults. *JAMA* 296(23):2805-2814.

Winocur, G., F. I. Craik, B. Levine, I. H. Robertson, M. A. Binns, M. Alexander, S. Black, D. Dawson, H. Palmer, T. McHugh, and D. T. Stuss. 2007. Cognitive rehabilitation in the elderly: Overview and future directions. *Journal of the International Neuropsychological Society* 13(1):166-171.

Zelinski, E. M., L. M. Spina, K. Yaffe, R. Ruff, R. F. Kennison, H. W. Mahncke, and G. E. Smith. 2011. Improvement in memory with plasticity-based adaptive cognitive training: Results of the 3-month follow-up. *Journal of the American Geriatrics Society* 59(2):258-265.

Zinke, K., M. Zeintl, A. Eschen, C. Herzog, and M. Kliegel. 2012. Potentials and limits of plasticity induced by working memory training in old-old age. *Gerontology* 58(1):79-87.

Zinke, K., M. Zeintl, N. S. Rose, J. Putzmann, A. Pydde, and M. Kliegel. 2014. Working memory training and transfer in older adults: Effects of age, baseline performance, and training gains. *Developmental Psychology* 50(1):304-315.

5

Health Care Response to Cognitive Aging

As a result of the aging of the population, older adults constitute an increasingly larger portion of the patients seen by health care professionals both in acute and ambulatory care settings. Moreover, with increased public awareness of and concern about cognitive impairment and dementia in older age, individuals and families are turning to health care professionals for information and advice about brain health. Approximately one in three American adults identifies Alzheimer's disease as the disease they fear most (MetLife Foundation and Harris Interactive Inc., 2011). An American Society on Aging-MetLife survey (ASA et al., 2006) found that a majority of American adults view having a memory checkup as being as important as having routine physical checkups; that 76 percent of women and 68 percent of men identify doctors as the best resource for information about brain fitness; and that more than 74 percent would advise a close friend or a family member who is concerned about memory to see a general practitioner. With individuals and families seeking assistance from practitioners to understand and manage cognitive aging, the health care system must be prepared to respond effectively.

This chapter focuses on the health care response to cognitive aging, including attitudes and practices of health care professionals and the health system, needs for improving the health care response through provider education and training, and opportunities for using medical visits to assess and to address cognitive aging.

ATTITUDES AND PRACTICES OF HEALTH PROFESSIONALS AND THE HEALTH SYSTEM

Despite the increasing frequency of concerns regarding memory and cognitive aging in routine care, few studies have examined physician practices and attitudes regarding advising patients about cognitive aging and reducing the risks for cognitive impairment or dementia. A survey of 1,000 primary care physicians and internists found that 40 percent of providers reported discussing issues related to preventing and reducing the risk of cognitive impairment and dementia with their adult patients (those with no known dementia) "often" or "very often" during the prior 6 months (Day et al., 2012). Approximately 20 percent reported "rarely" discussing this topic. Day and colleagues found that providers' recommendations depended on their perception of the strength of the evidence regarding cognitive health. While a slight majority (54 percent) rated the evidence for reducing cognitive impairment as "moderate" to "very strong," 39 percent rated it as "weak" or "very weak." When physicians reported giving advice about preventing or delaying cognitive impairment and dementia, their most commonly reported recommendations (reported by more than 50 percent of respondents) were be physically active, get intellectual stimulation, eat a healthy diet, be socially active, limit the use of alcohol, and attain/maintain a healthy weight.

Health care practitioners view addressing prevention and risk reduction concerning cognitive impairment and dementia in clinical practice as a challenge. As is the case with addressing prevention in routine care for other conditions, the major barriers include a lack of reimbursement and finding enough time to address both behavioral counseling and patients' more immediate health issues (Day et al., 2012; Yarnall et al., 2009). The main barriers to cognitive health counseling specifically are the perceived limited availability of scientific evidence or proven treatments in the field and the presence of inconclusive research (Day et al., 2012; Warren-Findlow et al., 2010).

A small number of studies have examined the sources of providers' information and evidence about cognitive health and aging, and their preferences for education and training. In a qualitative study that included focus groups and interviews with physicians, physician assistants, and nurse practitioners, continuing medical education (CME) was viewed as perhaps the easiest way to disseminate cognitive health information to providers (Warren-Findlow et al., 2010), CME can be offered through journals, online services, and in-person opportunities in order to reach providers in different settings. Online professional websites or services were identified by physicians, but not by non-physician participants, as a source of information.

Popular media, while recognized as having an impact on the public awareness of preventive behavior for some diseases, was not endorsed as a means for educating health care professionals (Warren-Findlow et al., 2010). In a survey, providers identified the following as important sources of information about new evidence and practice guidelines related to cognitive impairment or dementia: professional journals (42 percent), CME (17 percent), and professional websites or listservs (16.5 percent) (Day et al., 2012). Other sources endorsed infrequently included brochures and booklets, scientific meetings or conferences, information accessible by phone, popular media, and drug or pharmaceutical representatives.

IMPROVING THE HEALTH CARE RESPONSE

Several key national initiatives launched over the past decade address cognitive aging and the various health behaviors that can reduce risk (CDC and Alzheimer's Association, 2007). In addition, the research establishment has worked to produce the evidence needed to support public health and health care efforts to promote cognitive and emotional health in older adults (Hendrie et al., 2006). These efforts have emphasized the need for resources, tools, and education to aid providers in translating evidence into public health and practice. For health care providers, the primary needs include practice recommendations to guide assessment and counseling regarding cognitive aging, access to tools for evaluating cognition and advising patients regarding normal aging performance patterns, knowledge of effective interventions and recommendations for patient and family counseling, and decision aids to help identify when to refer patients for further evaluation and diagnosis or intervention. For health care systems and private and public health insurance companies there are numerous opportunities to provide educational materials and programs for older adults and family members and training for health care professionals to discuss cognitive aging and to promote cognitive health.

Education and Training for Providers in Cognitive Aging

One way to increase health care providers' preparedness for treating an aging population's cognitive health challenges is to provide formal education and training. To that end, new initiatives need to be designed and implemented aimed at increasing providers' awareness, knowledge, and skills for addressing the public's concerns regarding cognitive aging. Several health care disciplines specialize in aging and cognition (e.g., physicians, nurses, and others who specialize in geriatrics and geriatric neuropsychology), and these practitioners receive formal coursework and practice-based training in cognitive aging. However, because cognitive changes with age are a commonly identified concern among older adults, it is not just these specialists who need to have basic competencies in cognitive aging but rather the broad spectrum of professionals and disciplines working with adult and older adult populations. In addition, because cognition in later life is affected by life exposures and risk factors across the life span, efforts should be made to help practitioners serving all age groups understand potential cognitive impacts, even if little immediate harm is evident.

Several training programs and CME courses are designed to educate health care professionals in cognitive aging. For example, Eckstrom and colleagues (2008) designed a faculty CME workshop in which teaching faculty at two internal medicine training programs attended a 1-day workshop on geriatric knowledge and assessment of cognition and function. Kovacich and colleagues (2006) described a certificate program on cognitive vitality offered by the Meharry Consortium Geriatric Education Center. The program focuses on dispelling myths that dementia is a normal part of the aging process. Williams and colleagues (2007) reported on the Collaborative Centers for Research and Education in the Care of Older Adults Initiative, sponsored by John A. Hartford Foundation and administered by the Society for General Internal Medicine, which brings geriatricians and internists together to discuss the care of older adults.

In addition, a number of websites have been established as resources for improving training for health care professionals in the topics of aging populations and clinical practice. These websites include some content on cognition and aging, although it is not always the core focus. Examples include

- The Portal of Geriatrics Online Education (ADGAP, 2014), which was established on behalf of the Association of Directors of Geriatric Academic Programs, provides training modules on a broad spectrum of topics, including cognitive aging. One program related to cognitive aging is directed toward medical students, with specific learning objectives that include distinguishing between normal and abnormal aging changes in the brain, and systematic methods for assessing patients presenting with memory loss (Overbeck et al., 2014).
- Aging Q3, an initiative described by Moran and colleagues (2012), was developed to improve internal medicine residents' knowledge, skills, and clinical care capabilities relating to older adults. The training employs multiple intervention strategies—including a didactic curriculum and tools that can be accessed online, rounds, and health system interventions (e.g., electronic health record prompts)—designed to change how physicians practice. Although

cognitive aging is not a designated subject within the curriculum, cognition appears as a topic in the practice-based experience.
- Geri-EM (Melady et al., 2013) is a continuing education website begun in Ontario, Canada, that provides free information about improving care for older patients that is aimed at health care providers and interested members of the general public. By completing the website's modules, providers can earn CME credits through the College of Family Physicians of Canada, the Royal College of Physicians and Surgeons of Canada, or the American Medical Association. The website offers six modules covering medication management, trauma and falls, atypical presentations, functional assessment, end-of-life care, and cognitive impairment.

Reviewing the available literature and electronic resources reveals that a number of important steps have been taken toward designing content to increase health care professionals' awareness of and education in cognition and aging. However, the variability in the topics and scope of coverage indicates a need to identify core competencies in cognitive aging as part of the development and dissemination of educational strategies in this area.

Education and Training for Providers in Reversible Contributors to Cognitive Decline

While many medical risk factors for cognitive decline were identified in Chapter 4B, recommended interventions for most of these risk factors remain premature or uncertain at this time. However, there are two essential areas where the role of the health care professional is unequivocal; the prevention of delirium and medication monitoring. Given the high incidence of delirium, its preventable nature, and its contributions to cognitive decline (Inouye et al., 2014; see also Chapter 4B), health care professionals play a critical role in identifying patients at moderate to high risk for delirium, particularly in such high-risk clinical settings as pre-surgery, intensive care, and post-acute care. Screening for the well-established delirium risk factors and implementing delirium-prevention strategies as soon as possible after admission are important responsibilities of health care professionals caring for vulnerable older patients (Inouye et al., 2014; NICE, 2010).

A clinical guideline for delirium issued by the National Institute for Health and Care Excellence (NICE) listed risk factors for delirium, including age greater than 65 years, chronic cognitive impairment or dementia, current hip fracture, and severe illness (NICE, 2010). Other risk factors commonly cited in studies include multimorbidity, depression, cerebrovascular disease, and alcohol abuse (Inouye et al., 2014). Older adults with one or more of these risk factors at baseline should receive non-pharmacologic delirium preventive strategies, such as those outlined in the Hospital Elder Life Program (HELP, 2015a) or NICE guidelines, including cognitive reorientation, non-pharmacologic sleep enhancement, early mobilization, vision and hearing adaptations, nutrition and fluid replenishment, pain management, medication monitoring for appropriate use, adequate oxygenation, and prevention of constipation (see also Chapter 4B). In addition, these guidelines direct that, during their hospitalization, high-risk patients should receive daily cognitive screenings that assess attention and orientation (HELP, 2015b; Marcantonio et al., 2014).

Monitoring medications in older adults—and, avoiding the use of inappropriate medications—is a critical role for health care professionals, particularly primary care providers. Such medication reviews should be performed at each appointment, and especially at times of transition of care, such as post-surgery or post-hospital discharge. As noted in Chapter 4B, older individuals take an average of 14 prescription drugs per year (ASCP, 2015), which leads to a heightened risk of adverse drug reactions as well as drug–drug and drug–disease interactions. Health care professionals should regularly review their patients' comprehensive medication listings, including over-the-counter medications and herbal remedies. Assessing for any potentially inappropriate medication use is an essential task for the health care professional (AGS, 2012), particularly in the case of high-risk psychoactive medications, such as anticholinergic drugs, tricyclic antidepressants, benzodiazepines, antipsychotics, oral corticosteroids, H2 blockers, meperidine, and sedative hypnotic drugs. The involvement of a clinical pharmacist to review potential interactions is an important strategy for assuring the optimal management of more complex drug regimens.

Practice Guidelines and Core Competencies

A review of the resources necessary for minimum geriatric competencies in various health disciplines, including medicine, nursing, and social work, finds few competencies that are specific to normal cognitive aging. Some physician and nursing organizations include practice recommendations about working with older adults and about issues of cognition; however, the knowledge and skills necessary for addressing cognitive aging are often not delineated (POGOe, 2014).

The current practice guidelines and competencies that have been developed on cognition and aging can be used to inform core competencies for the broad spectrum of health care providers. Guidelines from organizations such as the American Psychological Association (APA) and the American Occupational Therapy Association (AOTA) provide standards and recommendations for conducting cognitive assessment of older adults, counseling older adults about cognitive changes, and working with older adults on functional changes associated with cognitive aging. Box 5-1 lists examples of resources for cognitive aging–related practice guidelines and competencies. Although many of the guidelines focus on dementia, they may have relevance to cognitive aging.

Core competencies should incorporate key information reflecting the current state of evidence about cognitive aging, as is reported in Chapters 4A, 4B, and 4C. In general, cognitive aging competency should include what is known about such topics as patterns of changes in cognition with

---

BOX 5-1
Examples of Practice Guidelines for Health Care Professionals Relevant to Cognitive Aging

American Association of Colleges of Nursing
- *Older Adult Care Competencies.* This briefly mentions that nursing personnel should be prepared to assess and treat cognition (among other functional domains), but it does not detail the specific knowledge or skills needed for this practice (AACN et al., 2010; Thornlow et al., 2006).

American Geriatrics Society
- *Clinical Practice Guideline for Postoperative Delirium in Older Adults* (AGS, 2014).
- *Best Practices Statement for Prevention and Treatment of Postoperative Delirium* (AGS Expert Panel, 2014).

American Occupational Therapy Association
- *Cognition, Cognitive Rehabilitation, and Occupational Performance.* This describes the scopes of practice of occupational therapy practitioners for assessing and intervening on cognition and cognitive dysfunction for the purpose of improving the performance of everyday activities. Older adults are included as one target population for such interventions (Giles et al., 2012).
- *Occupational Therapy Practice Guidelines for Productive Aging Community-Dwelling Older Adults* (Leland et al., 2012).

American Psychological Association
- *Guidelines for the Evaluation of Dementia and Age-Related Cognitive Changes.* These practice guidelines focus on assessing age-related cognitive change and dementia and include information on the rationale and applications, the domains of competence for conducting evaluations, ethical considerations, and processes and procedural issues for the conduct of evaluations (APA, 2012).

Royal Australian College of General Practitioners
- *Preventive Activities in Older Age* published in *Guidelines for Preventive Activities in General Practice, 8th Edition* (Royal Australian College of General Practitioners, 2012).

aging, risk and protective factors, implications for functioning, and assessment tools. Such competency would help move the health care system toward more effective response to cognitive aging.

Core competencies should encompass:

- The importance of cognitive health in basic medical care across all settings of care;
- The features and typical trajectories of cognitive aging, including an understanding of the differences between expected changes and those that may signal deficits related to disease and also an acknowledgment of the wide variability in changes in cognitive function over time among older adults;
- Assessment methods;
- Monitoring the effects of medications and combinations of medications on delirium and cognitive decline;
- Reversible conditions that contribute to cognitive deficits and declines, including depression, thyroid disease, and delirium;
- Interventions to minimize cognitive decline associated with medical conditions such as stroke, diabetes, head trauma, renal insufficiency, vision and hearing losses, and cardiac disease;
- Screening for delirium risk factors and implementing delirium prevention strategies for older persons in high-risk settings, such as preadmission or pre-surgery;
- Vulnerabilities associated with daily living, including driving, health care management and decision making, and financial responsibility, as well as strategies to mitigate those vulnerabilities;
- Health-promoting behaviors that may reduce the risks of cognitive decline, including exercise and social and intellectual engagement;
- Unhealthy behaviors that increase the risk of cognitive decline, such as cigarette smoking, excessive alcohol consumption, and a sedentary lifestyle;
- Evidence-based information regarding products that may be harmful or without benefit, including nutraceuticals and other interventions; and
- Perceptions, fears, and common misunderstandings about aging and cognitive decline.

The coordination of care takes on increasing importance in older individuals, particularly in the presence of cognitive aging and multimorbidity. As the older individual's needs and number of providers increase, care becomes quite complex, with multiple medications and a greater risk for fragmentation and errors. Care coordination has been identified as a priority for health care quality improvement (AHRQ, 2014; IOM, 2003).

USING MEDICAL VISITS TO ADDRESS COGNITIVE AGING

Currently, there is no consensus regarding the benefits of screening for cognitive aging in the general population of older adults. In a 2014 report, the U.S. Preventive Services Task Force (USPSTF) examined the benefits and harms of screening for cognitive impairment and concluded that, for the population of community-dwelling people over 65 years of age who are not experiencing symptoms of cognitive impairment, there is insufficient evidence to assess whether screening is helpful, and thus the task force did not issue a recommendation (Moyer, 2014). The USPSTF acknowledged that clinical decisions are needed on the individual level. Within the health care setting, which is designed to meet the needs of a diverse population of patients, there are opportunities to respond to the varying concerns of individuals and their families and to address cognitive aging through screening, diagnostic assessment, and patient education and counseling.

The Medicare Annual Wellness Visit

The Medicare Annual Wellness Visit (CMS, 2014b) was instituted in 2011 as an opportunity for preventive care that includes a provider assessment of cognitive aging. As part of a national priority on prevention included in the Affordable Care Act, all Medicare beneficiaries are eligible for this visit, which is available at no out-of-pocket cost (Koh and Sebelius, 2010). During the visit, preventive screenings are to be conducted and they are meant to result in the development of a personalized prevention plan to prevent or reduce disease and disability that is based on the individual's assessed health risk factors, including his or her medical and exposure history. A formal cognitive assessment is required for the detection of cognitive impairment. In developing a personalized prevention plan, providers are to offer feedback and educate the patient about risks, including risks for cognitive aging, when indicated. Providers can access a quick reference guide to the components of the visit and procedures (CMS, 2015).

There are limitations to the impact the Annual Wellness Visit can have in promoting cognitive aging and the early detection of cognitive impairment. In 2013, of the more than 35 million enrollees in Medicare Part B nationally, only 11 percent used the Annual Wellness Visit (CMS, 2014a). Although the detection of cognitive impairment is a required assessment component of the annual visit, no cognitive assessment procedures were specifically indicated or recommended to guide providers. Given the complexity of the issues pertaining to cognitive assessment in primary care, Cordell and colleagues (2012) conducted a review of the available tools and recommended a cognitive assessment toolkit, with provider training modules, for the Annual Wellness Visit and for other health visits. Other tools and resources are available as well (see Box 5-2). However, there have been no reports concerning the providers' awareness of, use of, or satisfaction with these cognition assessment recommendations and procedures. Moreover, data from Annual Wellness Visits have not been aggregated and reported in order to determine the cognitive status of Medicare beneficiaries seeking these preventive services or to gauge the effectiveness of the visits in addressing the cognitive aging needs of these individuals.

Resources for Cognitive Aging Assessment in Health Care

Older adults and their families frequently share with health care providers their complaints and concerns about changes in cognition and questions about whether the changes they perceive are normal or are a sign of dementia. Answering these questions requires an evaluation of the reported symptoms and the patient's cognitive performance and function to determine whether the individual's cognitive and functional patterns meet the established criteria for mild cognitive impairment or dementia. Health care professionals encounter questions of when and how to assess, which instruments to use, and when to refer the patient for a further comprehensive evaluation and workup. Box 5-2 provides some examples of resources intended to answer such questions and help equip practitioners with tools and instruments.

Cognitive Self-Assessment Tools for Use by Patients

Because the public has an interest in ascertaining cognitive functional status and dementia risk, tools and technologies are being investigated that will allow individuals to conduct cognition self-assessments to identify risk factors related to cognitive aging and to test discreet cognitive skills such as memory, and that will help guide discussions with their health care providers (e.g., Brandt et al., 2013, 2014). While self-assessment may have certain advantages, such as enabling large numbers of interested people to have easy access to cognitive evaluation, significant cautions should be kept in mind. For instance, the reliability and validity of these tests and the interpretations of their results are greatly improved when appropriately trained health care professionals administer them (AERA et al., 2014). While such cautions pertain to any cognitive testing, self-assessment may be particularly vulnerable to mishandling. Given the known potential disadvantages, cognition self-assessment products will require a great deal of research, monitoring, and long-term evaluation. Among the issues concerning self-assessment that require thorough exploration are the degree of accuracy of the self-assessment tools within and across diverse populations and groups (such as varying levels of educational achievement); the rates

BOX 5-2
Examples of Resources Addressing Cognitive Assessment Procedures and Tools for Use by Health Care Providers

Alzheimer's Association
- *Recommendations for Operationalizing the Detection of Cognitive Impairment During the Medicare Annual Wellness Visit in a Primary Care Setting* (Cordell et al., 2012). This provides a critical review of the most commonly used screening tools and assessment instruments available for determining cognitive performance and dementia risk in people age 65 years and older. It recommends an evaluation battery suitable for use during primary care visits (not limited to the Medicare Annual Wellness Visit).
- *Health Care Professionals' Cognitive Assessment Toolkit.* This provides tools and provider education for conducting a cognitive assessment during a time-limited office visit and includes patient, informant, and instructional videos for conducting the assessment (Alzheimer's Association, 2015).

American Occupational Therapy Association
- *Occupational Therapy's Role in Adult Cognitive Disorders.* It provides information on how occupational therapists can assist in the case of cognitive decline for older adults and their caregivers (AOTA, 2011).

American Psychiatric Association
- *Diagnostic and Statistical Manual of Mental Disorders, Fifth Edition* (APA, 2013). This resource lists and defines various cognitive domains and provides the tools for assessment of mild cognitive deficiencies.

American Psychological Association
- *Part III. Procedural Guidelines: Conducting Evaluations of Dementia and Age-Related Cognitive Change* (APA, 2012). These guidelines review testing principles and standards specific to conducting assessment, interpretation, and feedback related to age-related changes in cognition and dementia.

Hospital Elder Life Program
- This website provides tools to assist clinicians in screening for delirium in high-risk settings and includes instruments and step-by-step instructions (HELP, 2015a).

National Institute on Aging
- *Assessing Cognitive Impairment in Older Adults: A Quick Guide for Primary Care Physicians.* The topics include why cognitive assessment is important in older adults and when it is indicated, barriers such as the time to perform cognitive evaluations, and recommendations for assessment in primary care (NIA, 2014a).

of false positives (i.e., people whose cognitive performance does not represent abnormal change, but who are informed it is abnormal); the rates of false negatives (i.e., people whose cognitive performance does represent abnormal change, but who are informed it is normal); and the effects of the inaccurate interpretation of cognitive status on clinical, functional, and quality-of-life outcomes. Ultimately, this research will need to yield reliable, well-validated tools that aid concerned individuals and families as well as their health care providers.

Resources for Educating and Counseling Patients on Cognitive Aging

Although each medical encounter potentially is an opportunity to discuss cognitive aging and to address prevention and risk and protective factors, a survey of health care providers discussed earlier in the chapter indicates that these discussions often do not occur (Day et al., 2012). Box 5-3 gives examples of some of the resources available for patient education specifically on brain health and implications of cognitive aging on functioning and safety in older adults. To date the literature has not addressed the

---

BOX 5-3
Examples of Resources for Patient Counseling and Education About Cognitive Aging and Related Concerns

Alzheimer's Association
- *10 Early Signs and Symptoms of Alzheimer's.* This resource compares and contrasts normal age-related changes in cognition with signs of dementia; it identifies 10 warning signs of Alzheimer's disease (Alzheimer's Association, 2009).
- *Brain Health.* Patient education resources about cognitive aging and protective factors for maintaining brain health (Alzheimer's Association, 2014).

American Psychological Association
- *Older Adults' Health and Age-Related Changes: Reality Versus Myth.* This guide discusses myths and facts about age-related changes in cognition, physical health, and psychological health (APA, 2014).

National Institute on Aging
- *Talking with Your Older Patient: A Clinician's Handbook.* This handbook provides information and techniques to aid providers in counseling older adult patients and caregivers on topics including cognition concerns and problems ("Talking with Patients About Cognitive Problems") and risk reduction for unhealthy cognitive aging ("Encouraging Wellness") (NIA, 2008).

impact of provider counseling about cognitive aging on patient and family decision making, functioning, or quality of life.

One of the important roles of health care professionals is to counsel patients about safe medication use and the need to avoid long-term use of psychoactive medications, if possible, and to enable patients to monitor and report any potential cognitive side effects of the medications they use. In particular, patients need to know that episodes of acute confusion, memory loss, falls, motor vehicle accidents, and agitation may represent side effects of medications. Patients also need to know to avoid over-the-counter medications, such as antihistamines (diphenhydramine) found in allergy, sinus, and sleep (PM) formulations as much as possible because they may have important cognitive side effects that are readily overlooked. Resources for safe medication use in older adults are outlined in Chapter 6 (see Box 6-1).

In addition to the resources available to increase and improve counseling about the effects of aging on cognition, there are patient education resources aimed at teaching patients how to achieve healthy lifestyles, which can protect against poor cognitive aging. One example is the American Heart Association's Life's Simple 7® (AHA and ASA, 2014). The National Institute on Aging's Toolkit on provider and patient communication provides booklets to aid providers ("Talking with Your Older Patient: A Clinician's Handbook") and to aid patients ("Talking with Your Doctor: A Guide for Older Adults") with discussions in the health care setting. The toolkit also contains a presentation for small group learning, materials focused on memory and thinking changes with age, and recommendations for collaborative decision making (NIA, 2014b).

RECOMMENDATIONS

Recommendation 6: *Develop and Implement Core Competencies and Curricula in Cognitive Aging for Health Professionals*
The Department of Health and Human Services, the Department of Veterans Affairs, and educational, professional, and interdisciplinary associations and organizations involved in the health care of older adults (including, but not limited to, the Association of American Medical Colleges, the American Association of Colleges of Nursing, the National Association of Social Workers, the American Psychological Association, and the American Public Health Association) should develop and disseminate core competencies, curricula, and continuing education opportunities, including for primary care providers, that focus on cognitive aging as distinct from clinical cognitive syndromes and diseases, such as dementia.

Recommendation 7: *Promote Cognitive Health in Wellness and Medical Visits*

Public health agencies (including the Centers for Disease Control and Prevention and state health departments), health care systems (including the Veterans Health Administration), the Centers for Medicare & Medicaid Services (CMS), health insurance companies, health care professional schools and organizations, health care professionals, and individuals and their families should promote cognitive health in regular medical and wellness visits among people of all ages. Attention should also be given to cognitive outcomes during hospital stays and post-surgery.

Specifically, health care professionals should use patient visits to:
- identify risk factors for cognitive decline and recommend measures to minimize risk; and review patient medications, paying attention to medications known to have an impact on cognition;
- provide patients and families with information on cognitive aging (as distinct from dementia) and actions that they can take to maintain cognitive health and prevent cognitive decline; and
- encourage individuals and family members to discuss their concerns and questions regarding cognitive health.

In addition, other components of the health care system have a cognitive health promotion role:
- CMS should develop and implement demonstration projects to identify best practices for clinicians in assessing cognitive change and functional impairment and in providing appropriate counseling and prevention messages during, for example, the Medicare Annual Wellness Visit or other health care visits.
- Health care systems and private and public health insurance companies should develop evidence-based programs and materials on cognitive health across the life span.
- During and after hospital stays and post-surgery, health care providers, patients, and families should be alert to potential cognitive changes and delirium.

REFERENCES

AACN (American Association of Colleges of Nursing), The John A. Hartford Foundation Institute for Geriatric Nursing, and the National Organization of Nurse Practioner Faculties. 2010. *Adult-gerontology primary care nurse practitioner competencies.* http://www.aacn.nche.edu/geriatric-nursing/adultgeroprimcareNPcomp.pdf (accessed December 15, 2014).

ADGAP (Association of Directors of Geriatric Academic Programs). 2014. *POGOe: The Portal of Geriatrics Online Education.* http://www.pogoe.org (accessed January 27, 2015).

AERA, APA, and NCME (American Educational Research Association, American Psychological Association, and National Council on Measurement in Education). 2014. *Standards for educational and psychological testing.* Washington, DC: AERA Publications.

AGS (American Geriatrics Society). 2012. *AGS Beers criteria for potentially inappropriate medication use in older adults.* http://www.americangeriatrics.org/files/documents/beers/PrintableBeersPocketCard.pdf (accessed January 8, 2015).

———. 2014. *American Geriatrics Society clinical practice guideline for postoperative delirium in older adults.* http://geriatricscareonline.org/ProductAbstract/american-geriatrics-society-clinical-practice-guideline-for-postoperative-delirium-in-older-adults/CL018 (accessed January 29, 2015).

AGS Expert Panel on Postoperative Delirium in Older Adults. 2014. Postoperative delirium in older adults: Best practice statement from the American Geriatrics Society. *Journal of the American College of Surgeons* 220(2):136-148.

AHA and ASA (American Heart Association and American Stroke Association). 2014. *Life's simple 7: Heart health factors.* http://mylifecheck.heart.org/Multitab.aspx?NavID=3&CultureCode=en-US (accessed December 15, 2014).

AHRQ (Agency for Healthcare Research and Quality). 2014. *Care coordination.* http://www.ahrq.gov/professionals/prevention-chronic-care/improve/coordination (accessed February 13, 2015).

Alzheimer's Association. 2009. *10 early signs and symptoms of Alzheimer's.* http://www.alz.org/alzheimers_disease_10_signs_of_alzheimers.asp (accessed December 15, 2014).

———. 2014. *Brain health.* http://www.alz.org/we_can_help_brain_health_maintain_your_brain.asp (accessed December 15, 2014).

———. 2015. *Health Care Professionals and Alzheimer's.* http://www.alz.org/health-care-professionals/cognitive-tests-patient-assessment.asp (accessed February 2, 2015).

AOTA (American Occupational Therapy Association). 2011. *Occupational therapy's role in adult cognitive disorders.* http://www.aota.org/-/media/Corporate/Files/AboutOT/Professionals/WhatIsOT/PA/Facts/Cognition%20fact%20sheet.pdf (accessed February 11, 2015).

APA (American Psychological Association). 2012. Guidelines for the evaluation of dementia and age-related cognitive change. *American Psychologist* 67(1):1-9. http://www.apa.org/practice/guidelines/dementia-age.pdf (accessed December 12, 2014).

———. 2014. *Older adults' health and age-related changes: Reality versus myth.* http://www.apa.org/pi/aging/resources/guides/older-adults.pdf (accessed December 15, 2014).

APA (American Psychiatric Association). 2013. *Diagnostic and statistical manual of mental disorders, fifth ed.* Arlington, VA: American Psychiatric Publishing.

ASA (American Society on Aging), MetLife Foundation, and Harris Interactive Inc. 2006. *Attitudes and awareness of brain health poll.* http://www.paulnussbaum.com/metlifedoc.pdf (accessed December 15, 2014).

ASCP (American Society of Consultant Pharmacists). 2015. *ASCP fact sheet.* https://www.ascp.com/articles/about-ascp/ascp-fact-sheet (accessed January 28, 2015).

Brandt, J., C. Sullivan, I. L. E. Burrell, M. Rogerson, and A. Anderson. 2013. Internet-based screening for dementia risk. *PLoS ONE* 8(2):e57476.

Brandt, J., J. Blehar, A. Anderson, and A. L. Gross. 2014. Further validation of the internet-based Dementia Risk Assessment. *Journal of Alzheimer's Disease* 41(3):937-945.

CDC (Centers for Disease Control and Prevention) and Alzheimer's Association. 2007. *The Healthy Brain Initiative: A national public health road map to maintaining cognitive health.* http://www.alz.org/national/documents/report_healthybraininitiative.pdf (accessed December 15, 2014).

CMS (Centers for Medicare & Medicaid Services). 2014a. *Beneficiaries in original Medicare utilizing free preventative services by state. January-November 2013.* http://downloads.cms.gov/files/Preventive_Services_Utilization_by_State_Jan-Nov_2013.pdf (accessed December 15, 2014).

———. 2014b. *Quick reference information: The ABCs of providing the Annual Wellness Visit (AWV).* http://www.cms.gov/Outreach-and-Education/Medicare-Learning-Network-MLN/MLNProducts/downloads/AWV_Chart_ICN905706.pdf (accessed December 15, 2014).

———. 2015. *Preventative visit and yearly wellness exam.* http://www.medicare.gov/coverage/preventive-visit-and-yearly-wellness-exams.html (accessed January 8, 2015).

Cordell, C. B., S. Borson, M. Boustani, J. Chodosh, D. Reuben, J. Verghese, W. Thies, L. B. Fried, and Medicare Detection of Cognitive Impairment Workgroup. 2012. Alzheimer's Association recommendations for operationalizing the detection of cognitive impairment during the Medicare Annual Wellness Visit in a primary care setting. *Alzheimer's and Dementia* 9(2):141-150.

Day, K. L., D. B. Friedman, J. N. Laditka, L. A. Anderson, R. Hunter, S. B. Laditka, B. Wu, L. C. McGuire, and M. C. Coy. 2012. Prevention of cognitive impairment: Physician perceptions and practices. *Journal of Applied Gerontology* 31(6):743-754.

Eckstrom, E., S. S. Desai, A. J. Hunter, E. Allen, C. E. Tanner, L. M. Lucas, C. L. Joseph, M. R. Ririe, M. N. Doak, L. L. Humphrey, and J. L. Bowen. 2008. Aiming to improve care of older adults: An innovative faculty development workshop. *Journal of General Internal Medicine* 23(7):1053-1056.

Giles, G. M., M. V. Radomski, T. Champagne, M. A. Corcoran, G. Gillen, H. M. Kuhaneck, M. T. Morrison, B. Nadeau, I. Obermeyer, J. Toglia, and T. J. Wolf. 2012. *Cognition, cognitive rehabilitation, and occupational performance.* https://www.aota.org/-/media/Corporate/Files/AboutAOTA/OfficialDocs/Statements/Cognition%20Cognitive%20Rehabilitation%20and%20Occupational%20Performance.pdf (accessed December 15, 2014).

HELP (Hospital Elder Life Program). 2015a. *Hospital Elder Life Program (HELP) for prevention of delirium.* http://www.hospitalelderlifeprogram.org (accessed January 8, 2015).

———. 2015b. *Delirium instruments.* http://www.hospitalelderlifeprogram.org/delirium-instruments (accessed January 9, 2015).

Hendrie, H. C., M. S. Albert, M. A. Butters, S. Gao, D. S. Knopman, L. J. Launer, K. Yaffe, B. N. Cuthbert, E. Edwards, and M. V. Wagster. 2006. The NIH Cognitive and Emotional Health Project (CEHP): Report of the critical evaluation study committee. *Alzheimer's and Dementia* 2(1):12-32.

Inouye, S. K., R. G. J. Westendorp, and J. S. Saczynski. 2014. Delirium in elderly people. *Lancet* 383(9920):911-922.

IOM (Institute of Medicine). 2003. *Priority areas for national action: Transforming health care quality.* Washington, DC: The National Academies Press.

Koh, H. K., and K. G. Sebelius. 2010. Promoting prevention through the Affordable Care Act. *New England Journal of Medicine* 363(14):1296-1299.

Kovacich, J., R. Garrett, and E. M. Forti. 2006. New learning programs in cognitive vitality, Alzheimer's disease, and related dementias. *Gerontology and Geriatrics Education* 26(4):47-61.

Leland, N., S. J. Elliot, and K. Johnson. 2012. *Occupational therapy practice guidelines for productive aging community-dwelling older adults.* Bethesda, MD: AOTA Press.

Marcantonio, E. R., L. H. Ngo, M. O'Connor, R. N. Jones, P. K. Crane, E. D. Metzger, and S. K. Inouye. 2014. 3D-CAM: Derivation and validation of a 3-minute diagnostic interview for CAM-defined delirium: A cross sectional diagnostic test study. *Annals of Internal Medicine* 161(8):554-561.

Melady, D., Mount Sinai Emergency Associates, and LeaderLine Studios, Inc. 2013. *Geri-EM: Personalized e-learning in geriatric emergency medicine.* http://geri-em.com (accessed January 27, 2015).

MetLife Foundation and Harris Interactive Inc. 2011. *What America thinks: MetLife Foundation Alzheimer's survey.* https://www.metlife.com/assets/cao/foundation/alzheimers-2011.pdf (accessed December 15, 2014).

Moran, W. P., J. Zapka, P. J. Iverson, Y. Zhao, M. K. Wiley, P. Pride, and K. S. Davis. 2012. Aging Q3: An initiative to improve internal medicine residents' geriatrics knowledge, skills, and clinical performance. *Academic Medicine* 87(5):635-642.

Moyer, V. A. 2014. Screening for cognitive impairment in older adults: U.S. Preventive Services Task Force recommendation statement. *Annals of Internal Medicine* 160(11):791-797.

NIA (National Institute on Aging). 2008. *Talking with your older patient: A clinician's handbook.* NIH 08-7105. http://www.nia.nih.gov/sites/default/files/talking_with_your_older_patient.pdf (accessed December 15, 2014).

———. 2014a. *Assessing cognitive impairment in older patients: A quick guide for primary care physicians.* http://www.nia.nih.gov/alzheimers/publication/assessing-cognitive-impairment-older-patients (accessed February 2, 2015).

———. 2014b. *Health and aging: Talking with your doctor presentation toolkit.* http://www.nia.nih.gov/health/publication/talking-your-doctor-presentation-toolkit (accessed December 15, 2014).

NICE (National Institute for Health and Care Excellence). 2010. *Delirium: Diagnosis, prevention and management.* https://www.nice.org.uk/guidance/cg103 (accessed January 8, 2015).

Overbeck, K., A. Chopra, P. Basehore, and R. Nagele. 2014. *Medical student curriculum: Cognitive and behavioral disorders domain.* http://www.pogoe.org/productid/21303 (accessed December 15, 2014).

POGOe (The Portal of Geriatrics Online Education). 2014. *Geriatrics competencies by specialty.* http://www.pogoe.org/geriatrics-competencies (accessed December 15, 2014).

Royal Australian College of General Practitioners. 2012. Preventive activities in older age. In *Guidelines for preventative activities in general practice, Eighth ed.* East Melbourne: Royal Australian College of General Practitioners. Pp. 28-33.

Thornlow, D. K., C. Auerhahn, and J. Stanley. 2006. A necessity not a luxury: Preparing advanced practice nurses to care for older adults. *Journal of Professional Nursing* 22(2):116-122.

Warren-Findlow, J., A. E. Price, A. K. Hochhalter, and J. N. Laditka. 2010. Primary care providers' sources and preferences for cognitive health information in the United States. *Health Promotion International* 25(4):464-473.

Williams, B. C., V. Weber, S. F. Babbott, L. M. Kirk, M. T. Heflin, E. O'Toole, M. M. Schapira, E. Eckstrom, A. Tulsky, A. M. Wolf, and S. Landefeld. 2007. Faculty development for the 21st century: Lessons from the Society of General Internal Medicine-Hartford Collaborative Centers for the Care of Older Adults. *Journal of American Geriatrics Society* 55(6):941-947.

Yarnall, K. S., T. Østbye, K. M. Krause, K. I. Pollak, M. Gradison, and J. L. Michener. 2009. Family physicians as team leaders: "Time" to share the care. *Preventing Chronic Disease* 6(2):A59. http://www.cdc.gov/pcd/issues/2009/apr/08_0023.htm (accessed December 15, 2014).

6

Community Action: Health, Financial Management, Driving, Technology, and Consumer Decisions

Cognitive aging can affect judgment in a wide variety of situations, from choosing when to make a left turn while driving a car through a busy intersection to deciding whether a new investment is a wise choice or a financial scam to determining the best way to take care of one's health. People make these kinds of decisions every day. Thus, there is a need for local and national communities to provide sound, unbiased information to those who need it; there is a need for programs to help people compensate for their cognitive changes; and there is a need for policies to protect those having trouble making decisions on their own. Many public and private organizations already make valuable contributions in these areas. This chapter provides a brief overview of these topics, includes a sample of available resources, and identifies areas in which resources need to be developed or expanded. Extra attention is given to issues surrounding financial decision making since this area is frequently not addressed in discussions about cognitive aging.

SUPPORTING AND MAINTAINING THE PUBLIC'S COGNITIVE HEALTH

As discussed in Chapter 4C and detailed in Recommendation 3, there is evidence that individuals and their families can make changes to reduce cognitive decline and promote healthy cognitive aging. Individuals vary widely in their cognitive capacity and in the extent to which these actions will affect their cognitive function. Nevertheless, the committee recommends that individuals make an effort to promote their own cognitive health and that communities—small and large, local and national—play a significant role in developing partnerships and programs to promote and sustain these changes. Community organizations, senior centers, state and local public health departments, and public–private partnerships can play a significant role in identifying and disseminating evidence-based information and best practices and developing, implementing, and evaluating programs and resources. In fact, many programs are already in place. For example, the Healthy Brain Initiative has brought together a number of partners to develop local, state, and national initiatives (Alzheimer's Association and CDC, 2013).

The three health- and behavior-related actions identified by the committee with the strongest evidence for effectiveness in positively affecting cognitive aging are

- engaging in physical activity,
- reducing cardiovascular disease risk factors, and
- managing medications effectively.

The following sections describe a number of local and national programs that support older adults making these changes in their lives. The World Health Organization has a website with information on international cities that are working to be more age-friendly (WHO, 2015). As discussed in Chapters 4A, 4B, and 4C, other actions have shown positive cognitive benefits in some studies amid other positive health outcomes.

Learning more about what interventions are successful, what other risk factors are linked to cognitive aging, and what programs are most effective will require that older adults participate in research efforts and in the evaluation of community programs. A new federal collaboration—Recruiting Older Adults into Research (ROAR) from the Administration for Community Living (ACL), the National Institute on Aging (NIA), and the Centers for Disease Control and Prevention (CDC)—is aimed at encouraging older adults to participate in research with an initial focus on studies in Alzheimer's disease and dementia (NIA, 2014c).

Engage in Physical Activity

Community support for increasing physical activity can take many forms, from offering varied and affordable physical activity classes to promoting more walkable communities with well-maintained sidewalks, safe parks, and accessible public transportation. Opportunities to provide information on or previews of physical activity programs can also be embedded in community group meetings. For example, civic or retiree groups, such as the Rotary, Kiwanis, or Lions clubs, or the National Active and

Retired Federal Employees Association, are often looking for interactive educational programs, and members may be interested in learning about community resources for physical activity and other healthy practices for cognitive aging.

In 2014, the CDC published guidelines for physical activity in older adults with a section on resources to support physical activity (CDC, 2014b). In 2007 the CDC Prevention Research Centers' Healthy Aging Research Network published *Moving Ahead*, a brief guide to develop and sustain effective community-based physical activity programs (Belza and the PRC-HAN Physical Activity Conference Planning Workgroup, 2007). Information resources available to promote physical activity in older adults include Go4Life®, an exercise and physical activity campaign from NIA (NIA, 2014a). Go4Life® helps adults age 50 years and older to keep fit and to add exercise into their daily routine. The program offers exercise instruction and success stories on its website, and it provides exercise guidebooks (available in both English and Spanish) and an exercise video that can be viewed online or delivered by mail free of charge.

SilverSneakers® is an example of a growing public–private partnership focused on encouraging and incentivizing older adults to become more physically active (Healthways, 2014). This program is offered by a private-sector company through health insurers that are part of the Medicare Supplement and Medicare Advantage programs. The health insurer, in cooperation with Medicare, agrees to pay for a gym membership for its Medicare beneficiaries to encourage and support regular physical activity and reduce the cost barriers to physical activity. Linking physical activity to health insurance highlights the importance of physical activity for improving older adult health outcomes.

Some organizations are promoting the development of senior-friendly communities by making communities more walkable and by supporting transportation alternatives to driving. For example, the National Center on Senior Transportation provides model community transportation programs (NCST, 2014). The Alzheimer's Society in the United Kingdom has a program that aims to create dementia-friendly communities, which has applicability to other community efforts aimed at responding to cognitive aging (Green and Lakey, 2013).

Reduce Cardiovascular Disease Risk Factors

The management of cardiovascular disease risk factors encompasses physical activity, healthy eating, healthy weight management, and smoking cessation. For example, the American Heart Association's (AHA's) Life's Simple 7® goals for health (AHA, 2014) are

1. Get active
2. Control cholesterol
3. Eat better
4. Manage blood pressure
5. Lose weight
6. Reduce blood sugar
7. Stop smoking

The AHA program encourages individuals to set tangible goals for improving cardiovascular health. Based on the data presented in Chapter 4B of this report, working toward these goals may help improve cognitive health.

Many community resources, programs, and opportunities are aimed at reducing cardiovascular disease risk factors. For example, the evidence-based Chronic Disease Self-Management Program for adults with chronic conditions, originally developed at Stanford University's School of Medicine, is now offered at sites around the United States (Stanford School of Medicine, 2014). The program helps people with chronic conditions learn to manage and improve their own health and has the additional benefit of reducing health care costs. Coordinated in most states through state divisions or departments of aging or public health, the program relies on a network of trained volunteer and professional leaders working through community recreation centers, senior centers, libraries, hospitals, and other locations. The RE-AIM framework (Reach, Efficacy, Adoption, Implementation, Maintenance) has also been proposed for evaluating the dissemination and diffusion of evidence-based chronic disease management and wellness and prevention programs for older adults (Glasgow et al., 1999). This framework may serve as a useful model for assessing cognitive aging programs as well. Results from a survey of 40 state aging and public health professionals showed that these stakeholders supported using the framework, although those with direct experience with RE-AIM mentioned some challenges, including the need for assistance with applying the framework (Ory et al., 2015). Examples of the many other relevant programs include the Million Hearts® program, a partnership between public and private organizations to focus on reducing the risk for heart attacks and stroke (HHS, 2014b).

Manage Medications

As described in Chapter 4B, a number of medications can have a negative effect on cognition when used alone or in combination with other medications. These effects can be temporary or long term. Organizations, such as senior centers, faith communities, and civic groups, can connect individuals and family members with evidence-based resources that include lists of medications that may affect cognition and can encourage the discussion of their use with health care providers and pharmacists (see Box 6-1).

Efforts to increase awareness and action on this issue should include changing the prescribing behaviors of health care professionals as well as helping consumers feel comfortable talking with their prescribers about the potential cognitive side effects of the medications they use. In response to the American Board of Internal Medicine's Choosing Wisely® campaign (ABIM Foundation, 2015), the American Geriatrics Society recommends against the use of benzodiazepines and other sedative hypnotics as the first choice for treating insomnia, delirium, or agitation in people 65 years or older due to the increased risk of motor vehicle accidents, falls, and hip fractures (AGS, 2012). The EMPOWER (Eliminating Medications through Patient Ownership of End Results) study found that it is possible to reduce the use of benzodiazepines in adults 65 years and older (Tannenbaum et al., 2014). Study participants were given information about the risks of using benzodiazepines, therapeutic alternatives, and a tapering protocol. The strategy encourages the older adult to gain control and take the initiative to wean off the medication or find safer substitutes. Additionally, community consultant pharmacists have a role to play in reducing the use of high-risk or potentially inappropriate medications (ASCP, 2014).

Public awareness and education about medication management is critical since older adults and their family members may notice cognitive changes that could be reversible with changes in medications. Potential adverse effects of medications are frequent topics of discussion at senior

---

BOX 6-1
Online Resources for Safe Medication Use in Older Adults

- American Geriatrics Society Beers Criteria (including public education resources) (AGS, 2012)
- American Geriatrics Society Foundation—*What to Do and What to Ask Your Healthcare Provider If a Medication You Take Is Listed in the Beers Criteria for Potentially Inappropriate Medications to Use in Older Adults* (AGS Foundation, 2014)
- CDC—*Adults and Older Adult Adverse Drug Events* (CDC, 2014c)
- FDA—*Medicines and You: A Guide for Older Adults* (FDA, 2014)
- Health in Aging—*Medications and Older Adults* (Health in Aging, 2012)
- Institute for Safe Medication Practices (ISMP, 2014)
- Institute of Medicine report *Preventing Medication Errors: Quality Chasm Series* (IOM, 2007)
- National Institute on Aging—*Safe Use of Medicines* (NIA, 2010)
- NIH Senior Health—*Taking Medications Safely* (NIH Senior Health, 2014b)

centers, senior housing communities, and older adult learning initiatives such as Osher Lifelong Learning Institutes, which is associated with universities and colleges across the United States (Bernard Osher Foundation, 2014). Needs in this area include the evaluation of medication awareness and education programs and materials.

Sustaining Behavior Changes in Habits That Promote Cognitive Health

Sustaining behavior change can be challenging. Although effective means to promote behavior maintenance receive less attention in the literature than effective means to promote behavior change (Rothman, 2000), studies with long-term follow-up have identified some factors that may be important for behavior maintenance. These factors include frequent contact, satisfaction with behavioral outcomes, realistic expectations, enjoyment of the activity, feeling responsible for positive outcomes, having social support, monitoring and coping with relapse, feeling self-efficacy, and perceiving opportunities for safe activity (Bellg, 2003; Look AHEAD Research Group and Wing, 2010; Rothman, 2000; Van Dyck et al., 2011; van Stralen et al., 2009; Wadden et al., 2011). Public health researchers and others are working to understand which incentives, programs, and supports will help individuals with transitioning a newly developed behavior to a permanent behavior. This section provides a brief discussion of ways to sustain changes in physical activity. Reducing cardiovascular risk factors and many other relevant lifestyle and health behaviors has been and continues to be the focus of efforts to sustain behavior change (see Chapters 4A and 4B).

Sustaining Behavior Changes in Physical Exercise

A 5-year follow-up study of a trial to promote exercise found that older adults who had more positive feelings toward exercise and higher self-efficacy at Year 2 of the study were more likely to still be active 3 years later (McAuley et al., 2007). People who make physical activities a habit may have greater sustained levels of activity over time (van Stralen et al., 2009). However, those with strong existing habits may be resistant to efforts to increase their level of activity (van Bree et al., 2013).

Making permanent changes to the built environment may facilitate the maintenance of physical activity over time. The Community Preventative Services Task Force (2004) recommended improving access to places for physical activity through urban design and land-use policies. The strategy of environmental and policy interventions is to increase opportunities for leisure- and transportation-related physical activities as a way of increasing the overall physical activity levels of the population. Improvements to the built environment can include creating walkways, bike paths, parks, and recreation centers or improving their usability, utility, aesthetics, accessibility, and safety (e.g., by adding lighting or crosswalks). Researchers have found positive relationships between these types of improvements to built environments and the amount of walking or cycling done by the general population (McCormack and Shiell, 2011). Studies in adults have shown that the amount of walking is correlated with safety improvements and mixed land use, and with having sidewalks, a nearby mall, or good recreation facilities, although there are fewer studies demonstrating this in older adults (Kerr et al., 2012). These authors also noted that older adults mentioned traffic control measures (e.g., traffic signals that allow enough time to cross the street at a slower gait, more frequent crosswalks, and additional stop signs) as critical issues to address (Kerr et al., 2012). Because existing infrastructures vary widely, it is important for communities to involve older adults in determining which elements of the built environment need improvement. A systematic review of programs that promote physical activity for all age groups found that creating community rail-trails was very cost-effective (Laine et al., 2014), although costs for changes to the built environment may vary from community to community, based on the existing infrastructure.

FINANCIAL DECISION MAKING

Financial decision making, including managing current financial affairs and planning for one's financial future, is an aspect of financial capacity that can be quite complex and that requires high levels of cognitive function. It reflects a balance between fluid and crystallized intelligences. In financial terms, fluid intelligence refers to the abilities to manipulate and transform financial data, while crystallized intelligence involves knowledge and experience with financial products. Older adults with declines in their fluid intelligence are more likely to experience declines in financial capacity, but these declines may be offset by greater degrees of crystallized intelligence, particularly financial knowledge and experience (Li et al., 2015). An additional but relatively understudied determinant of financial capacity is the ability to judge trustworthiness and risk, which may be processed differently as people age (Castle et al., 2012; Samanez-Larkin and Knutson, 2014).

Older adults may be vulnerable to financial fraud or abuse just at the time in their lives when substantial financial decisions and financial planning need to be made (e.g., due to the start of retirement, Social Security, or other life changes). Results from the Health and Retirement Study indicate that at least one-third of surveyed participants who were age 50 years or older lacked sufficient numeracy to understand debt risk, compound interest, inflation, or investment risk (Lusardi and Mitchell, 2011). The same authors described the concept of "financial frailty" in older adults, explaining that as people age, they understand less about key differences in defined benefit versus defined contribution or Individual Retirement Accounts for retirement income (Lusardi and Mitchell, 2013). Furthermore, in a study of 645 community-based adults without dementia, the older of these adults exhibited lower financial literacy for decision making than did the midlife adults (Boyle et al., 2013). Of note, the study authors measured financial literacy in practical terms of understanding Medicare financial options. They suggested that having diverse resources (e.g., education, memory, executive function, etc.) contributes to financial literacy, but they also suggested that as much as half of the effect of age on financial literacy is due to decrements in executive function and episodic memory (Boyle et al., 2013).

Older adults may rely more on strategies that use biases or heuristics to help them make decisions than do younger adults (Carpenter and Yoon, 2011). This poses obvious risks for financial decisions in which analysis of large amounts of complicated information may be needed. It has been suggested that providing more simple information about expected value can improve financial decision-making performance (Carpenter and Yoon, 2011). However, others have concluded that there is little evidence that additional disclosure and consumer education are by themselves sufficient to improve financial choices in the context of cognitive aging (Agarwal et al., 2009). As a result, older adults are more likely than middle-aged adults to make less-than-advantageous decisions across a range of scenarios involving financial transactions such as credit cards and mortgages—decisions that can result in increased costs to them (Agarwal et al., 2009).

In 2010 alone, victims of financial elder abuse lost an estimated $2.9 billion, which included direct loss of money and goods to legitimate businesses, scams, and family and friends, and indirect losses through medical insurance fraud (MetLife Mature Market Institute et al., 2011). Age-related changes in cognitive abilities may put older adults at risk for financial fraud or exploitation (NAPSA, 2014). The Financial Fraud Enforcement Task Force, established in 2009, defines elder fraud as "an act targeting older adults in which attempts are made to deceive with promises of goods, services, or financial benefits that do not exist, were never intended to be provided, or were misrepresented" (Financial Fraud Enforcement Task Force, 2014). It also defined financial exploitation as "the illegal or improper use of an older adult's funds or property." A self-reported survey of older adults showed that 20 percent of Americans age 65 years and older have been taken advantage of financially by means of unsuitable investments, inappropriately high fees for financial services, or blatant fraud (Investor Protection Trust, 2015). Another study found that among a sample of older adults, a subgroup showed poor performance on a measure of risk–reward processing, which was associated with poor recognition of deceptively advertised products and a greater willingness to purchase these products (Denburg et al., 2007).

Advance planning for financial decisions as a protective strategy merits the same attention as advance planning for health care decision making (Sabatino, 2011). Triebel and Marson (2012) and Widera and colleagues (2011) provided additional rationales for earlier attention to declines in financial capacity; described practical warning signs for risks of financial neglect, abuse, or exploitation; and emphasized the need to encourage planning for financial protections. According to the National Council on Aging, the top 10 financial scams targeting older adults include telemarketing, Internet scams, and sales of anti-aging products (NCOA, 2014). Strategies that address individual planning and monitoring should be accompanied by system-level strategies that allow financial institutions to identify and intervene in suspicious or concerning transactions. These include giving institutions the authority to place a short-term hold on a suspicious or unsuitable transaction to allow time for investigation and intervention, clarifying privacy laws to allow this reporting, creating a national database of those who commit financial abuse and exploitation of elders, and revising databases that record consumer complaints so that the reporting of suspected fraud or exploitation does not appear among complaints about a financial advisor or institution. In 2010, Washington State enacted a law allowing a 10-day hold on any suspicious transaction involving a vulnerable adult to allow time for investigation and possible intervention.[1] The law also includes requirements for the training of financial institution employees about the financial exploitation of vulnerable adults.[2] Furthermore, standards are needed for how to present financial information requiring a decision so that it can be understood by someone who has cognitive changes seen with aging and to verify that the consumer has made a decision that meets his or her financial means and objectives. For example, California enacted the Reverse Mortgage Elder Protection Act of 2009[3] to promote older adults making informed decisions about reverse mortgages and to ensure that those involved in the sale of reverse mortgages act in the consumer's best interest.

---

[1]Financial Exploitation of Vulnerable Adults, Washington State Legislature Revised Code of Washington (RCW) 74.34.215 c 133 § 3 (2010).
[2]Financial Exploitation of Vulnerable Adults–Training–Reporting, Washington State Legislature RCW 74.34.220 c 133 § 5 (2010).
[3]Reverse Mortgage Elder Protection Act of 2009, California State Assembly AB 329 c236 (October 11, 2009).

Programs to Increase Awareness and Education About Elder Financial Fraud and Exploitation

Many federal, local, nonprofit, and private organizations are responding to the changes in older adults' capacity to make financial decisions and to their vulnerability to financial abuse by creating programs to increase the public's awareness and access to information resources. The target audiences for these programs are not only older adults but also their families, bankers, and financial advisors. These programs alert families to red flags or signs of change in financial capacity that might indicate a need for assistance or supervision. The signs can include changes in the filing of important papers or taxes, stacks of paid and unpaid bills, uncharacteristic errors with checkbooks or tipping, or changes in investment interests (e.g., a conservative investor with a new unexplained interest in get-rich-quick schemes). These programs also can help people learn how to identify a potential scam. Furthermore, some large investment advising organizations are now routinely asking new clients for the names of proxy or surrogate decision makers. The U.S. Department of Justice and the Federal Bureau of Investigation both work to investigate and address financial crimes against older adults (DOJ, 2014; FBI, 2013), and financial fraud directed at older adults has been the subject of many congressional hearings (e.g., U.S. House of Representatives, 2013; U.S. Senate, 2003). Examples of these programs and others are listed in Box 6-2.

Many state attorneys general offices provide online resources, such as pamphlets and links, regarding fraud and financial safety. At least one state has a program that will give presentations to senior groups about crime prevention, safety, identity theft, and frauds and scams (Virginia Office of the Attorney General, 2014).

Senior Medicare Patrols are grant-funded projects that help Medicare beneficiaries and their families across the United States prevent, identify, and report errors, fraud, and abuse in their Medicare benefits (ACL, 2015). These projects provide counseling and education by working with individuals or giving presentations to groups. The projects are funded by ACL, and together they served more than 1 million people in 2013.

Next Steps: Financial Decision Making

Credible consumer financial education programs are offered through community and civic groups; retirement housing communities; faith communities; and state, regional, and county aging networks. Few of these programs have been rigorously tested or in place long enough to measure outcomes. Educational programs or materials targeting older adults may be more effective with proactive language such as "savvy saving" rather than negative or

> **BOX 6-2**
> **Examples of Federal and Community Programs to Increase Awareness and Education About Elder Financial Abuse**
>
> Federal, local, nonprofit, and commercial organizations are responding to older adults' risk of financial abuse from international and national sources, community services, and even family members. Examples include
>
> **AARP:** AARP partners with local police and sheriff's departments in many states to hold "Scam Jams," which are information sessions for older adults about financial risks and protections. The organization has a free "Fraud Watch Network" that sends alerts and news about scams, fraud, and identity theft to those who sign up for the service (AARP, 2014c).
>
> **Consumer Financial Protection Bureau (CFPB):** The Dodd-Frank Wall Street Reform and Consumer Protection Act of 2010[a] established the CFPB which has the mission of "watching out for American consumers in the market for consumer financial products and services" (CFPB, 2015a). Within the Bureau, there is an Office of Financial Protection for Older Americans. This office provides a curriculum on preventing financial exploitation of older adults, as well as guides for various agents responsible for financial caregiving of older adults (e.g., powers of attorney, court-appointed guardians, trustees, and government fiduciaries). The downloadable guides explain in lay language the responsibilities of a fiduciary (CFPB, 2015b).
>
> **Federal Trade Commission (FTC):** FTC's financial fraud campaign, "Pass It On," is a consumer education program aimed at older adults which discusses identity theft, imposter scams, charity fraud, health care scams, paying too much, and "You've won!" scams (FTC, 2014). Grounded in an empowerment message, this program encourages older adults to share what they have learned about financial fraud with their friends and family, regardless of whether they themselves have been the target of a financial scam.
>
> **Wells Fargo Investment:** Elder Client Initiatives is a program that provides information for its network of advisors to help them recognize suspicious financial decision making or possible fraud in their clients' accounts (Braswell, 2014).
>
> **Additional online resources:**
> - Consumer Federation of America: *Nation's Top Ten Consumer Complaints* (CFA, 2014)
> - Federal Bureau of Investigation (FBI): *Fraud Target: Senior Citizens* (FBI, 2014)
> - Financial Fraud Enforcement Task Force: *Protect Yourself: Elder Fraud and Financial Exploitation* (Financial Fraud Enforcement Task Force, 2014)
> - National Council on Aging: *Top 10 Scams Targeting Seniors* (NCOA, 2014)
>
> ---
> [a]Dodd-Frank Wall Street Reform and Consumer Protection Act of 2010, U.S. Congress, Dodd-Frank § 1021 (enacted July 21, 2011).

stigmatizing language such as "victim," which can imply a loss of control or independence. The challenge for most programs aimed at financial advisors or directed to consumers is that new scams and threats to financial security of older adults outpace the capacity to keep the public and financial and law enforcement professionals adequately informed. Ongoing public–private partnerships and collaborations will be essential to reach specific targeted groups and diverse communities at a sufficiently fast pace.

Education and empowerment are essential tools for addressing the challenges of cognitive aging on older adults' financial security. However, systems-level revisions are needed as well. These could include developing and disseminating approaches that compensate for the cognitive changes seen with aging by verifying that the consumer has made a decision that meets his or her financial means and objectives. These approaches should include using layperson, everyday language that considers financial literacy. Techniques, such as using interview questions to assess a person's ability to make a financial decision or solve a financial problem (e.g., Lai and Karlawish, 2007; Marson et al., 2000), could also help increase the likelihood that a consumer understands and appreciates the financial choice he or she has made.

Furthermore, financial institutions should also be able to identify and intervene in suspicious or concerning transactions. Strategies to consider include giving financial institutions the authority to place a short-term hold on a suspicious or unsuitable transaction to allow time for investigation and intervention, enacting clear privacy laws to allow this type of reporting, creating a national database of those who commit elder abuse and financial exploitation, and revising databases that record consumer complaints so that a financial advisor's or institution's reporting of suspected fraud or exploitation does not appear as a complaint about the advisor or institution.

DRIVING

Driving an automobile safely relies on several elements of cognition, such as processing speed, decision making, and multitasking. Memory, visuospatial skills, and executive functioning are also crucial (NHTSA, 2014b). Furthermore, various sensory (e.g., hearing and vision) and physical abilities (e.g., neck flexibility in turning to look to the side and behind) are needed. All of these faculties can decline in older age. On the other hand, older drivers often bring decades of driving experience and lessons learned to bear on their driving. For individuals and their families who must make decisions about when and whether to limit driving or to stop driving altogether, the weighing of the risks and benefits of age-related cognitive and physical changes on driving skills can be a difficult process.

Restricting an older person's driving affects independent living, self-esteem, and safety for older adults and the public, which only adds to the importance of communities and society as a whole addressing this issue (Connell et al., 2013; Curl et al., 2014). Drivers who were age 70 or older were more likely to be involved in two-vehicle crashes than drivers between the ages of 30 and 69 years (NHTSA, 2011). Drivers who were age 80 or older posed more risk of death to themselves and their passengers than did drivers between the ages of 40 and 70 years (Tefft, 2008). These statistics raise the question of how best to simultaneously promote both autonomy and safety for older adults. Fortunately, there is a range of community resources focused on older adult driving that offers tools, information, and support for training programs, raising awareness, and assistance in considering when to limit driving.

Defensive driving courses are available for older adults, often with hands-on practice in behind-the-wheel strategies. For example, the American Automobile Association offers a course called RoadWise Drive (AAA, 2011), while AARP offers a Smart Driver Course (AARP, 2014b). Laws in 34 states and the District of Columbia require that auto insurance companies offer discounts to those who participate in these types of classroom safety courses. Twenty-three of those states and the District of Columbia require that online classes be covered in these discounts as well. The discounts can vary by age, location, driving record, etc. (AARP, 2014a). The Insurance Institute for Highway Safety has reported that evaluating the impact of these courses is difficult because "drivers who choose to take these courses are not representative of all drivers in their age group. Typically, they have lower crash rates before taking the course than those who do not choose to take them" (IIHS, 2014). The ACTIVE study showed that those trained to enhance visual processing speed were significantly less likely to be involved in at-fault crashes (Ball et al., 2010). Researchers have also found that older adults who receive driver training using a simulator improve their scanning behavior at intersections (Romoser, 2013).

A range of driving assessment tools is available to provide older drivers and their families with feedback on driving issues and concerns. For example, the California Department of Motor Vehicles provides a 15-question online self-assessment (California DMV, 2014). The University of Florida has developed the online tool, Fitness to Drive Screening Measure (University of Florida, 2013), which helps proxy raters (caregivers, friends, or family members) or occupational therapists determine whether an older adult is potentially able to drive safely; based on the results of the screening, recommendations may be provided for further instruction or resources. Resources are also available to assist health care providers in determining driving risk. A retrospective cohort study found that a screening tool called the 4Cs could be helpful in assessing driving competence (O'Connor et al., 2010). It is an interview-based tool for health providers to identify someone who is at risk for unsafe driving by examining the individual in regard to four domains: crash history, family concerns, clinical condition, and cognitive function. Regardless of the format of the assessment tool, driving assessments should be carefully validated before they are widely disseminated to ensure that they are providing the intended benefit to driver safety (Bedard et al., 2013; Gifford, 2013; Woolnough et al., 2013).

State departments of motor vehicles, insurance companies, and community organizations often take an active role in providing information to older adults and their families and in developing safety plans focused on older adult drivers (examples in Box 6-3). Efforts at the community, state, and national levels are under way to make communities more accessible and walkable, with transportation options for older adults that do not involve driving. One research agenda for aging and transportation identified several key areas for further work: screening and assessment, remediation and rehabilitation, vehicle design and modification, technological advancements, roadway design, transitioning to not driving, and alternative transportation options (Dickerson et al., 2007). For example, Michigan has developed a Senior Mobility and Safety Action Plan with the goal of reduc-

---

BOX 6-3
Online Resources for Older Adult Driving

- AAA Foundation: *How to Help an Older Driver* (AAA Foundation, 2014)
- NHTSA:
  - *Traffic Safety Plan for Older Drivers* (NHTSA, 2014a)
  - *How to Understand and Influence Older Drivers* (NHTSA, 2013)
- NIA: *Older Drivers* (NIA, 2014b)
- NIH's Senior Health: *Older Drivers: How Aging Affects Driving* (NIH Senior Health, 2014a)
- Examples of state resources:
  - Maryland Motor Vehicle Administration: *Additional Resources* (Maryland MVA, 2014)
  - Massachusetts Registry of Motor Vehicles: *Mature Drivers* (Massachusetts RMV, 2014)
  - New York State Office for the Aging: *Understanding and Helping an Older Driver* (NYSOFA, 2014)
  - Pennsylvania Department of Transportation: *Talking with Older Drivers: A Guide for Family and Friends* (Pennsylvania DOT, 2014)
  - Vermont Department of Motor Vehicles: *Mature Drivers* (Vermont DMV, 2014)
  - Virginia Grand Driver: *Driver Safety Tips* (Virginia Grand Driver, 2014)
  - Washington Department of Licensing: *Safe Driving for Seniors* (Washington State Department of Licensing, 2014)

ing the rate and severity of road accidents for older adults (Senior Mobility Work Group, 2013). The plan includes short- and long-term objectives for research and for making driving on roadways in Michigan safer for older drivers, such as by adding back plates to traffic lights facing east-west so that lights are easier to see.

CONSUMER DECISIONS

Many consumer products are being developed and marketed in response to consumers' interest in methods to prevent, slow, or reverse cognitive aging as well as its effects on people's daily lives. The challenge for consumers—including both middle-aged adults hoping to prevent cognitive aging and older adults and their families—is to sort through product claims and identify which products or actions are evidence-based and effective and which are not.

The large number of adults from middle to older age who are concerned about losing their cognitive abilities has created a vast potential marketplace for cognition-related products. Since older adults are an increasing proportion of the U.S. and world population (see Chapter 1), this marketplace will only grow over time. The potential for a lucrative market, coupled with the steadily growing number of research findings in this area and accentuated by the cognitive vulnerabilities that may affect some older adults, makes this a particularly important area in which to have independent, authoritative sources of information and regulatory oversight. Consumers need to be able to make informed choices among products that have evidence of effectiveness. Furthermore, because many of these products are not free, the need to make informed choices becomes even more important as many older adults have fixed incomes and may not be able to afford spending their limited financial resources on products with potentially false claims of improving cognitive function.

Many groups need independent and evidence-based information: individuals and their families; professionals in the health care, public health, and long-term care areas; and senior centers, exercise facilities, and numerous other locations. Chapter 7 provides details on communication strategies that may be effective for disseminating this type of information to the appropriate audiences.

Product Evaluation Criteria

To assist consumers in evaluating product advertisements and claims, the committee recommends developing an authoritative source of information and providing criteria for product evaluation. Consumer evaluations of the wide array of cognition-related products—ranging from pharmacologics and DNA testing to games and computer applications for self-testing cognition—could be informed by clear product evaluation criteria. Knowing which questions to ask, which issues to consider, and the potential pitfalls and trade-offs of one product versus another is a good starting point for consumers trying to make well-informed decisions. Recommendation 8 (later in this chapter) calls for the development of product evaluation criteria for cognition-related products. Questions and issues that may be considered include:

- *Real-world effectiveness:* Has the product demonstrated its effectiveness for real-world tasks that are of concern to the consumer (e.g., driving safety, living independently, etc.)?
- *Research quality:* Has the product been evaluated by comparing an experimental group with a control group, both of which have individuals with the same expectations of cognitive benefit?
- *Length of effectiveness:* Does the product demonstrate long-term benefits?
- *Other factors that affect the product's effectiveness:* Are there factors (e.g., age, health, motivation, general cognition ability) that moderate the benefit of the product?
- *Independent verification:* Have the benefits of the product been replicated by independent groups that do not benefit in any way (financially or otherwise) from the research findings?
- *Comparative effectiveness:* Have the benefits of the product been compared to the benefits of other products or lifestyle choices, such as physical activity, intellectual engagement, social interaction, or diet, that may impact cognitive health?

Information Gateway or Portal

An independent trusted online source of cognitive aging information is needed. Although information about cognitive aging is indeed available (as discussed throughout this report), the information is spread across numerous websites of government agencies, nonprofit organizations, research facilities, and private-sector corporations. An authoritative online gateway or portal could include evidence-based lay summaries of recent research findings in cognitive aging as well as links to resources from validated sources, advice on where to obtain additional information, and fact sheets on evaluating consumer products, understanding and using new technologies, and many additional topics. Such an information gateway would need to provide information in a clear and concise manner that meets health literacy standards. Keeping the website up to date would be of paramount importance. Furthermore, older adults without online access should in some way be able to have access to these same information resources.

Information gateways have been set up as resource tools for a variety of public health concerns. For example, the Child Welfare Information Gateway is a joint effort of the Department of Health and Human Services' Children's Bureau and the Administration for Children and Families that offers an extensive website of resources, information, and a toll-free information phone line to help protect children (HHS, 2014a). The Environmental Protection Agency provides the Pollution Prevention Information Clearinghouse as a free information service which is focused on "reducing and eliminating industrial pollutants through technology transfer, source reduction, education and public awareness" (EPA, 2014).

Several federal agencies have websites that could serve as information gateways for cognitive aging. Examples include the CDC's Healthy Brain Initiative website (CDC, 2014a), ACL's Brain Health website (ACL, 2014), and the website of the National Institutes of Health's National Center for Complementary and Integrative Health, which is updated regularly with evidence-based reports on products and practices (NIH, 2015). The gateway should be reviewed periodically to ensure that useful information is presented in a meaningful way. An example of an appropriate review is the evaluation of the Agency for Healthcare Research and Quality's National Guidelines Clearinghouse™ (AFYA, Inc., and The Lewin Group, 2011).

TECHNOLOGY

At the same time that the number of older adults is growing rapidly, technology is becoming ubiquitous and integrated into many aspects of everyday life. Technology innovations offer both promise and potential pitfalls for cognitive aging. On the one hand, new technologies can provide older adults with ways to adapt to and compensate for cognitive changes and help them maintain their independence and active lifestyles. For example, the availability of numerous online courses on a myriad of topics increases opportunities for older adults to engage in new learning, while technologies such as e-mail and social network tools can foster social connectivity and help alleviate social isolation and loneliness. Social networking site use among older adults has increased substantially over the past few years (Zickuhr and Madden, 2012).

On the other hand, new technologies are often not intuitive to older adults, and they are complicated to use, so older adults may avoid using them or, if they do use them, they may become frustrated by the technologies. In fact, an age-related digital divide remains despite an increased uptake of technology among older adults. This divide is especially evident when looking at technology use among adults who are age 75 or older and among older adults of lower socioeconomic status (Smith, 2014). To help bridge this divide, system designers need to perceive older adults as an important user group and to consider their needs, preferences, and abilities in the design process. Strategies to ensure that older adults have "meaningful access" to technology are also needed (Sharit et al., 2009). Extensive community and private-sector resources are already focused on addressing these areas. Because technology is such a broad topic with so many applications, this report highlights just a few examples where technology may be useful to or adapted for older individuals who are experiencing cognitive changes.

Smart Homes

Environmental adaptations and "smart homes" have been developed as a way to keep older adults safer at home, maintain or enhance their independence, improve early recognition of signs of illness, and improve quality of life. Many of these interventions consist of technologies that are integrated into the home environment to assist older adults by interpreting their needs and alerting providers or family members of possible emergencies or changes in physical or mental functioning. These technologies are able to monitor mobility, daily activity patterns, and physiologic parameters such as oxygen and glucose levels. They often employ home sensors or video cameras that detect such things as motion, the opening of the refrigerator door, or the toilet flushing or that assess such things as gait or walking speed (Jacelon and Hanson, 2013; Kang et al., 2010; Rantz et al., 2013).

Studies have also begun to test portable wearable devices that can track mobility and activity (Mudge et al., 2007). These studies have not examined the use of smart homes for the enhancement or maintenance of cognitive outcomes for older adults without cognitive impairment. Although these technologies do not directly measure cognition, they do monitor other elements of health that one may be less aware of as cognition changes. To be useful, the data from the sensors need not only to be collected and monitored but also to be interpreted and used to improve outcomes. These interventions have the potential to lessen the likelihood of illness and injury and to allow older individuals to live independently longer.

Teaching Older Adults to Use Technology

Not knowing how to use technology, or having a fear of using it, could stop older adults from wanting to incorporate technology into their daily lives. Older adults are interested in using, and capable of learning to use, technology applications, but it may take them longer to learn, and they may need more support than younger adults (Czaja et al., 2013). Older Adults Technology Services (OATS) is a nonprofit organization that receives funding from corporations, foundations, and government agencies to teach and support older adults in using technology. It has technology laboratories across New York City and serves more than 20,000 people each year (OATS, 2014). Analyses have shown that OATS training increases older adults' confidence, ability, and use of technology; increases access to information, including health and medical information; and reduces social isolation (Gardner, 2010). OATS also has a pilot project to bring computer training, home Internet access, and electronic devices to minority and low-socioeconomic-status older adults in an attempt to combat the social isolation that can set in for many older adults. OATS is expanding to rural areas and adding online courses in Internet essentials as well as pilot courses on health and financial information. There are also guidelines available for design training and instructional programs for older adult learners (e.g., Czaja et al., 2013).

Improving Web Usability

While the Internet can be beneficial in terms of supporting older adults and providing a source of new learning and cognitive engagement, many websites have usability problems and are difficult to navigate. Many Internet applications can be adapted so that they are easier to use by broad and diverse groups. The World Wide Web Consortium (W3C) is an international organization that develops standards for making the Internet more accessible to all people, including those with cognitive limitations. Its membership includes government, academic, nonprofit, and commercial institutions. It has developed standards for how to make website content and the user interface easier to understand and use. Examples include increasing website readability by providing definitions for unfamiliar words and using clear language, increasing website ease of use with the consistent presentation of navigation tools and repeated components, increasing the ability to correct and avoid mistakes by being able to review submissions and receive information on correcting errors, and suggesting compatibility between browsers and across platforms to maintain stability even on an unfamiliar device. W3C has also recommended alternatives for typing, writing, and clicking through keyboard controls for mouse tasks, voice recognition, and touchscreen capabilities. It provides design recommendations, such as predictive text, for those who have difficulty remembering addresses, names, phone numbers, and so on (W3C, 2014). Furthermore, designers should take into account the credibility of information, privacy, trust, and ease of training (Czaja et al., 2012; Sharit et al., 2009).

Simple Technology

Technology does not have to be complicated or expensive to be helpful to a person with cognitive aging. Setting up a household utility account for automatic electronic bill payment may be a helpful alternative to remembering to pay bills on time. An online calendar can automatically send e-mail reminders for appointments and can be shared with family members. A global positioning system can be used while driving to prevent getting lost. These seemingly simple modifications may go a long way toward helping people maintain independence and confidence.

Technology holds great promise for aiding older adults with their daily activities, although it can be inaccessible to them due to cost or complexity. When developing new technologies to help those with cognitive aging, the end user should not be forgotten. It is important to remember those who are aging as well as their friends, families, and caregivers and to learn what they need most and what will be most useful to them (IOM and NRC, 2013), while also considering how to design devices so that they are simple to use, easy to understand, and available to those who need them.

SUMMARY

As described throughout this chapter, communities across the country have been working to improve accessibility, independence, health, and quality of life for older adults. Many positive outcomes have already been achieved, but these programs need to be expanded to reach more people, new programs need to continue to be developed, and current programs need to be evaluated to determine best practices. With the wide variety of programs and activities available to the public, there is the possibility that some programs could have unintended consequences, so program evaluation will be especially important. Positive outcomes can be reached via many mechanisms and with innovation from organizations big and small, public and private.

RECOMMENDATIONS

Recommendation 8: *Develop Consumer Product Evaluation Criteria and an Independent Information Gateway*
The Centers for Disease Control and Prevention, National Institutes of Health, and the Administration for Community Living, in conjunction with other health and consumer protection agencies, nonprofit organizations, and professional associations, should develop, test, and implement cognitive aging information resources and tools that can

help individuals and families make more informed decisions regarding cognitive health.

Specifically,
- A central, user-friendly, easily navigated website should be available to provide independent, evidence-based information and links relevant to cognitive aging, including information on the promotion of protective behaviors and links to effective programs and services. The information should be presented in a way that takes health literacy into account.
- Consumer-relevant criteria should be developed and widely disseminated to provide individuals and families with guidance on evaluating cognition-related products (e.g., cognitive training products, nutriceuticals, and medications).

Recommendation 9: *Expand Services to Better Meet the Needs of Older Adults and Their Families with Respect to Cognitive Health*
Relevant federal and state agencies (including the Administration for Community Living [ACL], the Centers for Disease Control and Prevention [CDC], the National Highway Traffic Safety Administration [NHTSA], and the Consumer Financial Protection Bureau), nonprofit organizations (such as the Financial Industry Regulatory Authority), professional associations, and relevant private-sector companies and consumer organizations should develop, expand, implement, and evaluate programs and services used by older adults relevant to cognitive aging with the goal of helping older adults avoid exploitation, optimize their independence, improve their function in daily life, and aid their decision making.

Specifically,
- Financial decision making:
  ○ The banking and financial services industries and state and federal banking and financial regulators should develop and disseminate banking and financial policies, services, and information materials that assist older adults and their families in making decisions that meet their financial means and objectives, that reduce the opportunities for unsuitable decisions, and that mitigate the harms of such decisions.
  ○ Surrogacy mechanisms, such as powers of attorney or multiparty accounts, should have appropriate safeguards to protect the interests of the older adult.
  ○ The financial services industries and relevant state and federal agencies should develop, strengthen, and implement systems approaches, best practices, training, and

laws and regulations to help verify that financial transactions are not fraudulent or the result of diminished capacity or undue influence.
- Systems should be strengthened for reporting or taking other protective actions against potential financial fraud, exploitation, or abuse to relevant enforcement and investigative officials. Laws and regulations should be revised to mitigate civil liability and professional harms resulting from such protective actions.
* Driving and transportation:
- NHTSA, states' departments of motor vehicles, and relevant professional and consumer organizations such as the American Automobile Association should expand, validate, and disseminate tools and informational materials to assist older adults in maintaining and assessing their driving skills and to assist older adults and their families in making decisions about safe driving.
- The automobile industry should expand and evaluate technologies that enhance decision making and safety for older drivers.
- State and local transportation authorities, local planning commissions, private developers, and community groups should expand efforts to develop and implement alternative transportation options to accommodate changes that occur with cognitive aging, including efforts to ensure safe and walkable communities.
* Technology:
- Technology industries should develop and adapt hardware, software, and emerging technologies to accommodate the needs of older adults that are related to cognitive aging.
- The CDC, ACL, and other relevant agencies, organizations, and private-sector companies should support evidence-based programs that educate older adults in the use of emerging technologies.
* Health information:
- Health information providers, including private-sector companies and government agencies, should ensure that their websites (including patient health portals), packaging (including medication packaging), and other consumer health information relevant to cognitive aging meet health literacy standards.

REFERENCES

AAA (American Automobile Association). 2011. *Driver improvement courses for seniors.* http://seniordriving.aaa.com/maintain-mobility-independence/driver-improvement-courses-seniors (accessed February 6, 2015).

AAA Foundation. 2014. *How to help an older driver: A guide for planning safe transportation.* https://www.aaafoundation.org/sites/default/files/ODlarge.pdf (accessed December 15, 2014).

AARP. 2014a. *Auto insurance discounts.* http://www.aarp.org/home-garden/transportation/info-05-2010/auto_insurance_discounts.html (accessed December 15, 2014).

———. 2014b. *Driver safety program.* http://www.aarp.org/home-garden/transportation/driver_safety (accessed December 15, 2014).

———. 2014c. *Fraud watch network.* http://www.aarp.org/money/scamsfraud/fraud/fraud-watch-network (accessed December 15, 2014).

ABIM (American Board of Internal Medicine) Foundation. 2015. *Choosing Wisely®.* http://www.abimfoundation.org/Initiatives/Choosing-Wisely.aspx (accessed February 11, 2015).

ACL (Administration for Community Living). 2014. *Brain health as you age: You can make a difference.* http://www.acl.gov/Get_Help/BrainHealth/Index.aspx (accessed December 15, 2014).

———. 2015. *Senior Medicare Patrol (SMP): What SMPs do.* http://www.smpresource.org/Content/What-SMPs-Do.aspx (accessed January 7, 2015).

AFYA, Inc., and The Lewin Group. 2011. *Evaluation of the National Guidelines Clearinghouse (NGC).* http://www.ahrq.gov/research/findings/final-reports/ngceval/ngcevaluation.pdf (accessed December 15, 2014).

Agarwal, S., J. Driscoll, X. Gabaix, and D. Laibson. 2009. *The age of reason: Financial decisions over the life cycle and implications for regulations.* Washington, DC: Brookings Institution. http://www.brookings.edu/~/media/Projects/BPEA/Fall%202009/2009b_bpea_agarwal.pdf (accessed March 23, 2015).

AGS (American Geriatrics Society). 2012. American Geriatrics Society updated Beers criteria for potentially inappropriate medication use in older adults. *Journal of the American Geriatrics Society* 60(4):616-631.

AGS Foundation. 2014. *What to do and what to ask your healthcare provider if a medication you take is listed in the Beers criteria for potential inappropriate medications to use in older adults.* http://www.healthinaging.org/files/documents/Medications/Beers_Criteria_Public_QandA_Feb_2012.pdf (accessed December 15, 2014).

AHA (American Heart Association). 2014. *My life check: Life's simple 7™.* http://mylifecheck.heart.org/Multitab.aspx?NavID=3&CultureCode=en-US (accessed December 10, 2014).

Alzheimer's Association and CDC (Centers for Disease Control and Prevention). 2013. *The Healthy Brain Initiative: The public health road map for state and national partnerships, 2013-2018.* Chicago, IL: Alzheimer's Association. http://www.alz.org/national/documents/report_healthybraininitiative.pdf (accessed December 15, 2014).

ASCP (American Society of Consultant Pharmacists). 2014. *What is a consultant pharmacist?* https://www.ascp.com/articles/what-consultant-pharmacist (accessed December 15, 2014).

Ball, K., J. D. Edwards, L. A. Ross, and G. McGwin, Jr. 2010. Cognitive training decreases motor vehicle collision involvement of older drivers. *Journal of the American Geriatrics Society* 58(11):2107-2113.

Bedard, M., S. Gagnon, I. Gelinas, S. Marshall, G. Naglie, M. Porter, M. Rapoport, B. Vrkljan, and B. Weaver. 2013. Failure to predict on-road results. *Canadian Family Physician* 59(7):727.

Bellg, A. J. 2003. Maintenance of health behavior change in preventive cardiology: Internalization and self-regulation of new behaviors. *Behavior Modification* 27(1):103-131.

Belza, B., and the PRC-HAN Physical Activity Conference Planning Workgroup. 2007. *Moving ahead: Strategies and tools to plan, conduct, and maintain effective community-based physical activity programs for older adults.* Atlanta, GA: Centers for Disease Control and Prevention. http://www.cdc.gov/aging/pdf/community-based_physical_activity_programs_for_older_adults.pdf (accessed March 23, 2015).

Bernard Osher Foundation. 2014. *Osher Lifelong Learning Institutes.* http://www.osherfoundation.org/index.php?olli (accessed December 10, 2014).

Boyle, P. A., L. Yu, R. S. Wilson, E. Segawa, A. S. Buchman, and D. A. Bennett. 2013. Cognitive decline impairs financial and health literacy among community-based older persons without dementia. *Psychology and Aging* 28(3):614-624.

Braswell, M. 2014. Wells Fargo gets aggressive to help advisers protect assets of elderly clients. *InvestmentNews*, May 12. http://www.investmentnews.com/article/20140512/FREE/140519994 (accessed December 15, 2014).

California DMV (Department of Motor Vehicles). 2014. *Self-assessments.* http://apps.dmv.ca.gov/about/senior/senior_self_ess.html (accessed December 15, 2014).

Carpenter, S. M., and C. Yoon. 2011. Aging and consumer decision making. *Annals of the New York Academy of Sciences* 1235:e1-e12.

Castle, E., N. I. Eisenberger, T. E. Seeman, W. G. Moons, I. A. Boggero, M. S. Grinblatt, and S. E. Taylor. 2012. Neural and behavioral bases of age differences in perceptions of trust. *Proceedings of the National Academy of Sciences of the United States of America* 109(51):20848-20852.

CDC (Centers for Disease Control and Prevention). 2014a. *Healthy Brain Initiative.* http://www.cdc.gov/aging/healthybrain (accessed December 15, 2014).

———. 2014b. *How much physical activity do older adults need?* http://www.cdc.gov/physicalactivity/everyone/guidelines/olderadults.html (accessed December 15, 2014).

———. 2014c. *Medication safety program: Adults and older adult adverse drug events.* http://www.cdc.gov/MedicationSafety/Adult_AdverseDrugEvents.html (accessed December 15, 2014).

CFA (Consumer Federation of America). 2014. *Nation's top ten consumer complaints.* http://www.consumerfed.org/news/813 (accessed December 15, 2014).

CFPB (Consumer Financial Protection Bureau). 2015a. *Creating the consumer bureau.* http://www.consumerfinance.gov/the-bureau/creatingthebureau (accessed February 6, 2015).

———. 2015b. *Financial protection for older Americans.* http://www.consumerfinance.gov/older-americans (accessed February 6, 2015).

Community Preventive Services Task Force. 2004. *Environmental and policy approaches to increase physical activity: Street-scale urban design land use policies.* http://www.thecommunityguide.org/pa/environmental-policy/streetscale.html (accessed January 12, 2015).

Connell, C. M., A. Harmon, M. R. Janevic, and L. P. Kostyniuk. 2013. Older adults' driving reduction and cessation: Perspectives of adult children. *Journal of Applied Gerontology* 32(8):975-996.

Curl, A. L., J. D. Stowe, T. M. Cooney, and C. M. Proulx. 2014. Giving up the keys: How driving cessation affects engagement in later life. *Gerontologist* 54(3):423-433.

Czaja, S. J., C. C. Lee, J. Branham, and P. Remis. 2012. OASIS connections: Results from an evaluation study. *Gerontologist* 52(5):712-721.

Czaja, S. J., J. Sharit, C. C. Lee, S. N. Nair, M. A. Hernandez, N. Arana, and S. H. Fu. 2013. Factors influencing use of an e-health website in a community sample of older adults. *Journal of the American Medical Informatics Association* 20(2):277-284.

Denburg, N. L., C. A. Cole, M. Hernandez, T. H. Yamada, D. Tranel, A. Bechara, and R. B. Wallace. 2007. The orbitofrontal cortex, real-world decision making, and normal aging. *Annals of the New York Academy of Sciences* 1121:480-498.

Dickerson, A. E., L. J. Molnar, D. W. Eby, G. Adler, M. Bedard, M. Berg-Weger, S. Classen, D. Foley, A. Horowitz, H. Kerschner, O. Page, N. M. Silverstein, L. Staplin, and L. Trujillo. 2007. Transportation and aging: A research agenda for advancing safe mobility. *Gerontologist* 47(5):578-590.
DOJ (Department of Justice). 2014. *Fraud section.* http://www.justice.gov/civil/fraud-section (accessed December 16, 2014).
EPA (Environmental Protection Agency). 2014. *Pollution Prevention Information Clearinghouse (PPIC).* http://www.epa.gov/ppic (accessed December 10, 2014).
FBI (Federal Bureau of Investigation). 2013. *The FBI's efforts to combat elder fraud.* http://www.fbi.gov/news/testimony/the-fbis-efforts-to-combat-elder-fraud (accessed December 16, 2014).
———. 2014. *Fraud target: Senior citizens.* http://www.fbi.gov/scams-safety/fraud/seniors (accessed December 15, 2014).
FDA (Food and Drug Administration). 2014. *Medicines and you: A guide for older adults.* http://www.fda.gov/Drugs/ResourcesForYou/ucm163959.htm (accessed December 15, 2014).
Financial Fraud Enforcement Task Force. 2014. *Protect yourself: Elder fraud and financial exploitation.* http://www.stopfraud.gov/protect-yourself.html (accessed November 4, 2014).
FTC (Federal Trade Commission). 2014. *Pass it on.* http://www.consumer.ftc.gov/features/feature-0030-pass-it-on (accessed December 15, 2014).
Gardner, P. J. 2010. *Older adults and OATS computer training: A social impact analysis findings report.* New York: The New York Academy of Medicine.
Gifford, R. 2013. Flawed conclusion. *Canadian Family Physician* 59(7):726-727.
Glasgow, R. E., T. M. Vogt, and S. M. Boles. 1999. Evaluating the public health impact of health promotion interventions: The RE-AIM Framework. *American Journal of Public Health* 89(9):1322-1327.
Green, G., and L. Lakey. 2013. *Building dementia-friendly communities: A priority for everyone.* Alzheimer's Society. http://www.actonalz.org/sites/default/files/documents/Dementia_friendly_communities_full_report.pdf (accessed March 23, 2015).
Health in Aging. 2012. *Medications and older adults.* http://www.healthinaging.org/medications-older-adults (accessed December 15, 2014).
Healthways. 2014. *Healthways SilverSneakers Fitness.* https://www.silversneakers.com (accessed December 10, 2014).
HHS (Department of Health and Human Services). 2014a. *Child welfare information gateway.* https://www.childwelfare.gov (accessed December 10, 2014).
———. 2014b. *Million Hearts®.* http://millionhearts.hhs.gov/index.html (accessed December 10, 2014).
IIHS (Insurance Institute for Highway Safety). 2014. *Older drivers.* http://www.iihs.org/iihs/topics/t/older-drivers/qanda (accessed December 10, 2014).
Investor Protection Trust. 2015. *IPT activities: 06.15.2010—IPT elder investor fraud survey: 1 out of 5 older Americans are financial swindle victims.* http://www.investorprotection.org/pt-activities/?fa=research (accessed February 19, 2015).
IOM (Institute of Medicine). 2007. *Preventing medication errors: Quality chasm series.* Washington, DC: The National Academies Press.
IOM and NRC (National Research Council). 2013. *Fostering independence, participation, and healthy aging through technology: Workshop summary.* Washington, DC: The National Academies Press.
ISMP (Institute for Safe Medication Practices). 2014. *Home page.* http://www.ismp.org (accessed December 15, 2014).
Jacelon, C. S., and A. Hanson. 2013. Older adults' participation in the development of smart environments: An integrated review of the literature. *Geriatric Nursing* 34(2):116-121.

Kang, H. G., D. F. Mahoney, H. Hoenig, V. A. Hirth, P. Bonato, I. Hajjar, and L. A. Lipsitz. 2010. In situ monitoring of health in older adults: Technologies and issues. *Journal of the American Geriatrics Society* 58(8):1579-1586.

Kerr, J., D. Rosenberg, and L. Frank. 2012. The role of the built environment in healthy aging: Community design, physical activity, and health among older adults. *Journal of Planning Literature* 27(1):43-60.

Lai, J. M., and J. Karlawish. 2007. Assessing the capacity to make everyday decisions: A guide for clinicians and an agenda for future research. *American Journal of Geriatric Psychiatry* 15(2):101-111.

Laine, J., V. Kuvaja-Kollner, E. Pietila, M. Koivuneva, H. Valtonen, and E. Kankaanpaa. 2014. Cost-effectiveness of population-level physical activity interventions: A systematic review. *American Journal of Health Promotion* 29(2):71-80.

Li, Y., J. Gao, A. Z. Enkavi, L. Zaval, E. U. Weber, and E. J. Johnson. 2015. Sound credit scores and financial decisions despite cognitive aging. *Proceedings of the National Academy of Sciences of the United States of America* 112(1):65-69.

Look AHEAD Research Group and R. R. Wing. 2010. Long-term effects of a lifestyle intervention on weight and cardiovascular risk factors in individuals with type 2 diabetes mellitus: Four-year results of the Look AHEAD trial. *Archives of Internal Medicine* 170(17):1566-1575.

Lusardi, A., and O. S. Mitchell. 2011. Financial literacy and planning: Implications for retirement and wellbeing. *National Bureau of Economic Research Working Paper Series*, Working Paper No. 17078. http://www.dartmouth.edu/~alusardi/Papers/Financial Literacy.pdf (accessed March 17, 2015).

———. 2013. Older adult debt and financial frailty. *University of Michigan Retirement Research Center Working Paper Series*, Working Paper No. 2013-291. http://www.mrrc.isr.umich.edu/publications/papers/pdf/wp291.pdf (accessed March 17, 2015).

Marson, D. C., S. M. Sawrie, S. Snyder, B. McInturff, T. Stalvey, A. Boothe, T. Aldridge, A. Chatterjee, and L. E. Harrell. 2000. Assessing financial capacity in patients with Alzheimer disease: A conceptual model and prototype instrument. *Archives of Neurology* 57(6):877-884.

Maryland MVA (Motor Vehicle Administration). 2014. *Additional resources.* http://www.mva.maryland.gov/safety/older/additional-resources.htm (accessed December 15, 2014).

Massachusetts RMV (Registry of Motor Vehicles). 2014. *Mature drivers.* http://www.massrmv.com/rmv/seniors (accessed December 15, 2014).

McAuley, E., K. S. Morris, R. W. Motl, L. Hu, J. F. Konopack, and S. Elavsky. 2007. Long-term follow-up of physical activity behavior in older adults. *Health Psychology* 26(3):375-380.

McCormack, G. R., and A. Shiell. 2011. In search of causality: A systematic review of the relationship between the built environment and physical activity among adults. *International Journal of Behavioral Nutrition and Physical Activity* 8:125.

MetLife Mature Market Institute, National Committee for the Prevention of Elder Abuse, and Virginia Tech. 2011. *The MetLife study of elder financial abuse: Crimes of occasion, desperation, and predation against America's elders.* New York: MetLife Mature Market Institute. https://www.metlife.com/assets/cao/mmi/publications/studies/2011/mmi-elder-financial-abuse.pdf (accessed March 17, 2015).

Mudge, S., N. S. Stott, and S. E. Walt. 2007. Criterion validity of the stepwatch activity monitor as a measure of walking activity in patients after stroke. *Archives of Physical Medicine and Rehabilitation* 88(12):1710-1715.

NAPSA (National Adult Protective Services Association). 2014. *National Adult Protective Services Association.* http://www.napsa-now.org (accessed November 4, 2014).

NCOA (National Council on Aging). 2014. *Top 10 scams targeting seniors.* http://www.ncoa.org/enhance-economic-security/economic-security-Initiative/savvy-saving-seniors/top-10-scams-targeting.html (accessed December 10, 2014).

NCST (National Center on Senior Transportation). 2014. *Your resource on senior transportation.* http://seniortransportation.net (accessed December 15, 2014).

NHTSA (National Highway Traffic and Safety Administration). 2011. *Intersection crashes among drivers in their 60s, 70s, and 80s.* http://www.nhtsa.gov/staticfiles/nti/pdf/811495.pdf (accessed February 8, 2015).

———. 2013. *How to understand and influence older drivers.* http://www.nhtsa.gov/people/injury/olddrive/UnderstandOlderDrivers (accessed December 15, 2014).

———. 2014a. *NHTSA announces new 5-year traffic safety plan and guidelines for older drivers and passengers.* http://www.nhtsa.gov/About+NHTSA/Press+Releases/NHTSA+Announces+New+5-Year+Traffic+Safety+Plan+and+Guidelines+for+Older+Drivers+and+Passengers (accessed December 15, 2014).

———. 2014b. *Physician's guide to assessing and counseling older drivers: Chapter 3: Formally assess function.* http://www.nhtsa.gov/people/injury/olddrive/olderdriversbook/pages/Chapter3.html (accessed December 10, 2014).

NIA (National Institute on Aging). 2010. *Safe use of medicines: Take your medicines the right way-each day!* http://www.nia.nih.gov/sites/default/files/_use_of_medicines_0.pdf (accessed December 15, 2014).

———. 2014a. *Go4life®.* http://go4life.nia.nih.gov (accessed December 10, 2014).

———. 2014b. *Older drivers.* http://www.nia.nih.gov/health/publication/older-drivers (accessed December 15, 2014).

———. 2014c. *Recruiting Older Adults into Research (ROAR) toolkit.* http://www.nia.nih.gov/health/publication/roar-toolkit (accessed December 10, 2014).

NIH (National Institutes of Health). 2015. *National Center for Complementary and Integrative Health.* http://nccih.nih.gov (accessed February 11, 2015).

NIH Senior Health. 2014a. *Older drivers.* http://nihseniorhealth.gov/olderdrivers/howagingaffectsdriving/01.html (accessed December 15, 2014).

———. 2014b. *Taking medicines safely.* http://nihseniorhealth.gov/takingmedicines/takingmedicinessafely/01.html (accessed December 15, 2014).

NYSOFA (New York State Office for the Aging). 2014. *Resource guide for caregivers: Understanding and helping an older driver.* http://www.aging.ny.gov/Transportation/GuideForCaregivers/2010ResourceGuideForCaregivers.pdf (accessed January 11, 2015).

OATS (Older Adults Technology Services). 2014. *Our approach.* http://oats.org/approach (accessed December 15, 2014).

O'Connor, M. G., L. R. Kapust, B. Lin, A. M. Hollis, and R. N. Jones. 2010. The 4Cs (crash history, family concerns, clinical condition, and cognitive functions): A screening tool for the evaluation of the at-risk driver. *Journal of the American Geriatrics Society* 58(6):1104-1108.

Ory, M. G., M. Altpeter, B. Belza, J. Helduser, C. Zhang, and M. L. Smith. 2015. Perceptions about community applications of RE-AIM in the promotion of evidence-based programs for older adults. *Evaluation and the Health Professions* 38(1):15-20.

Pennsylvania DOT (Department of Transportation). 2014. *Talking with older drivers: A guide for family and friends.* http://www.dmv.state.pa.us/pdotforms/misc/Pub_345.pdf (accessed January 11, 2015).

Rantz, M. J., M. Skubic, C. Abbott, C. Galambos, Y. Pak, D. K. Ho, E. E. Stone, L. Rui, J. Back, and S. J. Miller. 2013. In-home fall risk assessment and detection sensor system. *Journal of Gerontological Nursing* 39(7):18-22.

Romoser, M. R. 2013. The long-term effects of active training strategies on improving older drivers' scanning in intersections: A two-year follow-up to Romoser and Fisher (2009). *Human Factors* 55(2):278-284.

Rothman, A. J. 2000. Toward a theory-based analysis of behavioral maintenance. *Health Psychology* 19(1 Suppl):64-69.

Sabatino, C. P. 2011. Damage prevention and control for financial incapacity. *JAMA* 305(7): 707-708.

Samanez-Larkin, G. R., and B. Knutson. 2014. Reward processing and risky decision making in the aging brain. In *The neuroscience of risky decision making*, edited by V. F. Reyna and V. Zayas. Washington, DC: American Psychological Association. Pp. 123-142.

Senior Mobility Work Group. 2013. *Michigan senior mobility and safety action plan 2013-2016*. Governor's Traffic Safety Advisory Commission. http://www.michigan.gov/documents/msp/Senior_Mobilty_Action_Plan_September_2013-2_Reviewed_11-7-13_JH_439560_7.pdf (accessed March 17, 2015).

Sharit, J., S. J. Czaja, M. A. Hernandez, and S. N. Nair. 2009. The employability of older workers as teleworkers: An appraisal of issues and an empirical study. *Human Factors and Ergonomics in Manufacturing* 19(5):457-477.

Smith, A. 2014. *Older adults and technology use*. http://www.pewinternet.org/2014/04/03/older-adults-and-technology-use (accessed February 20, 2015).

Stanford School of Medicine. 2014. *Chronic Disease Self-Management Program (Better Choices, Better Health® workshop)*. http://patienteducation.stanford.edu/programs/cdsmp.html (accessed December 15, 2014).

Tannenbaum, C., P. Martin, R. Tamblyn, A. Benedetti, and S. Ahmed. 2014. Reduction of inappropriate benzodiazepine prescriptions among older adults through direct patient education: The EMPOWER cluster randomized trial. *JAMA Internal Medicine* 174(6):890-898.

Tefft, B. C. 2008. Risks older drivers pose to themselves and to other road users. *Journal of Safety Research* 39(6):577-582.

Triebel, K. L., and D. Marson. 2012. The warning signs of diminished financial capacity in older adults. *Generations* 36(2):39-45.

University of Florida. 2013. *Fitness-to-drive screening measure online*. http://ftds.phhp.ufl.edu (accessed December 10, 2014).

U.S. Congress, House of Representatives. Committee on Energy and Commerce, Subcommittee on Commerce, Manufacturing, and Trade. *Fraud on the elderly: A growing concern for a growing population*. 113th Cong. 1st Sess. May 16, 2013.

U.S. Congress, Senate. Committee on Health, Education, Labor, and Pensions, Subcommittee on Aging. *Elder justice and protection: Stopping the financial abuse*. 108th Cong. 1st Sess. October 30, 2003.

van Bree, R. J., M. M. van Stralen, C. Bolman, A. N. Mudde, H. de Vries, and L. Lechner. 2013. Habit as moderator of the intention-physical activity relationship in older adults: A longitudinal study. *Psychology & Health* 28(5):514-532.

Van Dyck, D., K. De Greef, B. Deforche, J. Ruige, C. E. Tudor-Locke, J. M. Kaufman, N. Owen, and I. De Bourdeaudhuij. 2011. Mediators of physical activity change in a behavioral modification program for type 2 diabetes patients. *International Journal of Behavioral Nutrition and Physical Activity* 8:105.

van Stralen, M. M., H. De Vries, A. N. Mudde, C. Bolman, and L. Lechner. 2009. Determinants of initiation and maintenance of physical activity among older adults: A literature review. *Health Psychology Review* 3(2):147-207.

Vermont DMV (Department of Motor Vehicles). 2014. *Mature drivers*. http://dmv.vermont.gov/licenses/mature_drivers (accessed December 15, 2014).

Virginia Grand Driver. 2014. *Driver safety tips.* http://granddriver.net/seniors/driver-safety-tips (accessed December 17, 2014).

Virginia Office of the Attorney General. 2014. *Seniors: Virginia Triad resources.* http://www.oag.state.va.us/index.php/programs-initiatives/triad-seniors (accessed December 15, 2014).

W3C (World Wide Web Consortium). 2014. *Web Accessibility Initiative: Accessibility principles.* http://www.w3.org/WAI/intro/people-use-web/principles#alternatives (accessed December 15, 2014).

Wadden, T. A., R. H. Neiberg, R. R. Wing, J. M. Clark, L. M. Delahanty, J. O. Hill, J. Krakoff, A. Otto, D. H. Ryan, and M. Z. Vitolins. 2011. Four-year weight losses in the Look AHEAD study: Factors associated with long-term success. *Obesity* 19(10):1987-1998.

Washington State Department of Licensing. 2014. *Safe driving for seniors.* http://www.dol.wa.gov/driverslicense/seniors.html (accessed December 15, 2014).

WHO (World Health Organization). 2015. *Age-friendly world: Adding life to years.* http://agefriendlyworld.org/en (accessed February 27, 2015).

Widera, E., V. Steenpass, D. Marson, and R. Sudore. 2011. Finances in the older patient with cognitive impairment: "He didn't want me to take over." *JAMA* 305(7):698-706.

Woolnough, A., D. Salim, S. C. Marshall, K. Weegar, M. M. Porter, M. J. Rapoport, M. Man-Son-Hing, M. Bedard, I. Gelinas, N. Korner-Bitensky, B. Mazer, G. Naglie, H. Tuokko, and B. Vrkljan. 2013. Determining the validity of the AMA guide: A historical cohort analysis of the assessment of driving related skills and crash rate among older drivers. *Accident Analysis and Prevention* 61:311-316.

Zickuhr, K., and M. Madden. 2012. *Older adults and internet use: For the first time, half of adults ages 65 and older are online.* Washington, DC: Pew Research Center. http://www.pewinternet.org/files/old-media/Files/Reports/2012/PIP_Older_adults_and_internet_use.pdf (accessed March 17, 2015).

7

Public Education and Key Messages

Meeting the public health goal of maintaining cognitive health requires clear and effective communication featuring accurate, up-to-date, and consistent messages that resonate with individuals and their communities. Attention needs to be paid to whether different segments of the population are exposed to relevant information, persuaded to act accordingly, and have the environmental supports in place to change and maintain behaviors that are supportive of cognitive health. Because new research findings are constantly becoming available, stakeholders also need reliable means of keeping up with this rapidly changing field.

This chapter covers what is known about public knowledge, attitudes, and beliefs about cognitive aging (as distinct from Alzheimer's disease or dementia); how the public currently receives and could receive information about cognitive aging; and effective public health messaging. The chapter concludes with key messages to be disseminated on cognitive aging and recommendations for next steps.

PUBLIC PERCEPTIONS AND BELIEFS ABOUT COGNITIVE AGING

The term "cognitive aging" is relatively new, and therefore the public is less familiar with it than with terms for brain diseases such as dementia and Alzheimer's disease. The level of awareness of Alzheimer's disease is very high. In 2006, 93 percent of Americans age 45 or older said they had heard of Alzheimer's disease (MetLife MMI and LifePlans, 2006). Public communication about cognitive aging will need to cover its definition and scope (see Chapters 1 and 2), explain how it differs from brain disease, describe the range of cognitive abilities and how they change with age (some improve, some decline), highlight the variability among individuals in cognitive changes with age, and underscore the ways in which maintaining cognitive health preserves an individual's relationships, independence, sense of autonomy, and enjoyment of favorite activities.

When trying to influence health behavior change, such as the adoption of behaviors that protect and enhance cognitive health, it is important to understand the motives that people have for their actions, their perceptions about the efficacy of the actions and their ability to perform them, and the environmental factors that support or hinder the behaviors (Ajzen, 1991; Bandura, 1986; Fisher and Fisher, 2002; Sallis et al., 2008). Past public communication campaigns aimed at preventing negative health outcomes have made an impact on middle-aged and older adults (Snyder and LaCroix, 2013), meaning that public efforts to change the behavior of middle-aged and older individuals related to cognitive aging may be more successful than such interventions at earlier ages, when people may believe the issue is less personally relevant. Understanding how middle-aged and older adults feel about cognitive health and decline is essential.

In surveys and focus groups, midlife and older adults express significant widespread fears and concerns about cognitive decline and the loss of decision-making capacity (AARP, 2012; Anderson et al., 2009; CDC, 2013; Friedman et al., 2013; Laditka et al., 2011; Price et al., 2011). Studies in 2002 and 2006 found that more than 60 percent of the adult population feared memory loss when they were older (Cutler et al., 2002; PARADE and Research!America, 2006). In 2009, 73 percent of adults over 18 years of age reported that they were concerned or very concerned "that their memory may worsen with age," a concern that was highest among women and those of middle age (Friedman et al., 2013). A substantial proportion of adults (66 percent) is also concerned about needing to take care of a loved one with Alzheimer's disease in the future, while 44 percent currently have a family member or friend with Alzheimer's disease (MetLife MMI et al., 2011). Sixty percent of people over 50 years of age would like to know their own risk of developing Alzheimer's disease someday (Roberts et al., 2014). Most people over 50 years old (89 percent in a recent survey) understand that genetics can play a role in Alzheimer's disease risk; fewer (55 percent) realize that stress can play a role in its development (Roberts et al., 2014).

A number of studies highlight older Americans' greater fear of dementia and memory loss, compared with other health and financial worries. In 2013 a YouGov survey supported by the Alzheimer's Association and the Centers for Disease Control and Prevention (CDC) found that Americans age 60 and older were more afraid of Alzheimer's disease or dementia than of cancer, heart disease, stroke, or diabetes (Alzheimer's Association, 2014). The primary reasons why people are afraid of Alzheimer's disease are forgetting family, becoming a burden to the family, and not being able to take care of oneself. Additional reasons are the fear of losing their personality and who they are, and having had experience with someone who had the disease (Alzheimer's Association, 2014). Similarly, a small nonrepresentative survey found that people over 50 years of age were more afraid of "losing my mental sharpness" than other risks, which included, in declining order, "losing my overall health," "a family member losing their overall health," "not being able to take care of myself," "running out of money," "getting a terminal illness," and "losing a spouse" (AARP, 2014).

The relatively high level of worry among older Americans about maintaining their own and their loved one's cognitive health as they age gives public education campaigns a motivator for behavior change that they should be able to tap into.

Perceptions of Actions to Maintain Cognitive Health

Surveys indicate that most members of the general public are aware of behaviors that they believe can help safeguard their cognition as they age. One survey found that 88 percent of respondents who were 42 years old or older said they believed that there was something they could do to keep their brains fit, such as doing mental challenges and eating a healthy diet (ASA and MetLife Foundation, 2006).

A large national 2010 survey that asked adults over 50 years of age about Alzheimer's disease found that most believed that keeping mentally active (93 percent), eating a healthy diet (87 percent), keeping physically active (88 percent), and taking vitamins or dietary supplements (71 percent) are very or somewhat effective in preventing the disease (Roberts et al., 2014). People who were older or were African American were more likely to endorse physical activity as a protective factor; women, African Americans, and those with lower education were more likely to endorse eating a healthy diet; and those who were 65 to 74 years old, Hispanics, African Americans, those with less education, and those who did not know anyone or who did not have a first-degree relative or spouse with Alzheimer's disease were more likely to profess a belief in taking vitamins or supplements as a preventive measure (Roberts et al., 2014).

In 2009 Friedman and colleagues (2013) added questions to a large nationally representative survey (HealthStyles Consumer Survey) that addressed beliefs about memory worsening with age, activities that may benefit abilities to think and remember, preferred sources of information, and whether health professionals had spoken to consumers about ways to "stay sharp." Adults age 18 and older agreed with statements that they could prevent or delay cognitive impairment through intellectual stimulation (87 percent), physical activity (83 percent), a healthy diet (83 percent), maintaining a healthy weight (65 percent), social involvement (64 percent), taking vitamins or supplements (64 percent), avoiding smoking (52 percent), and taking prescribed medicines (31 percent). In contrast, slightly fewer said they actually engaged in these activities and behavior: 74 percent said they engaged in intellectually stimulating activities, 72 percent in physical activity, 65 percent in a healthy diet, 55 percent in maintaining a healthy weight, 52 percent in social involvement, 61 percent in taking vitamins or supplements, 59 percent in avoiding smoking, and 38 percent in taking prescribed medicines (Friedman et al., 2013). In another survey, conducted online in 2008, 50 percent of the African Americans surveyed said they engaged in behavior aimed at maintaining brain health (Alzheimer's Association, 2008).

Misunderstandings About Cognitive Aging

Misunderstandings about cognitive aging are common. First, brain health is often seen as limited to preserving memory, perhaps because of the devastating and observable effect of Alzheimer's disease (e.g., Laditka et al., 2013). However, as discussed in Chapters 1 and 2, cognition encompasses many brain functions.

Second, people do not generally understand that aging can have both positive and negative effects on cognition. Wisdom and expertise can increase as people age. The ability to think logically and solve problems is maintained over time in healthy adults. Overall, older adults are more likely to be satisfied with their lives in general, and they report experiencing negative emotions, such as anger and worry, less often than people in young adulthood and midlife (Carstensen et al., 2011; Charles et al., 2001; Stone et al., 2010). Older adults may be better able than younger counterparts to regulate their emotions in the face of stress (e.g., Brose et al., 2011; Neupert et al., 2007; NRC, 2006; Schilling and Diehl, 2014; Uchino et al., 2006). Older adults tend to have a more secure and complex view of themselves than do younger people (Perlmutter, 1988). Focusing only on the negative effects of aging on cognition may be inappropriately stigmatizing.

Third, the preventive actions that people should take to preserve or enhance their cognitive function are often misunderstood. Many people mistakenly believe that vitamins and supplements are effective in maintaining cognitive health (Friedman et al., 2013; Roberts et al., 2014), even though there is no compelling evidence that, in the absence of individual deficits in specific vitamin levels, such dietary additions are beneficial (see Chapter 4A). Sales of online cognitive games and training suggest that individuals see these products as beneficial to their cognitive health, although much remains to be learned about the extent to which the skills learned through games and cognitive training can transfer to activities of daily life (see Chapter 4C). Qualitative research suggests that people rely on anecdotal evidence, such as observing that a physically active friend developed Alzheimer's disease, to assess the efficacy of preventive actions, which can result in misleading conclusions (Wu et al., 2009). Messages for the public should emphasize the cognitive health actions that (1) have the strongest research evidence indicating that they improve cognitive health and preventing declines; or (2) have scientific evidence indicating that they are likely to be beneficial for cognitive health and also are proven to be beneficial for health overall.

Fourth, misperceptions exist about the science of the brain and how it works and ages. The gaps in current understanding are not surprising given the rapid gains in neuroscience knowledge in recent decades. People may believe that brain neurons die as they age and that neuron death is inevitable. In fact, neurons may lose synapses as an individual ages, but in the absence of neurodegenerative disorders such as Alzheimer's disease, neuron death is minimal (Morrison and Baxter, 2012). Mistaken understandings of brain mechanisms of cognitive decline may block people from seeing any reason to invest in prevention efforts.

Sociocultural Differences in Perceptions of Cognitive Aging

Understanding the variations in how people perceive cognitive aging is important in order to inform the development of appropriate and well-targeted public education programs. Both quantitative and qualitative data show some differences and some commonalities among diverse sociocultural groups. Other studies, although focused on risk of cognitive impairment and prevention of Alzheimer's disease, provide important information about misinformation, concerns, motivations, and current actions.

Ethnicity

Enough ethnic and racial groups differences in perceptions about cognitive aging exist to require careful testing of public campaigns among different audiences (IOM, 2002). Some surveys have suggested that African American and Latino survey participants worry slightly less about dementia than do white participants (Connell et al., 2009; Friedman et al., 2013; Roberts et al., 2003), but more recent data do not show significant ethnic differences in worry about Alzheimer's disease (Roberts et al., 2014).

Building on earlier ethnographic and qualitative studies (e.g., Fox et al., 1999; Hashmi, 2009), the Healthy Aging Research Network, which is funded by the CDC, conducted focus groups throughout the United States in order to examine perceptions of cognitive aging (see, Laditka, J. N., et al., 2009, for a description). All ethnic groups expressed fears about memory loss and used similar terms to talk about the state of decline. Many commonalities were seen across ethnicities in their perceptions of what it means to age well, including being cognitively alert and maintaining a positive outlook, having a good memory, being socially active and engaged, living to an advanced age, and having good physical health (Friedman et al., 2011; Laditka, S. B., et al., 2009). Beliefs about efficacious strategies to stay mentally sharp—such as being active socially and connected to the community, having mental stimulation such as reading, and being physically active—were also similar across groups (Friedman et al., 2011; Wilcox et al., 2009).

However, there were differences among the ethnic groups' views about the attributed causes and symptoms of people with cognitive impairment, as well as their level of concern about stigma and family reactions to cognitive impairment. These differences suggest ways in which messages may need to be tailored (Laditka et al., 2011, 2013). In addition, there may be differences in beliefs about the inevitability of dementia, which could point to differences in individuals' motivation to perform actions to prevent cognitive decline. Researchers developing messages will need to assess beliefs about the inevitability of disease.

When asked about the efficacy of prevention efforts, African American and white participants are more likely than other ethnic groups (Chinese American, Latino, and Vietnamese American) to endorse mental exercises and puzzles (Friedman et al., 2011). Other differences in beliefs about prevention behaviors, including beliefs that particular foods and supplements promote cognitive health, may need to be addressed in public communication efforts aimed at promoting evidence-based behavior (Friedman et al., 2011; Laditka, J. N., et al., 2009; Wilcox et al., 2009).

Public education efforts should begin with an exploration of the attitudes and beliefs of the particular population segments that a given program or campaign is attempting to reach. Given the wide variation in perceptions about cognitive health and dementia throughout the world (Hashmi, 2009; Henderson and Traphagan, 2005), new immigrant groups may have views that are significantly different from those of the U.S. resident populations studied in surveys to date. Furthermore, wide variations in views will exist among individuals within the broad ethnic groups surveyed.

Gender

Some studies find that women are more concerned than men about cognitive aging (Friedman et al., 2013; Wu et al., 2009), but other studies do not find a difference (Roberts et al., 2014). Women are more likely than men to know that having a first-degree relative with Alzheimer's disease increases their risk for the disease and to believe that a healthy diet can be a protective factor against Alzheimer's disease (Roberts et al., 2014). In a qualitative comparison of rural men and women, women were more likely to search for information about cognitive health and to consider reducing stress, adopting a healthier diet, and increasing their social engagement to promote cognitive health (Wu et al., 2009).

Education and Income

People with fewer economic resources and less education often have a high burden of disease and less knowledge about health promotion and disease prevention than those with more education and income. For example, people with fewer economic resources and less education are more likely to believe that there are prescription drugs, vitamins, and supplements that can help prevent cognitive impairment (Roberts et al., 2014). This is particularly concerning given that they may spend limited household resources on unproven measures instead of on physical activity and reducing cardiovascular risks, which are known to be efficacious (Chapters 4A and 4B).

People of lower socioeconomic status are less likely to have a healthy lifestyle, and they face numerous environmental barriers to changing their physical activity and dietary habits. Well-designed educational campaigns and programs will be sensitive to the contexts in which people live and to their personal resources, available and preferred ways of learning about health issues, the sources they trust for health information, and their literacy levels (see section below).

Summary

The knowledge and motivation to engage in behavior that promotes cognitive health may vary by gender, ethnicity, income, and education level, and thus educational strategies and materials need to be relevant to the needs of specific target groups. If there is evidence that broad public campaigns are not successful, it will be advantageous to target each segment of the population separately (IOM, 2002).

INFORMATION ENVIRONMENT

Efforts to educate the public about cognitive aging and to promote particular types of behavior will need to take into account the information-rich environment in the United States and how best to reach middle-aged and older adults. The existence of information in the environment hardly guarantees that people pay attention to it; there is a long tradition in communication research of studying the conditions under which information in the media has an impact and how people use the media (e.g., Bryant and Oliver, 2009). Additional studies will be needed to understand when and for whom cognitive aging information in the environment makes a difference. As one example, qualitative studies suggest that at the oldest ages people rely more on health professionals and people in their social network than on media sources to keep them up to date on information (e.g., Williamson and Asla, 2009).

News Media and Magazines

U.S. adults age 65 years and older rely more on television and newspapers for their news than do other age groups (Pew Research Center, 2015). However, the committee was unable to identify studies examining the coverage of cognitive aging in traditional news and information media (including broadcast and print).

The issue has been addressed in magazine coverage. A content analysis of articles in the top eight women's and men's magazines in 2006–2007 found an average of four messages related to cognitive health per magazine in 2006, and three in 2007, with the most common recommendations for maintaining cognitive health relating to diet, followed by vitamins and supplements, cognitive exercises, physical activity, and social interactions (Friedman et al., 2010). No mention was made of hypertension and diabetes as risk factors for cognitive health, and magazines targeting African Americans had very little cognitive health information (Friedman et al., 2010). An analysis of the top five magazines among people 50 years and older had similar findings (Mathews et al., 2009) with only a small portion of the articles promoting physical activity for brain health. In another assessment of magazines targeting U.S. older adults, the recommended amount of physical activity per week varied widely, only half of the stories explained the link between physical activity and cognitive health, and few cited the empirical evidence for the relationships (Price et al., 2011). More research is needed to understand how cognitive aging is covered in television news and newspapers in the United States, including in Spanish-language and other news media targeting specific cultural groups.

Internet and Social Media

For many people seeking health information, the Internet has become a major resource. The digital divide has shrunk, with people of most ethnicities and ages using the Internet, with the least likely users being adults 80 years and older (although 37 percent of this group was found to use the Internet) and those who have little education (Pew Research Center, 2014). About half of adults who are 65 years and older and who use the Internet say that getting health information is one of their top motivations for going online (Pew Research Center, 2014).

Studies have examined the coverage of cognitive health on websites of news organizations, health systems, state and city health departments, and senior centers. From 2007 to 2010, the top three cable news websites included about 230 stories related to cognitive health, with an emphasis on maintaining function and preventing decline through lifestyle choices (Vandenberg et al., 2012). The study authors estimated that only 18 percent of the stories were aimed at older adults and that 20 percent featured vitamins and supplements (Vandenberg et al., 2012). Not surprisingly, cognitive function and impairment were not well defined in the stories (Vandenberg et al., 2012). After reviewing the websites of 156 large health systems and health departments and 181 senior centers, Laditka and colleagues (2012) found that large health systems were more likely to promote cognitive health than were senior centers, but promotion of physical activity represented only 20 percent of the website content.

Although active monthly Twitter users are predominantly younger (only 3 percent of adults who are 65 years and older use Twitter regularly), it can be an important channel for people already interested in a topic, including activists, policy makers, and public health officials (Pew Research Center, 2014). There are studies focused on dementia as a topic of conversations on Twitter, but the committee did not find studies looking at the topics of cognitive health or cognitive aging. One content analysis of a sample of information about dementia on Twitter found that news about recent research studies was the most common type of content and that only a small number of those studies were about the prevention of dementia (Robillard et al., 2013). Most tweets about dementia were posted by health professionals, health information sites, news organizations, and commercial entities. Consistent with the way that Twitter is often used—to push readers to websites or videos with more information—most tweets about dementia contained a link to a major news outlet or health information site (Robillard et al., 2013).

About half of older adults who are online use social networking sites such as Facebook, which increases their social connections with family and friends (Pew Research Center, 2014). It is unknown how often they share information and provide encouragement for behaviors that support or undermine cognitive health.

In summary, information is available online about cognitive health and it has been covered to some degree in magazines, but it is unknown how much cognitive aging has appeared in the news sources that older adults most often use—television and newspapers. More information is needed about how people of different ages learn about cognitive aging, including which sources they actively use, features they prefer or avoid, and their ability to evaluate the quality of the information.

Entertainment Media

Knowing the extent to which entertainment fare on television and in movies depict healthy older adults engaged in behavior relevant to promoting cognitive health would be valuable information for public education efforts. Research has shown that people can become motivated and learn new skills through the modeling provided by fictional accounts as long as the actions result in positive consequences for the character (Bandura, 1986; Singhal and Rogers, 1999). Although it cannot be said for sure because of the lack of research, it is likely that the topic is not well covered, given that the entertainment media tends to underrepresent older adults compared to their presence in the U.S. population. Older adults are underrepresented in prime-time television (Signorielli, 2004), video games (Williams et al., 2009), prime-time medical dramas (Hetsroni, 2009), and children's programs (Bond and Drogos, 2008).

In a 2006 study of children's programming, older adults tended to be portrayed as healthy, morally good, attractive, and satisfied with life, but only 36 percent of older adult characters were women and only 14 percent were people of color (Bond and Drogos, 2008). Disney animated movies similarly underrepresent older women and people of color, and a study found that overall, 42 percent of older characters were portrayed negatively (e.g., grumpy, evil, helpless, or "crazy"), with almost half of the villains in the stories being older adults (Robinson et al., 2007).

Given the general lack of attention to cognitive health in past studies of entertainment fare, and the likelihood that content may have changed since existing studies were conducted, it would be beneficial to systematically study the current depiction of cognitive aging in entertainment media.

Current Public Education Campaigns and Resources

Media campaigns are needed that focus on cognitive aging and that convey the range of non-dementia cognitive issues faced by older adults and their families as well as the wide variability in cognitive function among older adults. Much of the outreach to date has concerned dementia or has addressed only a particular risk factor prevention strategy. Although some messages and materials are relevant—as reviewed below—there remains a strong need for campaigns that focus squarely on healthy cognitive aging.

In addition to its goals relevant to people diagnosed with dementia and their caregivers, the Healthy Brain Initiative seeks to improve the cognitive health of the American population (Alzheimer's Association and CDC, 2013). One goal is to support state and local needs assessments to identify disparities and ensure that educational materials are culturally appropriate (Alzheimer's Association and CDC, 2013). To date, the CDC

Healthy Aging Research Network has used qualitative methods to assess the public understanding of cognitive aging and to make recommendations about public messages, such as the need to make messages more salient to people with diverse backgrounds. Much of that research is cited earlier in this chapter. A number of the objectives related to public awareness and improved access to information and resources are relevant to healthy cognitive aging, including

- coordinating national and state efforts to disseminate evidence-based messages about risk reduction for preserving cognitive health;
- working to ensure the consistency of cognitive health messages across national, state, and local levels;
- decreasing stigma and promoting strategies for the public to learn how to communicate appropriately with people with dementia;
- promoting early diagnosis of cognitive impairment; and
- promoting research on cognitive health promotion.

As of 2011, the CDC had improved the information infrastructure relating to cognitive health for professionals by creating lesson plans for middle- and high-school science teachers, making improvements to its website, adding items related to cognitive impairment to the Behavioral Risk Factor Surveillance System survey (see Chapter 3), giving presentations at professional organizations, and publishing scientific literature on the topic (Alzheimer's Association and CDC, 2013). In 2014 the initiative funded five prevention research centers at leading universities to establish a research network to monitor attitudes and health status over time, to create and test messages and interventions to improve or maintain cognitive function, and to use that knowledge to support effective programs and practices in states and communities (CDC, 2014).

Using workshops, events, and mass media, the CDC and the Alzheimer's Association ran a demonstration project through local Alzheimer's Association chapters in Atlanta and Los Angeles aimed at increasing awareness of cognitive health, physical activity, and cardiovascular health among African American baby boomers. The evaluation found that people who had participated in the workshops had increased knowledge about brain health and were more motivated to engage in preventive behaviors related to screening for chronic cardiovascular disease risks (Fuller et al., 2012). However, the workshops and events reached only a small number of people in the target group, and it is unclear how many people were exposed to the modest media presence (Fuller et al., 2012). Furthermore, the extent to which people in the workshops or at the events changed their behavior is unknown, as is whether attendees inspired others to change their behavior. While the

> **BOX 7-1**
> **Examples of Information Resources on Cognitive Aging**
>
> - **AARP, Dana Foundation, and MetLife Foundation:** These organizations print and distribute a series of booklets in English, Mandarin, and Spanish on recent advances in brain studies titled *Staying Sharp*. They offer related videos on their websites. Topics include successful cognitive aging, memory loss and aging, cognition and chronic diseases, and learning throughout life (AARP, 2015b; Dana Foundation, 2015). AARP also has a dedicated webpage, the Brain Health Center, with information, tips, news, and blogs (AARP, 2015a).
> - **Administration for Community Living:** *Brain Health as You Age* fact sheets are available as a one-page document and in greater detail through Web links. The website provides a PowerPoint presentation that can be used by senior centers and other organizations reaching out to older adults, family members, and caregivers (ACL, 2015).
> - **Alzheimer's Association:** The association provides resources on risk factors and prevention and a flyer, *Know the 10 Signs: Early Detection Matters* (Alzheimer's Association, 2015).
> - **American College of Sports Medicine:** Brochures can be downloaded that deal with specifics of exercise, including balance training for older adults, how to hydrate effectively, using a heart monitor, lowering blood pressure, and starting a walking program (ACSM, 2014).
> - **CDC:** The CDC provides information on the Healthy Brain Initiative, including the fact sheet, *What Is a Healthy Brain? New Research Explores Perceptions of Cognitive Health Among Diverse Older Adults* (CDC, 2015).
> - **Easter Seals:** Information is available for the public on brain health for youth and adults, with online screening tools for developmental delays in youth and an online driver skills training program for older adults (Easter Seals, 2015).

project showed that community partners can be engaged within a relatively short period of time to promote cognitive health and that workshops on cognitive health designed with local partners and targeted to a specific age and ethnicity can affect knowledge and some behavioral intentions, a greater media presence will be necessary to reach large numbers of people.

Federal agencies and nongovernmental organizations have made information available for interested members of the public and for public health and health care professionals to use with their patients or clients. Examples are listed in Box 7-1.

RELEVANT COMMUNICATIONS STRATEGIES AND MESSAGES

Communication and public education efforts pertinent to cognitive aging can benefit from and build on the public health improvement efforts

- **HHS Office of Disease Prevention and Health Promotion:** The office provides information for older adults on target amounts of physical activity (HHS, 2015), for example, the brochure *Be Active Your Way*.
- **The Hospital Elder Life Program:** The program provides information for older adults undergoing surgery and hospitalization, with the goal of preventing delirium (HELP, 2015).
- **National Heart, Lung, and Blood Institute (NHLBI):** NHLBI provides resources for promoting heart health that are also relevant to addressing cardiovascular risk factors for cognitive health. Programs include the Aim for a Healthy Weight, Heart Truth, and Stay in Circulation (for peripheral arterial disease) campaigns. Heart healthy recipes and physical activity programs are also available, with an emphasis on information for various ethnic groups (NHLBI, 2015a,b).
- **National Institute on Aging:** Information on age-related cognitive change is available through the Alzheimer's Disease Education & Referral Center website. The NIA also sponsors the Go4Life exercise and physical activity campaign that includes an informational website aimed at older adults as well as tipsheets, and the guide *Exercise & Physical Activity: Your Everyday Guide* from the National Institute on Aging, which is available in English and Spanish (NIA, 2014). The campaign has many partners that may distribute the original or co-brand the messages and materials, link to the campaign website, and host events.
- **U.S. Department of Agriculture:** Resources are available to personalize a food plan and use an interactive tool to set goals, track diet and activity levels, and receive feedback (SuperTracker) (USDA, 2015).
- **Washington University School of Medicine:** The school's website hosts an interactive tool that helps people calculate their risk of developing heart disease, diabetes, and stroke, among other conditions (Washington University School of Medicine, 2013).

by federal, state, and local agencies, nonprofit organizations, community initiatives, foundations, and private-sector companies.

Physical Activity

Physical activity is recommended for all age groups because of its health benefits in a variety of domains, including cognitive health (see Chapter 4A). However, the concerted efforts to improve physical activity levels in the general population over the past 40 years have not managed to counter the rising levels of inactivity (Brownson et al., 2005). Most older adults are inactive, and among the very old the rate of decline in activity levels is more rapid each year (Buchman et al., 2014). Interventions to improve physical activity among older adults achieve, on average, incremental improvements, but generally the increase is not enough to meet recommended levels (Conn et al., 2003, 2012). Because people who were more active when they were younger often continue to be more active as they age (e.g., Dohle and Wansink, 2013), it might be useful if future efforts to improve cognitive health target younger age groups. Numerous strategies have been explored for increasing physical activity levels (Prohaska and Peters, 2007), and, as discussed in Box 7-2 and Chapter 6, a combination of strategies will likely be most useful in sustaining behavior change. Evaluations will continue to be needed to determine the most effective approaches to long-term behavior change.

Although evidence to recommend media campaigns as a standalone approach to increase physical activity is lacking (Brown et al., 2012; Kahn et al., 2002), targeted campaigns with links to community-based opportunities for physical activity can be an effective strategy for some population groups (Heath et al., 2012). Note that because limited-duration media campaigns may not result in sustained behavior change, they may be most effective

---

BOX 7-2
Strategies for Increasing Physical Activity

Counseling and small group sessions: Counseling can happen in many settings, from a clinician's office to recreation facilities, gyms, libraries, and even at home. Evidence suggests that counseling by a trained layperson can be as effective as counseling by physicians (Moyer and U.S. Preventive Services Task Force, 2012). One review found that physical activity programs with high and moderate intensity of counseling efforts (e.g., 3 to 24 phone sessions or 1 to 8 in-person sessions) resulted in increased activity, but programs lasting 30 minutes or less were not effective. The behavior change techniques that were found to be most successful in increasing physical activity in older adults were identifying barriers and problem solving, providing rewards contingent on successful behavior, and modeling the behavior (French et al., 2014).

Individually tailored programs: Programs can be individualized to teach skills related to the increase and maintenance of physical activity, such as goal setting and self-monitoring, building social support, self-rewards and positive self-talk, and problem solving to maintain behavior change and prevent relapses (Kahn et al., 2002; Task Force on Community Prevention Services, 2002). These programs can be delivered in person, over the phone, through the mail, or over the Internet, and have been shown to be effective (e.g., Noar et al., 2007; Snyder and LaCroix, 2013).

Online programs: Meta-analyses have shown positive effects on adults' physical activity from Internet-based programs (Vandelanotte et al., 2007) as well as text-messaging programs (Head et al., 2013), and both may be appropriate for tech-savvy seniors. For example, a 6-week randomized controlled trial of motivational text messages increased step count in a target group of urban African Americans ages 60 to 85 years (Kim and Glanz, 2013).

over the long term when tied with efforts that keep people engaged, such as social support approaches.

Medication Adherence and Review

Proper medication adherence is critical for preventing many of the risk factors for cognitive decline. As detailed in Chapter 4B, some medications can impair cognition in older adults, and all older adults should have careful and periodic review of their medications, including supplements, by a clinician. Of the 67 million U.S. adults with hypertension, an estimated 54 percent are not controlling it, even though most have a source of health care and insurance (CDC, 2012b; Johnson et al., 2014; Ritchey et al., 2014). Older adults may find it difficult to adhere to their medication regimens, particularly when they need to take many medications. Many older adults,

---

Social support for exercise: The Task Force on Community Prevention Services (2002) found strong evidence for effectiveness of social support programs, such as urging people to find exercise buddies or join a walking group. A recent meta-analysis found that interventions for older adults that promote walking in groups increased physical activity (Kassavou et al., 2013). Such interventions also have the advantage of promoting social engagement, which may further contribute to cognitive health (see Chapter 4A).

Improving the built environment: Many communities are improving the walkability of their neighborhoods and are increasing the number and quality of parks and community spaces with the goal of increasing residents' physical activity levels (see Chapter 6). Public messaging should announce improvements to the environment, promote existing opportunities and resources in the community, and disseminate such tools as walking route maps (Heath et al., 2006; Hobbs et al., 2013; Task Force on Community Prevention Services, 2002). Reminders at point-of-decision moments can be an effective way to promote small functional changes in everyday living, such as taking the stairs instead of an elevator (Soler et al., 2010).

Products to incentivize physical activity: Pedometers and other self-monitoring products are useful to some individuals for monitoring and promoting physical activity; however, only a fraction of the people who start using pedometers or other monitoring technologies use them long term (Teyhen et al., 2014).

Comprehensive community interventions: The most effective approach may be "all-of-the-above"—that is, comprehensive community interventions that combine media promotion, support and self-help groups, counseling, risk screening, events, and enhancing the environment for physical activity. The social ecological model has been a useful framework in which to integrate intervention strategies. An example is the Active for Life program, which combines paid advertising, direct mail, media relations with testimonials and events, a tailored 12-week activity program, pedometer use promotion, and advocacy for environmental changes and pedestrian safety (Wilcox et al., 2009).

however, do recognize their own memory limits and use memory aids, and sometimes they are more conscientious than middle-aged adults about taking their medications (Park et al., 1999).

Recent reviews have suggested that educational and other interventions can promote adherence to medication regimens if they improve knowledge about the relevant medical condition, provide ongoing counseling and accountability, provide appropriate tools and strategies to help patients self-monitor, and increase access to memory aids that help people remember to take and refill their medications (Frazee et al., 2014; Zullig et al., 2013). A meta-analysis of interventions to improve anti-hypertensive medication adherence among older adults found that these interventions successfully improved adherence and knowledge and also helped improve diastolic blood pressure (Conn et al., 2009). The interventions were more effective among women and those taking three to five medications. Interventions targeting adherence plus another behavior had the same impact as interventions targeting adherence alone, which suggests that cognitive aging campaigns could focus on adherence alone or adherence and other goals, such as physical activity. Neither the mode of delivery (e.g., media, face-to-face counseling, or both) nor the type of professional conducting the counseling made any difference in the results. A meta-analysis of pharmacist-delivered interventions, which most often included medication management providing information for the patient and frequent follow-ups, found improvements in adherence and in blood pressure (Morgado et al., 2011).

Some of the more effective interventions for medication adherence among adults 60 years and older are tailoring (changing the message based on information about the individual patients), face-to-face counseling, and rehearsal of medication taking (Xu, 2014). Clinicians offering interventions should consider targeting multiple family members with high blood pressure at once; research with African Americans found that older parents were better at taking anti-hypertension medications than their adult children and that when the adult children had conversations with their parents about hypertension, the adult children had higher adherence levels too (Warren-Findlow et al., 2011). Despite the efficacy of face-to-face communication strategies, it can be difficult to recruit people to participate in small group interventions (Robare et al., 2011), so additional channels should be considered.

Financial Responsibility, Driving, and Health Decisions

The risks related to cognitive changes with age that require the greatest attention may be those related to health and financial decision making and also skills requiring complex judgment and quick reactions in high-risk situations, such as driving; these risks require attention even in the absence of Alzheimer's or related diseases (see Chapter 6) (Agarwal et al., 2009; Boyle et al., 2012; Carpenter and Yoon, 2011; James et al., 2012; Klein and Karlawish, 2010; Sabatino, 2011; Triebel and Marson, 2012; Widera et al., 2011). Efforts need to be made to improve and increase the development, testing, and evaluating of the messages that older adults and their families need on these issues.

In terms of financial decision making, surveys show a gap between people's estimates of their ability to make financial decisions and their actual financial literacy, and this gap widens with age (Lusardi and Mitchell, 2011). As discussed in Chapter 6, a number of efforts are under way to assist older adults and their families in making sound financial decisions. Messages targeted to older adults could: emphasize the need for periodic financial reviews and the steps to take to consult with financial advisors who are legally required to represent the client's financial interests, are registered, and have not violated the law in the past; alert people to common scams and unscrupulous sales practices; and identify methods for finding trustworthy information with which to raise financial literacy, if they so choose. Tools to help people select reliable and trustworthy brokers and to avoid fraud, such as the Financial Industry Regulatory Authority's (FINRA's) "BrokerCheck," "RiskMeter," and "ScamMeter" developed by FINRA, could be promoted more widely (FINRA, 2015). At the same time, more research is needed on the types and efficacy of financial education (including the value of these online tools) in improving decision making (Agarwal et al., 2009).

As in the case with financial literacy, older drivers often do not recognize when they need coaching to improve their skills or when to stop driving. The decision to stop driving can be emotionally laden, because driving is often linked with independence (NRC, 2006). Messages aimed at older adults, their families, and health care providers can promote older driver training programs, local transportation alternatives, warning signs of diminished driving ability, and assessments of driving skills. Older adults may be motivated to reevaluate their driving by a desire to not harm others or by the rising cost of their automobile insurance. The availability of periodic confidential driving assessments may ameliorate the fear of losing driving privileges for unwarranted reasons. Public campaigns aimed at older drivers and families could help connect people with assessment and training programs in their communities and online (see Chapter 6).

When faced with decisions on medical procedures, older adults may benefit from messages telling them where to learn more about specific treatment options and informing them of the need to review decisions with trusted others. For people of all ages, decision making is more difficult under stress, such as after a diagnosis (Keinan, 1987). Information about care options for older adults should be carefully pretested to ensure that the population can use and understand them. Communication skills training can be beneficial for both families and health professionals (Heaney and Israel, 2009; Kurtz et al., 2009; Wolff and Roter, 2011; Wolff et al., 2014).

In sum, families and people who work with older adults should be made aware of the potential challenges to health, driving, and financial decision making that may occur with age and be alert for signs indicating a need for greater involvement in decisions. Families may benefit from messages suggesting strategies for communicating with their older relatives about specific decisions and decision making in general.

CHALLENGES FOR PUBLIC EDUCATION CAMPAIGNS

Combating Stigma and Prejudice

Studies have shown that in many countries, the United States included, cognitive impairment is stigmatized, and this stigma has been a barrier to early detection and treatment (Wahl, 2012; WHO, 2012). By extension, people with healthy cognitive aging may be reluctant to seek a professional assessment of their cognitive status. Stigma may block people from communicating about their fear of cognitive decline with family and friends, making it less likely they will learn about preventive measures or ways to reverse treatable causes of decline. For example, if a memory lapse is met by ridicule or visible impatience, a person may be embarrassed or feel shame, and psychological research suggests that shame often results in escaping and avoiding the shame-inducing situations (Tangney, 2013). There is also the potential that fear and stigma will lead an individual to shy away from social interactions, and the resulting diminished social connections, support, and stimulation in turn could contribute to further cognitive decline.

Older adults with more positive views of themselves and of aging in general have better health and are less likely to be depressed (Coleman et al., 1993). At the same time, negative stereotypes about older adults in general—such as that they are losing their cognitive, physical, and communication abilities—may affect how older adults perceive themselves and also affect interactions between generations (Caporael and Culbertson, 1986; Levy et al., 1999; Pasupathi et al., 1995; Williams and Nussbaum, 2001). Negative stereotypes can affect various physical measures—increasing blood pressure and heart rate and decreasing walking speed—as well as such cognitive and attitudinal outcomes as memory decline, and even the will to live (Hausdorff et al., 1999; Hess et al., 2003; Levy et al., 1999, 2000).

Cognitively healthy older adults who experience patronizing attitudes from young adults are more likely to perceive themselves as impaired (e.g., Kemper et al., 1996). As a result, older people may avoid situations in which they may be the target of prejudice (NRC, 2006; Shelton et al., 2005). This can reduce older adults' opportunities to engage in some of the recommended behaviors that are useful in maintaining cognitive health. If, for example, older adults avoid going to the gym for fear of not "measuring up," they may get less physical activity than they need. If they avoid social interactions with younger people, they may be missing the benefits of social engagement.

Evaluations of programs specifically related to stigma against people with cognitive aging are sparse, and this topic should be explored in future research. In the absence of research on what works to counter stigma for cognitive aging, it is useful to consider programs that counter other types of stigma and prejudices. The experiences, both positive and negative, with programs that have attempted to combat stigma against aging in general as well as those countering stigma against dementia or other mental illnesses can point to a number of strategies that could be employed.

Promote Positive Interactions

Research shows that good quality contact between individuals can help dispel a person's negative attitudes toward another group (Knox et al., 1986), and this phenomenon has been used in interventions against ageism and mental health stigmas. Meta-analyses of programs designed to reduce stigma against mental illness in the general population have found that in-person contact is an efficacious approach among adults (Corrigan et al., 2012; Griffiths et al., 2014). For example, the campaign *Time to Change in the U.K.* aimed to reduce mental illness stigma by fostering social contact at mass events and in places with a lot of foot traffic, such as malls and community centers (Evans-Lacko et al., 2012). The evaluation of this program found that mere contact was not enough—people needed to feel they were working together to improve conditions for people with mental illness. When they had a sense of common goals, they improved their intention to have greater social contact in the future with people with mental illnesses, even 4 to 6 weeks after the interaction (Evans-Lacko et al., 2012).

A meta-analysis of mental health stigma interventions aimed at health care workers found that the key elements of effective interventions were emphasizing the possibility of recovery from mental illness and having multiple forms of social contact with people who have experienced it (Knaak et al., 2014). On average, those programs had at least a short-term effect on stigma; the long-term effects are unknown (Knaak et al., 2014). These insights suggest an emphasis on messages that stress the importance of prevention measures relevant to cognitive aging as well as the importance of positive intragenerational contacts.

Use Real-Life Exemplars

Because reaching a large percentage of the population with in-person contact interventions can be expensive and difficult to implement, media-based approaches may be more useful in reaching larger numbers of people. Research studies have found that stereotypes can be combated through exposure to positive exemplars that run counter to the stereotype (Duval et al., 2000). Both information-oriented media programs and entertainment-oriented media programs should be considered. News and other information media should provide accurate and appropriate messages that will overcome and not reinforce stereotypes. Organizations concerned about the portrayal of cognitive aging in the media could monitor the extent to which the coverage is biased and push for change.

Public education campaigns can also put a positive face on cognitive aging. Analyses of media interventions for mental health stigma found that media messages that contain first-person testimonials—but not third-person accounts—about mental illness were successful in combating prejudice (Clement et al., 2013). An example of such a program is a current UK effort, Dementia Friends, which seeks to improve public knowledge of dementia by using news stories about real individuals living with the condition and focusing on what people can do to assist those in their community (Dementia Friends, 2015). People who want more information can watch video testimonials about the experience of dementia, attend local information sessions, or receive a free package of materials, including a booklet with tips on actions. To destigmatize dementia, the campaign employs additional tactics, including naming famous people who have had dementia and speaking about dementia's commonalities with other chronic health conditions. The campaign also uses celebrities—such as the prime minister—to gain coverage. A similar campaign has been launched in New Zealand with a famous television personality and a sports star as "champions for dementia," with an emphasis on preventive behaviors, including physical activity, diet, and not smoking (Alzheimers New Zealand, 2012). In the United States, examples of similar efforts include the documentary *I'll Be Me* about a famous musician. Evaluations of these first-person campaigns will provide valuable information on the influence of media coverage.

Portray Older Adults Positively in Entertainment

To combat the stigma of cognitive aging, entertainment media can provide stories featuring older adults, incorporate accurate portrayals of people with various levels of cognitive health, and depict respectful interactions between people with and without cognitive impairments. Use of older characters who are portrayed as being engaged in complex cognitive analyses and decisions may help combat the stigma that can be associated with cognitive aging. Campaigns can also take advantage of movies and stories about cognitive health when they appear to provide timely and reliable information for the general public. Across a range of health topics, evaluations of "education-entertainment" that feature storylines related to health issues within dramas, music, games, or other entertainment fare have shown some success in increasing viewers' acceptance of people with a medical condition, as well as increasing knowledge about a condition and individuals' willingness to engage in preventive behavior (e.g., Kennedy et al., 2004; Movius et al., 2007; Singhal and Rogers, 1999). Organizations that provide health and medical information resources for television and movie writers (such as Hollywood, Health & Society) are valuable in improving the accuracy of programs and promoting the incorporation of health issues into storylines (Hollywood, Health & Society, 2014). Content analyses are helpful in documenting the state of entertainment media depictions to understand where improvements are needed; however, existing studies are out of date (e.g., Gerbner et al., 1980; Signorielli, 2004).

Overcoming Communication Barriers

Communication aimed at older adults will need to take into account those adults' physical declines in hearing and vision and their possible problems with literacy and number skills (numeracy). Almost two-thirds of adults who are more than 70 years of age experience some degree of hearing loss (Lin et al., 2011). With normal age-related declines in hearing, spoken words can become difficult to understand, particularly when there is background noise (Gordon-Salant, 2006). Vision may also decline with age and exacerbate communication challenges.

Public education messages should encourage the use of appropriate technologies to correct for impairments (e.g., hearing aids, glasses) so that people may continue to participate in social interactions, have an easier time learning new things, and move about more safely. Furthermore, it is critical that public communication campaigns focused on older adults take into account the potential hearing and vision declines and design their messages and communication strategies accordingly. Messages should be pretested to ensure that they can be seen and heard by older adults. For example, one group of researchers when designing an interactive program for older adults that checks for drug interactions, pretested prototypes in focus groups and adjusted their materials to incorporate larger type and bold lettering, large navigation buttons, and streamlined controls (Strickler and Neafsey, 2002).

Another potential communication barrier is low literacy, which is more common among older adults than among younger adults (Kutner et al.,

2007). According to the National Assessment of Adult Literacy, between one-quarter and one-third of adults 65 years and older in 2003 (the latest year with statistics for older adults) had below basic skills in at least one type of literacy (Kutner et al., 2007). At that time, 23 percent of older adults could not understand information from texts like news stories and brochures; 27 percent could not use documents like forms and applications, maps, tables, and food and drug labels; and 34 percent could not identify and make calculations using numbers in printed materials, such as balancing a checkbook, calculating a service tip, or understanding interest on a loan (Kutner et al., 2007).

Another important type of literacy is health literacy, which is "the degree to which individuals have the capacity to obtain, process, and understand basic health information and services needed to make appropriate health decisions" (IOM, 2004, p. 2, quoting Ratzan and Parker, 2000). Relevant areas of health knowledge include the prevention and self-management of health problems; navigating the health system; and clinical tasks such as filling out forms, understanding dosing instructions, and diagnostic testing. In 2003, researchers found that 29 percent of adults more than 65 years old had below basic health literacy skills (Kutner et al., 2006). Those with below basic health literacy skills were health-information poor and less likely than those with greater skills to obtain health information from almost any source, including friends and family, health professionals, newspapers, magazines, books or brochures, and the Internet. Their only consistent sources for health information were television and radio (Kutner et al., 2006).

Low health literacy has negative consequences on public health. People with lower health literacy rate their overall health as poorer, know less about their health, use fewer preventive services, have higher rates of hospitalization, and participate less in health promotion programs (IOM, 2004). Thus, programs to support cognitive health will need to take health literacy of their target populations into account. Strategies to deal with low literacy levels include

- careful development of materials (with appropriate visuals, simple messages, and specific actions) (CDC, 2009, 2011; Jacobson and Parker, 2014; Lipkus, 2007; Sheridan et al., 2011);
- pretesting material (including assessing whether people can explain the message in their own words and demonstrate behavioral skills) and refining the materials based on the feedback (CDC, 2009; Weinreich, 2010);
- teaching oral communication skills to health care workers (e.g., Green et al., 2014; Plimpton and Root, 1994); and

- promoting shared decision making between patients and clinicians (Durand et al., 2014).

DESIGNING PUBLIC EDUCATION CAMPAIGNS AND COMMUNICATION PROGRAMS

For public education about cognitive aging to succeed, it will be critical for public health planners to follow the principles of good communication design. Campaign planners can use the many tools available at the CDC's gateway website for health communication and social marketing practice (CDC, 2012a).

The initial phases of design involve specifying the goals and measurable objectives for each target group. This is typically an iterative process, during which the initial specifications are revised based on a variety of considerations: archival research; research into the current beliefs, behavior, and barriers faced by the target groups; analyses of the physical, organizational, political, and social environment; and consideration of resources. The main goals should be to change or maintain specific behaviors, such as following physical activity guidelines or adhering to blood pressure medications. The exact behavior (or products or services, depending on what is being promoted) should be selected and refined based on formative research. The goals should emphasize behavior change and maintenance rather than knowledge and awareness because research has repeatedly shown that what people know they should do and what they actually do are different (Andreasen, 1995). Given that the terminology for cognitive aging is new, initial campaigns might set intermediate knowledge goals focused on increasing the understanding of what cognitive aging is and is not and on ways to promote cognitive health.

Successful social marketing efforts segment the population into different groups and then strategically select target groups (Lee and Kotler, 2011). Designing a more effective communications strategy is easier when dealing with a specific, relatively homogeneous group (Slater, 1995). The criteria for segmenting groups may include risk status for cognitive decline, existing beliefs and openness to behavior change, current behaviors, environmental barriers and support, and communication patterns (Snyder, 2007). For example, a campaign focused on reducing cardiovascular disease risks might segment people into the following groups:

1. those known to be at low risk,
2. those at risk who are not taking preventive measures,
3. those at risk who are taking preventive measures,
4. those who have been diagnosed with cardiovascular disease but who are not adhering to medical advice, and

5. those who have been diagnosed with cardiovascular disease and who are adhering to medical advice.

From a public health standpoint, the priority groups would be groups 2 and 4. These segments may be further subdivided according to the barriers they face (i.e., cannot afford medications, do not trust the medical advice given, etc.) or the opportunities for communication (i.e., regular contact with a medical practice or clinic, integration into community organizations, media usage). As reviewed earlier in this chapter, individuals' behavior may vary according to their age, ethnicity, gender, and cultural groupings related to beliefs, risks, and practices or location within specific geographic areas. Such differences would affect how segments are defined.

Generally, campaigns also might try to reach individuals who have an important influence on the people in the primary target groups through their communication and actions (e.g., family members, health care professionals) or through policy and environmental changes (e.g., local transportation officials, parks and recreation departments). Ultimately, segments can be prioritized based on the organizational mission of the campaign or program sponsor, public health needs, and effort (time, cost, and resources).

Once the goals—including target behaviors and populations—have been selected, the next step is to determine the behavior change approach that will be used. Campaign designers map out the pathways and barriers to change and maintenance for each behavior. Logic models based on behavior change theories and research with the target groups may clarify this process, and many useful theories have been applied successfully across a wide range of health behaviors and populations (for a review, see Glanz et al., 2008). When thinking about how to change new types of behavior, planners may also consider the taxonomy of behavior change techniques, which cuts across theories (Abraham and Michie, 2008; Michie et al., 2013). For established intervention domains, planners should take into account any existing systematic reviews of the effectiveness of various techniques for changing and maintaining healthy behavior (e.g., see French et al., 2014). If the target behavior is hindered by environmental barriers, then advocacy with policy makers, professionals, businesses, and the general public may be necessary (Wallack et al., 1993).

The next step is to plan the communication approach, including message content, communication channels, and message presentation (Snyder, 2007). The message content, while based on the goals, should be adapted for the target group and the behavior change strategy. For example, messages striving to persuade people to do something they already know they need to do, such as be more physically active, may address issues such as the severity and likelihood of the consequences of not following the recommendation, the benefits of compliance with the recommendations, stereotypes of people at risk, norms surrounding compliance, and skills in setting and monitoring goals or engaging in the behavior. Messages should emphasize points that are new to the target group; there is little to gain from telling people what they already know (Snyder and Hamilton, 2002). Research suggests that older adults are constantly refining their goals as they age and are more likely than younger people to actively pursue goals to protect themselves from feared outcomes (Cross and Markus, 1991; Markus and Nurius, 1986). Older adults also tend to respond better to positive feedback that emphasizes progress, however small, toward goals, rather than negative feedback that may undermine self-confidence (West and Ebner, 2013).

The communication channels for a given campaign or program may include interpersonal sources of information (e.g., friends, family, and health professionals), traditional media (e.g., television and pamphlets), and new media (websites, social media, and interactive programs or games). Media formats to consider using include news stories, editorials, messages embedded in entertainment programs or games, advertisements, public service announcements, interactive tailored programs, and testimonials. Interpersonal communication may take the form of in-person, phone, or Web-based consultations, social media messaging, lectures, small group meetings, and other approaches. Campaign planners should select channels and formats based on the target groups' usage patterns and preferences; campaigns that use multiple channels often have greater impacts (Snyder, 2007).

Note that media use patterns change across the life span (Robinson et al., 2004) and potentially from one generation to the next. For example, baby boomers are much more likely to use the Internet than people who are now more than 85 years old (Pew Research Center, 2014). Behavior change across a population is more likely when a combination of channels is used and when media can be selected so as to maximize the number of people in the target population who are reached (Hornik, 2002; Snyder and Hamilton, 2002). At the same time, interpersonal sources may have greater credibility. An AARP (2012) survey of adults more than 50 years old found that they trusted health professionals more than "mass media" reports. They wanted a single reliable source of information to help them understand conflicting research reports, which supports the suggestion of an information gateway (see Recommendation 8). Both mass media and interpersonal channels may be useful in promoting different aspects of healthy cognitive aging.

In terms of the message presentation (or campaign "look and feel"), planners should aim for high levels of attention, memorability, and believability, and the sources of the messages should be perceived as highly credible and likable. Typically, messages that are of high quality and delivered in multiple versions attract greater attention and are more memorable (Snyder, 2007). Structured conversations, such as motivational interviewing or tailored interventions, may prove effective with people of all ages (Lustria et al., 2013; Miller and Rollnick, 2002; Noar et al., 2007). As noted above, the message presentations should take into account the target group's literacy and health literacy skills, their language preferences, and potential communication impairments.

Furthermore, the emotional tone of the messages needs to be appropriate to the target group and the context. For example, laboratory studies show that older people have a greater response to positive emotions and messages about benefits than do younger adults, and they have a lesser response to negative events (Mather and Carstensen, 2005; Reed et al., 2014; Samanez-Larkin et al; 2007; Shamaskin et al., 2010). Similarly, an intervention study found that framing messages in terms of the positive benefits of change (rather than losses associated with not changing) seems to be a more effective approach with older adults (Notthoff and Carstensen, 2014).

Pretesting preliminary versions of messages and presentations with the target populations is critical in refining the communication approach and increasing the likelihood of impact. Message timing is also critical, although it is currently not known how often cognitive aging messages need to be received in order to sustain behavior change over time. Finally, campaigns can use elements that increase messages' memorability, such as logos, jingles, slogans, and taglines.

In sum, cognitive aging programs and campaigns to reach members of the public will need to develop specific behavioral goals for each target population, behavior change strategy, and communication strategy—including channels, message content, and presentation. Most likely, the most effective programs will employ a comprehensive strategy that addresses environmental constraints, individual behavior change, and social influences on the target population. In addition, ongoing feedback during planning and implementation in the form of formative and outcomes evaluation can improve program designs over time. Evaluation results should be made available broadly to enable the field of communications regarding cognitive aging to advance.

KEY MESSAGES AND RECOMMENDATION

Based on the review of the evidence throughout this report, the committee has developed several key messages for the public (see Box 7-3). The first area of emphasis is promoting an understanding of cognitive aging (what it is and what it is not) with a focus on the wide variation among individuals in the nature and extent of cognitive changes with age. Additionally, people across the life span should be informed about the actions they can take in childhood, youth, young adulthood, middle age, and older age to preserve and enhance their cognitive health. Older adults and their families

> **BOX 7-3**
> **Key Messages**
>
> - **Cognitive health should be promoted across the life span.** Due to the complexity of the human brain, numerous risk and protective factors may affect cognitive abilities in ways that vary among individuals.
> - **Age affects all organ systems.** The brain ages, just like other parts of the body. The types and rates of change can vary widely among individuals.
> - **Cognitive changes are not necessarily signs of neurodegenerative disease (such as Alzheimer's disease) or other neurological diseases.**
> - **Actions can be taken by individuals to help maintain cognitive health.** These actions include
>   - Be physically active.
>   - Reduce and manage cardiovascular disease risk factors (including hypertension, diabetes, and smoking).
>   - Discuss and review your health conditions and your medications that might influence your cognitive health with your health care provider.
> - **Cognitive changes can affect daily activities (e.g., driving, medication management, financial decisions) and independent living.** Older adults and their families need to monitor for cognitive changes and make informed decisions.
> - **Aging can have positive effects on cognition** (e.g., wisdom learned from experience).
> - **Participation of individuals in cognitive aging research is important** to advance understanding of the causes, outcomes, and interventions for cognitive aging.

also need information both on the potential for cognitive aging to affect decision making in some individuals and on strategies to protect against poor decisions, and older adults and their families can be encouraged to talk with their health care provider if they have concerns. Because of the need for and importance of research into cognitive aging, participation in research to advance the science of cognitive aging should be encouraged.

Recommendation 10: *Expand Public Communication Efforts and Promote Key Messages and Actions*
The Centers for Disease Control and Prevention, the Administration for Community Living, the National Institutes of Health, other relevant federal agencies, state and local government agencies, relevant nonprofit and advocacy organizations and foundations, professional societies, and private-sector companies should develop, evaluate, and communicate key evidence-based messages about cognitive aging through social marketing and media campaigns; work to ensure accurate news and

storylines about cognitive aging through media relations; and promote effective services related to cognitive health in order to increase public understanding about cognitive aging and support actions that people can do to maintain their cognitive health.

Public communications efforts should:

- Reach the diverse U.S. population with campaigns and programs targeted to all relevant groups;
- Be sensitive to existing differences in knowledge, literacy, health literacy, perceived risk, cognitive aging–related behavior, communication practices, cultures and beliefs, speech and hearing declines, and skills and self-efficacy among target groups;
- Include evaluation components to assess outreach efficacy in the short and long term, and research the optimal communication strategies for the key messages among the target groups;
- Be updated as new evidence is gained on cognitive aging;
- Emphasize a lifelong approach to cognitive health;
- Promote succinct and actionable key messages that are understandable, memorable, and relevant to the target groups;
- Focus on sustaining changes in behaviors that promote cognitive health; and
- Promote effective evidence-based tools for maintenance of cognitive health and cognitive change assessment, as well as the information gateway on cognitive aging (see Recommendation 8).

REFERENCES

AARP. 2012. *Findings from AARP's 2012 Member Opinion Survey (MOS)*. http://www.aarp.org/content/dam/aarp/research/surveys_statistics/general/2013/Findings-from-AARP-2012-Member-Opinion-Survey-AARP.pdf (accessed January 12, 2015).

———. 2014. *Brain health: Understand the trends and drivers of brain health from the consumer point of view.* PowerPoint presented to the Committee on the Public Health Dimensions of Cognitive Aging by Sarah Lock, Washington, DC, February 3. Available by request through the National Academies' Public Access Records Office.

———. 2015a. *Brain health center.* http://www.aarp.org/health/brain-health (accessed January 5, 2015).

———. 2015b. *Staying sharp: Understanding and maintaining your brain.* http://www.aarp.org/about-aarp/nrta/info-2005/understand_maintain_brain.html (accessed January 5, 2015).

Abraham, C., and S. Michie. 2008. A taxonomy of behavior change techniques used in interventions. *Health Psychology* 27(3):379-387.

ACL (Administration for Community Living). 2015. *Brain health as you age: You can make a difference!* http://www.acl.gov/Get_Help/BrainHealth/Index.aspx (accessed January 5, 2015).

ACSM (American College of Sports Medicine). 2014. *Brochures.* http://www.acsm.org/access-public-information/brochures-fact-sheets/brochures (accessed January 5, 2015).

Agarwal, S., J. Driscoll, X. Gabaix, and D. Laibson. 2009. *The age of reason: Financial decisions over the life cycle and implications for regulations.* Washington, DC: Brookings Institution.

Ajzen, I. 1991. The theory of planned behavior. *Organizational Behavior and Human Decision Processes* 50:179-211.

Alzheimer's Association. 2008. *New survey shows African-Americans are concerned with heart health but unaware of link to brain health.* http://www.alz.org/news_and_events_12875.asp (accessed January 13, 2015).

———. 2014. 2014 Alzheimer's disease facts and figures. *Alzheimer's and Dementia* 10(2):e47-e92.

———. 2015. *Know the 10 signs.* http://www.alz.org/national/documents/checklist_10signs.pdf (accessed January 5, 2015).

Alzheimer's Association and CDC (Centers for Disease Control and Prevention). 2013. *The Healthy Brain Initiative: The public health road map for state and national partnerships, 2013-2018.* Chicago, IL: Alzheimer's Association. http://www.cdc.gov/aging/pdf/2013-healthy-brain-initiative.pdf (accessed February 19, 2015).

Alzheimers New Zealand. 2012. *Champions for Dementia.* http://www.alzheimers.org.nz/awareness/champions-for-dementia (accessed January 5, 2015).

Anderson, L. A., K. L. Day, R. L. Beard, P. S. Reed, and B. Wu. 2009. The public's perceptions about cognitive health and Alzheimer's disease among the U. S. population: A national review. *Gerontologist* 49(Suppl 1):S3-S11.

Andreasen, A. 1995. *Marketing social change: Changing behavior to promote health, social development, and the environment.* Somerset, NJ: Jossey-Bass.

ASA (American Society on Aging) and MetLife Foundation. 2006. *Attitudes and awareness of brain health poll.* San Francisco, CA: ASA.

Bandura, A. 1986. *Social foundations of thought and action: A social cognitive theory.* Englewood Cliffs, NJ: Prentice-Hall.

Bond, B., and K. Drogos. 2008. *Portrayals of the elderly on children's television programming: A content analysis.* Paper presented at the National Communication Association 94th Annual Convention, San Diego, CA. http://citation.allacademic.com/meta/p275229_index.html (accessed January 13, 2015).

Boyle, P. A., L. Yu, R. S. Wilson, K. Gamble, A. S. Buchman, and D. A. Bennett. 2012. Poor decision making is a consequence of cognitive decline among older persons without Alzheimer's disease or mild cognitive impairment. *PLoS ONE* 7(8):e43647.

Brose, A., F. Schmiedek, M. Lovden, and U. Lindenberger. 2011. Normal aging dampens the link between intrusive thoughts and negative affect in reaction to daily stressors. *Psychology and Aging* 26(2):488-502.

Brown, D. R., J. Soares, J. M. Epping, T. J. Lankford, J. S. Wallace, D. Hopkins, L. R. Buchanan, and C. T. Orleans. 2012. Stand-alone mass media campaigns to increase physical activity: A Community Guide updated review. *American Journal of Preventive Medicine* 43(5):551-561.

Brownson, R. C., T. K. Boehmer, and D. A. Luke. 2005. Declining rates of physical activity in the United States: What are the contributors? *Annual Review of Public Health* 26:421-443.

Bryant, J., and D. Oliver. 2009. *Media effects: Advances in theory and research.* New York: Taylor and Francis.

Buchman, A. S., R. S. Wilson, L. Yu, B. D. James, P. A. Boyle, and D. A. Bennett. 2014. Total daily activity declines more rapidly with increasing age in older adults. *Archives of Gerontology and Geriatrics* 58(1):74-79.

Caporael, L. R., and G. H. Culbertson. 1986. Verbal response modes of baby talk and other speech at institutions for the aged. *Language & Communication* 6(1-2):99-112.

Carpenter, S. M., and C. Yoon. 2011. Aging and consumer decision making. *Annals of the New York Academy of Sciences* 1235(1):E1-E12.

Carstensen, L. L., B. Turan, S. Scheibe, N. Ram, H. Ersner-Hershfield, G. R. Samanez-Larkin, K. P. Brooks, and J. R. Nesselroade. 2011. Emotional experience improves with age: Evidence based on over 10 years of experience sampling. *Psychology and Aging* 26(1):21-33.

CDC (Centers for Disease Control and Prevention). 2009. *Simply Put: A guide for creating easy-to-understand materials.* http://www.cdc.gov/healthcommunication/pdf/simply-put.pdf (accessed January 21, 2015).

———. 2011. *Older adults: Designing health information to meet their needs.* http://www.cdc.gov/healthliteracy/developmaterials/audiences/index.html (accessed January 6, 2015).

———. 2012a. *Gateway to health communication and social marketing practice.* http://www.cdc.gov/healthcommunication/ToolsTemplates (accessed January 12, 2015).

———. 2012b. Vital signs: Awareness and treatment of uncontrolled hypertension among adults—United States, 2003-2010. *Morbidity and Mortality Weekly Report* 61:703-709.

———. 2013. Self-reported increased confusion or memory loss and associated functional difficulties among adults aged ≥60 years—21 states, 2011. *Morbidity and Mortality Weekly Report* 62(18):347-350.

———. 2014. *CDC's Healthy Brain Initiative Research Network.* http://www.cdc.gov/aging/healthybrain/research-network/index.html (accessed February 6, 2015).

———. 2015. *What is a healthy brain? New research explores perceptions of cognitive health among diverse older adults.* http://www.cdc.gov/aging/pdf/perceptions_of_cog_hlth_fact sheet.pdf (accessed January 5, 2015).

Charles, S. T., C. A. Reynolds and M. Gatz. 2001. Age-related differences and change in positive and negative affect over 23 years. *Journal of Personality and Social Psychology* 80:136-151.

Clement, S., F. Lassman, E. Barley, S. Evans-Lacko, P. Williams, S. Yamaguchi, M. Slade, N. Rusch, and G. Thornicroft. 2013. Mass media interventions for reducing mental health-related stigma. *Cochrane Database of Systematic Reviews* 7:CD009453.

Coleman, P., A. Aubin, M. Robinson, C. Ivani-Chalian, and R. Briggs. 1993. Predictors of depressive symptoms and low self-esteem in a follow-up study of elderly people over 10 years. *International Journal of Geriatric Psychiatry* 8(4):343-349.

Conn, V. S., M. A. Minor, K. J. Burks, M. J. Rantz, and S. H. Pomeroy. 2003. Integrative review of physical activity intervention research with aging adults. *Journal of the American Geriatrics Society* 51(8):1159-1168.

Conn, V. S., A. R. Hafdahl, P. S. Cooper, T. M. Ruppar, D. R. Mehr, and C. L. Russell. 2009. Interventions to improve medication adherence among older adults: Meta-analysis of adherance outcomes among randomized controlled trials. *The Gerontologist* 49(4):447-462.

Conn, V. S., L. J. Phillips, T. M. Ruppar, and J. A. Chase. 2012. Physical activity interventions with healthy minority adults: Meta-analysis of behavior and health outcomes. *Journal of Health Care for the Poor and Underserved* 23(1):59-80.

Connell, C. M., J. Scott Roberts, S. J. McLaughlin, and D. Akinleye. 2009. Racial differences in knowledge and beliefs about Alzheimer disease. *Alzheimer Disease and Associated Disorders* 23(2):110-116.

Corrigan, P. W., S. B. Morris, P. J. Michaels, J. D. Rafacz, and N. Rusch. 2012. Challenging the public stigma of mental illness: A meta-analysis of outcome studies. *Psychiatric Services* 63(10):963-973.

Cross, S., and H. R. Markus. 1991. Possible selves across the life span. *Human Development* 34:230-255.

Cutler, N., N. W. Whitelaw, and B. L. Beattie. 2002. *American perspectives of aging in the 21st century.* Washington, DC: National Council on Aging.
Dana Foundation. 2015. *Seniors.* http://www.dana.org/seniors (accessed January 5, 2015).
Dementia Friends. 2015. *Become a dementia friend today.* https://www.dementiafriends.org.uk (accessed January 6, 2015).
Dohle, S., and B. Wansink. 2013. Fit in 50 years: Participation in high school sports best predicts one's physical activity after age 70. *BMC Public Health* 13:1100.
Durand, M. A., L. Carpenter, H. Dolan, P. Bravo, M. Mann, F. Bunn, and G. Elwyn. 2014. Do interventions designed to support shared decision-making reduce health inequalities? A systematic review and meta-analysis. *PLoS ONE* 9(4):e94670.
Duval, L. L., J. B. Ruscher, K. Welsh, and S. P. Catanese. 2000. Bolstering and undercutting use of the elderly stereotype through communication of exemplars: The role of speaker age and exemplar stereotypicality. *Basic and Applied Social Psychology* 22(3):137-146.
Easter Seals. 2015. *Welcome to the Easter Seals brain health center.* http://www.easterseals.com/our-programs/brain-health (accessed January 5, 2015).
Evans-Lacko, S., J. London, S. Japhet, N. Rusch, C. Flach, E. Corker, C. Henderson, and G. Thornicroft. 2012. Mass social contact interventions and their effect on mental health related stigma and intended discrimination. *BMC Public Health* 12:489.
FINRA (Financial Industry Regulatory Authority). 2015. *Avoid investment fraud.* http://www.finra.org/Investors/ProtectYourself/AvoidInvestmentFraud (accessed January 6, 2015).
Fisher, J. D., and W. A. Fisher. 2002. The information-motivation-behavioral skills model. In *Emerging theories in health promotion practice and research: Strategies for improving public health,* edited by R. J. DiClementi, R. A. Crosby, and M. C. Kegler. San Francisco: Jossey-Bass. Pp. 40-70.
Fox, K., W. L. Hinton, and S. Levkoff. 1999. Take up the caregiver's burden: Stories of care for urban African American elders with dementia. *Culture, Medicine and Psychiatry* 23(4):501-529.
Frazee, S. G., D. J. Muzina, and R. F. Nease. 2014. Strategies to overcome medication non-adherence. *JAMA* 311(16):1693.
French, D. P., E. K. Olander, A. Chisholm, and J. McSharry. 2014. Which behaviour change techniques are most effective at increasing older adults' self-efficacy and physical activity behaviour? A systematic review. *Annals of Behavioral Medicine* 48(2):225-234.
Friedman, D. B., J. N. Laditka, S. B. Laditka, and A. E. Mathews. 2010. Cognitive health messages in popular women's and men's magazines, 2006-2007. *Preventing Chronic Disease* 7(2):A32.
Friedman, D. B., S. B. Laditka, J. N. Laditka, B. Wu, R. Liu, A. E. Price, W. Tseng, S. J. Corwin, S. L. Ivey, R. Hunter, and J. R. Sharkey. 2011. Ethnically diverse older adults' beliefs about staying mentally sharp. *International Journal of Aging and Human Development* 73(1):27-52.
Friedman, D. B., I. D. Rose, L. A. Anderson, R. Hunter, L. L. Bryant, B. Wu, A. J. Deokar, and W. Tseng. 2013. Beliefs and communication practices regarding cognitive functioning among consumers and primary care providers in the United States, 2009. *Preventing Chronic Disease* 10:120249.
Fuller, F. T., A. Johnson-Turbes, M. A. Hall, and T. A. Osuji. 2012. Promoting brain health for African Americans: Evaluating the Healthy Brain Initiative, a community-level demonstration project. *Journal of Health Care for the Poor and Underserved* 23(1):99-113.
Gerbner, G., L. Gross, N. Signorielli, and M. Morgan. 1980. Aging with television: Images on television drama and conceptions of social reality. *Journal of Communication* 30(1):37-47.
Glanz, K., B. K. Rimer, and K. Viswanath. 2008. *Health behavior & health education,* 4th ed. Somerset, NJ: Jossey-Bass.

Gordon-Salant, S. 2006. Speech perception and auditory temporal processing performance by older listeners: Implications for real-world communication. *Seminars in Hearing* 27(4):264-268.
Green, J. A., A. M. Gonzaga, E. D. Cohen, and C. L. Spagnoletti. 2014. Addressing health literacy through clear health communication: A training program for internal medicine residents. *Patient Education and Counseling* 95(1):76-82.
Griffiths, K. M., B. Carron-Arthur, A. Parsons, and R. Reid. 2014. Effectiveness of programs for reducing the stigma associated with mental disorders: A meta-analysis of randomized controlled trials. *World Psychiatry* 13(2):161-175.
Hashmi, M. 2009. Dementia: An anthropological perspective. *International Journal of Geriatric Psychiatry* 24(2):207-212.
Hausdorff, J. M., B. R. Levy, and J. Y. Wei. 1999. The power of ageism on physical function of older persons: Reversibility of age-related gait changes. *Journal of the American Geriatrics Society* 47(11):1346-1349.
Head, K. J., S. M. Noar, N. T. Iannarino, and N. Grant Harrington. 2013. Efficacy of text messaging-based interventions for health promotion: A meta-analysis. *Social Science and Medicine* 97:41-48.
Heaney, C. A., and B. A. Israel. 2009. Social networks and social support. In *Health behavior and health education*, edited by K. Glanz, B. K. Rimer, and K. Viswanath. Piscataway, NJ: Jossey-Bass. Pp. 189-210.
Heath, G. W., R. C. Brownson, J. Kruger, R. Miles, K. E. Powell, and L. T. Ramsey. 2006. The effectiveness of urban design and land use and transport policies and practices to increase physical activity: A systematic review. *Journal of Aging and Physical Activity* 3:S55-S76.
Heath, G. W., D. C. Parra, O. L. Sarmiento, L. B. Andersen, N. Owen, S. Goenka, F. Montes, and R. C. Brownson. 2012. Evidence-based intervention in physical activity: Lessons from around the world. *Lancet* 380(9838):272-281.
HELP (Hospital Elder Life Program). 2015. *Healthy living: At the hospital.* http://www.hospitalelderlifeprogram.org/for-patients/healthy-living-at-the-hospital (accessed January 12, 2015).
Henderson, J. N., and J. W. Traphagan. 2005. Cultural factors in dementia: Perspectives from the anthropology of aging. *Alzheimer Disease and Associated Disorders* 19(4):272-274.
Hess, T. M., C. Auman, S. J. Colcombe, and T. A. Rahhal. 2003. The impact of stereotype threat on age differences in memory performance. *The Journals of Gerontology, Series B: Psychological Sciences and Social Sciences* 58(1):P3-P11.
Hetsroni, A. 2009. If you must be hospitalized, television is not the place: Diagnoses, survival rates and demographic characteristics of patients in TV hospital dramas. *Communication Research Reports* 26(4):311-322.
HHS (Department of Health and Human Services). 2015. *Physical activity guidelines for Americans.* http://www.health.gov/paguidelines/guidelines (accessed January 5, 2015).
Hobbs, N., A. Godfrey, J. Lara, L. Errington, T. D. Meyer, L. Rochester, M. White, J. C. Mathers, and F. F. Sniehotta. 2013. Are behavioral interventions effective in increasing physical activity at 12 to 36 months in adults aged 55 to 70 years? A systematic review and meta-analysis. *BMC Medicine* 11:75.
Hollywood, Health & Society. 2014. *Hollywood, Health & Society: Providing the entertainment industry with free, expert information for storylines on health and climate change.* https://hollywoodhealthandsociety.org (accessed January 6, 2015).
Hornik, R. C. 2002. *Public health communication: Evidence for behavior change.* Hillsdale, NJ: Lawrence Erlbaum Associates.
IOM (Institute of Medicine). 2002. *Speaking of health: Assessing health communication strategies for diverse populations.* Washington, DC: The National Academies Press.
———. 2004. *Health literacy: A prescription to end confusion.* Washington, DC: The National Academies Press.

Jacobson, K. L., and R. M. Parker. 2014. *Health literacy principles: Guidance for making information understandable, useful, and navigable: Discussion paper*. http://iom.edu/~/media/HealthLiteracyGuidance.pdf (accessed January 12, 2015).

James, B. D., P. A. Boyle, J. S. Bennett, and D. A. Bennett. 2012. The impact of health and financial literacy making in community-based older adults. *Gerontology* 58(6):531-539.

Johnson, N. B., L. D. Hayes, K. Brown, E. C. Hoo, and K. A. Ethier. 2014. CDC national health report: Leading causes of morbidity and mortality and associated behavioral risk and protective factors—United States, 2005-2013. *Morbidity and Mortality Weekly Report: Surveillance Summaries* 63(Suppl 4):3-27.

Kahn, E. B., L. T. Ramsey, R. C. Brownson, G. W. Heath, E. H. Howze, K. E. Powell, E. J. Stone, M. W. Rajab, and P. Corso. 2002. The effectiveness of interventions to increase physical activity. A systematic review. *American Journal of Preventive Medicine* 22(4 Suppl):73-107.

Kassavou, A., A. Turner, and D. P. French. 2013. Do interventions to promote walking in groups increase physical activity? A meta-analysis. *The International Journal of Behavioral Nutrition and Physical Activity* 10:18.

Keinan, G. 1987. Decision making under stress: Scanning of alternatives under controllable and uncontrollable threats. *Journal of Personality and Social Psychology* 52(3):639-644.

Kemper, S., M. Othick, J. Warren, J. Gubarchuk, and H. Gerhing. 1996. Facilitating older adults' performance on a referential communication task through speech accommodations. *Aging, Neuropsychology, and Cognition* 3(1):37-55.

Kennedy, M. G., A. O'Leary, V. Beck, K. Pollard, and P. Simpson. 2004. Increases in calls to the CDC National STD and AIDS hotline following AIDS-related episodes in a soap opera. *Journal of Communication* 54(2):287-301.

Kim, B. H., and K. Glanz. 2013. Text messaging to motivate walking in older African Americans: A randomized controlled trial. *American Journal of Preventive Medicine* 44(1):71-75.

Klein, E., and J. Karlawish. 2010. Challenges and opportunities for developing and implementing incentives to improve health-related behaviors in older adults. *Journal of the American Geriatrics Society* 58(9):1758-1763.

Knaak, S., G. Modgill, and S. B. Patten. 2014. Key ingredients of anti-stigma programs for health care providers: A data synthesis of evaluative studies. *Canadian Journal of Psychiatry* 59(10 Suppl 1):S19-S26.

Knox, V. J., W. L. Gekoski, and E. A. Johnson. 1986. Contact with and perceptions of the elderly. *The Gerontologist* 26(3):309-313.

Kurtz, S., J. Silverman, and J. Draper. 2009. *Teaching and learning communication skills in medicine*. London, UK: Radcliffe Publishing Ltd.

Kutner, M., E. Greenberg, Y. Jin, and C. Paulsen. 2006. *The health literacy of America's adults: Results from the 2003 National Assessment of Adult Literacy (NCES 2006-483)*. Washington, DC: National Center for Education Statistics.

Kutner, M., E. Greenberg, Y. Jin, B. Boyle, Y. Hsu, and E. Dunleavy. 2007. *Literacy in everyday life: Results from the 2003 National Assessment of Adult Literacy (NCES 2007-480)*. Washington, DC: National Center for Education Statistics.

Laditka, J. N., R. L. Beard, L. L. Bryant, D. Fetterman, R. Hunter, S. Ivey, R. G. Logsdon, J. R. Sharkey, and B. Wu. 2009. Promoting cognitive health: A formative research collaboration of the Healthy Aging Research Network. *The Gerontologist* 49(Suppl 1):S12-S17.

Laditka, J. N., S. B. Laditka, R. Liu, A. E. Price, B. Wu, D. B. Friedman, S. J. Corwin, J. R. Sharkey, W. Tseng, R. H. Hunter, and R. G. Logsdon. 2011. Older adults' concerns about cognitive health: Commonalities and differences among six United States ethnic groups. *Ageing and Society* 31(7):1202-1228.

Laditka, J. N., S. B. Laditka, and K. B. Lowe. 2012. Promoting cognitive health: A web site review of health systems, public health departments, and senior centers. *American Journal of Alzheimer's Disease and Other Dementias* 27(8):600-608.

Laditka, S. B., S. J. Corwin, J. N. Laditka, R. Liu, W. Tseng, B. Wu, R. L. Beard, J. R. Sharkey, and S. L. Ivey. 2009. Attitudes about aging well among a diverse group of older Americans: Implications for promoting cognitive health. *The Gerontologist* 49(Suppl 1):S30-S39.

Laditka, S. B., J. N. Laditka, R. Liu, A. E. Price, D. B. Friedman, B. Wu, L. L. Bryant, S. J. Corwin, and S. L. Ivey. 2013. How do older people describe others with cognitive impairment? A multiethnic study in the United States. *Ageing and Society* 33(3):369-392.

Lee, N. R., and P. A. Kotler. 2011. *Social marketing: Influencing behaviors for good.* 4th ed. Thousand Oaks, CA: Sage Publications, Inc.

Levy, B., O. Ashman, and I. Dror. 1999. To be or not to be: The effects of aging stereotypes on the will to live. *Omega* 40(3):409-420.

Levy, B. R., J. M. Hausdorff, R. Hencke, and J. Y. Wei. 2000. Reducing cardiovascular stress with positive self-stereotypes of aging. *The Journals of Gerontology, Series B: Psychological Sciences and Social Sciences* 55(4):P205-P213.

Lin, F. R., R. Thorpe, S. Gordon-Salant, and L. Ferrucci. 2011. Hearing loss prevalence and risk factors among older adults in the United States. *The Journals of Gerontology, Series A: Biological Sciences and Medical Sciences* 66(5):582-590.

Lipkus, I. M. 2007. Numeric, verbal, and visual formats of conveying health risks: Suggested best practices and future recommendations. *Medical Decision Making* 27(5):696-713.

Lusardi, A., and O. S. Mitchell. 2011. Financial literacy and planning: Implications for retirement and wellbeing. *National Bureau of Economic Research Working Paper Series* Working Paper No. 17078.

Lustria, M. L., S. M. Noar, J. Cortese, S. K. Van Stee, R. L. Glueckauf, and J. Lee. 2013. A meta-analysis of web-delivered tailored health behavior change interventions. *Journal of Health Communications* 18(9):1039-1069.

Markus, H. R., and P. Nurius. 1986. Possible selves. *American Psychologist* 41:954-969.

Mather, M., and L. L. Carstensen. 2005. Aging and motivated cognition: The positivity effect in attention and memory. *Trends in Cognitive Sciences* 9(10):496-502.

Mathews, A. E., S. B. Laditka, J. N. Laditka, and D. B. Friedman. 2009. What are the top-circulating magazines in the United States telling older adults about cognitive health? *American Journal of Alzheimer's Disease and Other Dementias* 24(4):302-312.

MetLife Mature Market Institute and LifePlans Inc. 2006. *The MetLife study of Alzheimer's disease: The caregiving experience.* https://www.metlife.com/assets/cao/mmi/publications/studies/mmi-alzheimers-disease-caregiving-experience-study.pdf (accessed January 12, 2015).

MetLife Mature Market Institute, National Committee for the Prevention of Elder Abuse, and Virginia Tech. 2011. *The MetLife study of elder financial abuse: Crimes of occasion, desperation, and predation against America's elders.* New York: MetLife Mature Market Institute. https://www.metlife.com/assets/cao/mmi/publications/studies/2011/mmi-elder-financial-abuse.pdf (accessed March 17, 2015).

Michie, S., M. Richardson, M. Johnston, C. Abraham, J. Francis, W. Hardeman, M. P. Eccles, J. Cane, and C. E. Wood. 2013. The behavior change technique taxonomy (v1) of 93 hierarchically clustered techniques: Building an international consensus for the reporting of behavior change interventions. *Annals of Behavioral Medicine* 46(1):81-95.

Miller, W. R., and S. Rollnick. 2002. *Motivational interviewing: Preparing people for change,* 2nd ed. New York: Guilford.

Morgado, M. P., S. R. Morgado, L. C. Mendes, L. J. Pereira, and M. Castelo-Branco. 2011. Pharmacist interventions to enhance blood pressure control and adherence to antihypertensive therapy: Review and meta-analysis. *American Journal of Health-System Pharmacy* 68(3):241-253.

Morrison, J. H., and M. G. Baxter. 2012. The ageing cortical synapse: Hallmarks and implications for cognitive decline. *Nature Reviews: Neuroscience* 13(4):240-250.

Movius, L., M. Cody, G. Huang, M. Berkowitz, and S. Morgan. 2007. Motivating television viewers to become organ donors. *Cases in Public Health Communication & Marketing*. http://publichealth.gwu.edu/departments/pch/phcm/casesjournal/volume1/peer-reviewed/cases_1_08.pdf (accessed March 24, 2015).

Moyer, V. A., and U.S. Preventive Services Task Force. 2012. Behavioral counseling interventions to promote a healthful diet and physical activity for cardiovascular disease prevention in adults: U.S. Preventive Services Task Force recommendation statement. *Annals of Internal Medicine* 157(5):367-371.

Neupert, S. D., D. M. Almeida, and S. T. Charles. 2007. Age differences in reactivity to daily stressors: The role of personal control. *The Journals of Gerontology, Series B: Psychological Sciences and Social Sciences* 62(4):P216-P225.

NHLBI (National Heart, Lung, and Blood Institute). 2015a. *Delicious heart healthy recipes*. https://healthyeating.nhlbi.nih.gov (accessed January 5, 2015).

———. 2015b. *Resources for the public*. https://www.nhlbi.nih.gov/health/resources#heart (accessed January 5, 2015).

NIA (National Institute on Aging). 2014. *Go4life*. http://go4life.nia.nih.gov (accessed December 10, 2014).

Noar, S. M., C. N. Benac, and M. S. Harris. 2007. Does tailoring matter? Meta-analytic review of tailored print health behavior change interventions. *Psychological Bulletin* 133(4):673-693.

Notthoff, N., and L. L. Carstensen. 2014. Positive messaging promotes walking in older adults. *Psychology and Aging* 29(2):329-341.

NRC (National Research Council). 2006. *When I'm 64*. Edited by L. L. Carstensen and C. R. Hartel. Washington, DC: The National Academies Press.

PARADE and Research!America. 2006. *America speaks! Poll data summary*. Volume 7. http://www.researchamerica.org/uploads/AmericaSpeaksV7.pdf (accessed January 13, 2015).

Park, D. C., C. Hertzog, H. Leventhal, R. W. Morrell, E. Leventhal, D. Birchmore, M. Martin, and J. Bennett. 1999. Medication adherence in rheumatoid arthritis patients: Older is wiser. *Journal of the American Geriatrics Society* 47(2):172-183.

Pasupathi, M., L. L. Carstensen, and J. L. Tsai. 1995. Ageism in interpersonal setttings. In *The social psychology of interpersonal discrimination*, edited by B. Lott and D. Maluso. New York: Guilford Press. Pp. 160-182.

Perlmutter, M. 1988. Cognitive potential throughout life. In *Emergent theories of aging*, edited by J. Birren and V. Bengtson. New York: Springer. Pp. 247-268.

Pew Research Center. 2014. *Older adults and technology use. Usage and adoption*. http://www.pewinternet.org/2014/04/03/usage-and-adoption (accessed February 19, 2015).

———. 2015. *Newspaper readership by age: Percentage nationally who read any daily newspaper yesterday*. http://www.journalism.org/media-indicators/newspaper-readership-by-age (accessed January 5, 2015).

Plimpton, S., and J. Root. 1994. Materials and strategies that work in low literacy health communication. *Public Health Reports* 109(1):86-92.

Price, A. E., S. J. Corwin, D. B. Friedman, S. B. Laditka, N. Colabianchi, and K. M. Montgomery. 2011. Older adults' perceptions of physical activity and cognitive health: Implications for health communication. *Health Education & Behavior* 38(1):15-24.

Prohaska, T. R., and K. E. Peters. 2007. Physical activity and cognitive functioning: translating research to practice with a public health approach. *Alzheimer's and Dementia* 3(2 Suppl):S58-S64.

Ratzan, S. C., and R. M. Parker. 2000. Introduction. In *National Library of Medicine current bibliographies in medicine: Health literacy*, edited by C. R. Selden, M. Zorn, S. C. Ratzan, and R. M. Parker. Bethesda, MD: National Institutes of Health, U.S. Department of Health and Human Services. Pp. v-vi.

Reed, A. E., L. Chan, and J. A. Mikels. 2014. Meta-analysis of the age-related positivity effect: age differences in preferences for positive over negative information. *Psychology and Aging* 29(1):1-15.

Ritchey, M. D., H. K. Wall, C. Gillespie, M. G. George, and A. Jamal. 2014. Million hearts: Prevalence of leading cardiovascular disease risk factors—United States, 2005-2012. *Morbidity and Mortality Weekly Report* 63(21):462-467.

Robare, J. F., C. M. Bayles, A. B. Newman, K. Williams, C. Milas, R. Boudreau, K. McTigue, S. M. Albert, C. Taylor, and L. H. Kuller. 2011. The "10 keys" to healthy aging: 24-month follow-up results from an innovative community-based prevention program. *Health Education and Behavior* 38(4):379-388.

Roberts, J. S., C. M. Connell, D. Cisewski, Y. G. Hipps, S. Demissie, and R. C. Green. 2003. Differences between African Americans and whites in their perceptions of Alzheimer disease. *Alzheimer Disease and Associated Disorders* 17(1):19-26.

Roberts, J. S., S. J. McLaughlin, and C. M. Connell. 2014. Public beliefs and knowledge about risk and protective factors for Alzheimer's disease. *Alzheimer's & Dementia* 10(5 Suppl):S381-S389.

Robillard, J. M., T. W. Johnson, C. Hennessey, B. L. Beattie, and J. Illes. 2013. Aging 2.0: Health information about dementia on Twitter. *PLoS ONE* 8(7):e69861.

Robinson, J. D., T. Skill, and J. W. Turner. 2004. Media usage patterns and portrayals of seniors. In *Handbook of communication and aging research*, 2nd ed., edited by J. F. Nussbaum and J. Coupland. Mahwah, NJ: Erlbaum. Pp. 423-450.

Robinson, T., M. Callister, D. Magoffin, and J. Moore. 2007. The portrayal of older characters in Disney animated films. *Journal of Aging Studies* 21(3):203-213.

Sabatino, C. P. 2011. Damage prevention and control for financial incapacity. *JAMA* 305(7): 707-708.

Sallis, J. F., N. Owen, and E. B. Fisher. 2008. Ecological models of health behaviors. In *Health behavior and health education*. 4th ed, edited by K. Glanz, B. K. Rimer, and K. Viswanath. Piscataway, NJ: Jossey-Bass.

Samanez-Larkin, G. R., S. E. Gibbs, K. Khanna, L. Nielsen, L. L. Carstensen, and B. Knutson. 2007. Anticipation of monetary gain but not loss in healthy older adults. *Nature Neuroscience* 10(6):787-791.

Schilling, O. K., and M. Diehl. 2014. Reactivity to stressor pile-up in adulthood: Effects on daily negative and positive affect. *Psychology and Aging* 29(1):72-83.

Shamaskin, A. M., J. A. Mikels, and A. E. Reed. 2010. Getting the message across: Age differences in the positive and negative framing of health care messages. *Psychology and Aging* 25(3):746-751.

Shelton, J. N., J. A. Richeson, and J. Salvatore. 2005. Expecting to be the target of prejudice: Implications for interethnic interactions. *Personality & Social Psychology Bulletin* 31(9):1189-1202.

Sheridan, S. L., D. J. Halpern, A. J. Viera, N. D. Berkman, K. E. Donahue, and K. Crotty. 2011. Interventions for individuals with low health literacy: A systematic review. *Journal of Health Communication* 16(Suppl 3):30-54.

Signorielli, N. 2004. Aging on television: Messages relating to gender, race, and occupation in prime time. *Journal of Broadcasting & Electronic Media* 48(2):279-301.

Singhal, A., and E. M. Rogers. 1999. *Entertainment-education: A communication strategy for social change.* Mahwah, NJ: Lawrence Erlbaum Associates.

Slater, M. D. 1995. Choosing audience segmentation strategies and methods for health communication. In *Designing health messages: Approaches from communication theory and public health practice,* edited by E. W. Maibach and R. L. Parrott. Thousand Oaks, CA: Sage. Pp. 186-198.

Snyder, L. B. 2007. Health communication campaigns and their impact on behavior. *Journal of Nutrition Education and Behavior* 39(2 Suppl):S32-S40.

Snyder, L. B., and M. A. Hamilton. 2002. Meta-analysis of U.S. health campaign effects on behavior: Emphasize enforcement, exposure, and new information, and beware the secular trend. In *Public health communication: Evidence for behavior change,* edited by R. C. Hornik. Hillsdale, NJ: Lawrence Erlbaum Associates.

Snyder, L. B., and J. M. LaCroix. 2013. How effective are mediated health campaigns? A synthesis of meta-analyses. In *Public communication campaigns,* edited by R. Rice and C. Atkin. Thousand Oaks, CA: Sage. Pp. 113-129.

Soler, R. E., K. D. Leeks, L. R. Buchanan, R. C. Brownson, G. W. Heath, and D. H. Hopkins. 2010. Point-of-decision prompts to increase stair use. A systematic review update. *American Journal of Preventive Medicine* 38(2 Suppl):S292-S300.

Stone, A. A., J. E. Schwartz, J. E. Broderick, and A. Deaton. 2010. A snapshot of the age distribution of psychological well-being in the United States. *Proceedings of the National Academy of Sciences of the United States of America* 107(22):9985-9990.

Strickler, Z., and P. Neafsey. 2002. Visual design of interactive software for older adults: Preventing drug interactions in older adults. *Visible Language* 36(1):4-29.

Tangney, J. P., J. Stuewig, E. T. Malouf, and K. Youman. 2013. Communicative functions of shame and guilt. In *Cooperation and its evolution,* edited by K. Sterelny, R. Joyce, B. Calcott, and B. Fraser. Cambridge, MA: MIT Press. Pp. 485-502.

Task Force on Community Prevention Services. 2002. Recommendations to increase physical activity in communities. *American Journal of Preventive Medicine* 22(4 Suppl):67-72.

Teyhen, D. S., M. Aldag, D. Centola, E. Edinborough, J. D. Ghannadian, A. Haught, T. Jackson, J. Kinn, K. J. Kunkler, B. Levine, V. E. Martindale, D. Neal, L. B. Snyder, M. A. Styn, F. Thorndike, V. Trabosh, and D. J. Parramore. 2014. Key enablers to facilitate healthy behavior change: Workshop summary. *Journal of Orthopaedic and Sports Physical Therapy* 44(5):378-387.

Triebel, K. L., and D. Marson. 2012. The warning signs of diminished financial capacity in older adults. *Generations* 36(2):39-45.

Uchino, B. N., C. A. Berg, T. W. Smith, G. Pearce, and M. Skinner. 2006. Age-related differences in ambulatory blood pressure during daily stress: Evidence for greater blood pressure reactivity with age. *Psychology and Aging* 21(2):231-239.

USDA (U.S. Department of Agriculture). 2015. *How much physical activity is needed?* http://www.choosemyplate.gov/physical-activity/amount.html (accessed January 5, 2015).

Vandelanotte, C., K. M. Spathonis, E. G. Eakin, and N. Owen. 2007. Website-delivered physical activity interventions: A review of the literature. *American Journal of Preventive Medicine* 33(1):54-64.

Vandenberg, A. E., A. E. Price, D. B. Friedman, G. Marchman, and L. A. Anderson. 2012. How do top cable news websites portray cognition as an aging issue? *The Gerontologist* 52(3):367-382.

Wahl, O. F. 2012. Stigma as a barrier to recovery from mental illness. *Trends in Cognitive Science* 16(1):9-10.

Wallack, L., L. Dorfman, D. Jernigan, and M. Themba. 1993. *Media advocacy and public health: Power for prevention.* Newbury Park, CA: Sage.

Warren-Findlow, J., R. B. Seymour, and D. Shenk. 2011. Intergenerational transmission of chronic illness self-care: Results from the caring for hypertension in African American families study. *Gerontologist* 51(1):64-75.

Washington University School of Medicine. 2013. *Your disease risk: The source on prevention.* http://www.yourdiseaserisk.wustl.edu/YDRDefault.aspx?ScreenScreenControl=YDRGeneral&ScreenName=YDRHome.htm (accessed January 5, 2015).

Weinreich, N. 2010. *A step-by-step guide to designing change for good,* 2nd ed. Thousand Oaks, CA: Sage.

West, R. L., and N. C. Ebner. 2013. Linking goals and aging: Experimental and lifespan approaches. In *New developments in goal setting and task performance,* edited by E. A. Locke and G. P. Latham. New York: Routledge. Pp. 439-459.

WHO (World Health Organization). 2012. *Dementia: A public health priority.* Geneva: WHO.

Widera, E., V. Steenpass, D. Marson, and R. Sudore. 2011. Finances in the older patient with cognitive impairment: "He didn't want me to take over." *JAMA* 305(7):698-706.

Wilcox, S., M. Dowda, S. Wegley, and M. G. Ory. 2009. Maintenance of change in the Active-for-Life Initiative. *American Journal of Preventive Medicine* 37(6):501-504.

Williams, A., and J. F. Nussbaum. 2001. *Intergenerational communication across the lifespan.* Mahwah, NJ: Lawrence Erlbaum Associates.

Williams, D., N. Martins, M. Consalvo, and J. D. Ivory. 2009. The virtual census: Representations of gender, race and age in video games. *New Media & Society* 11(5):815-834.

Williamson, K., and T. Asla. 2009. Information behavior of people in the fourth age. *Library and Information Science Research* 31(2):76-83.

Wolff, J. L., and D. L. Roter. 2011. Family presence in routine medical visits: A meta-analytical review. *Social Science and Medicine* 72(6):823-831.

Wolff, J. L., D. L. Roter, J. Barron, C. M. Boyd, B. Leff, T. E. Finucane, J. J. Gallo, P. V. Rabins, D. L. Roth, and L. N. Gitlin. 2014. A tool to strengthen the older patient-companion partnership in primary care: Results from a pilot study. *Journal of the American Geriatrics Society* 62(2):312-319.

Wu, B., R. T. Goins, J. N. Laditka, V. Ignatenko, and E. Goedereis. 2009. Gender differences in views about cognitive health and healthy lifestyle behaviors among rural older adults. *The Gerontologist* 49(Suppl 1):S72-S78.

Xu, A., T. Chomutare, and S. Iyengar. 2014. Persuasive attributes of medication adherence interventions for older adults: A systematic review. *Technology and Health Care* 22(2):189-198.

Zullig, L. L., E. D. Peterson, and H. B. Bosworth. 2013. Ingredients of successful interventions to improve medication adherence. *JAMA* 310(24):2611-2612.

8

Opportunities for Action

Aging is inevitable, but individuals, families, communities, and society can take actions that may help prevent or ameliorate the impact of aging on cognition, create greater understanding about its impact, and help older adults live fuller and more independent lives. One of the major concerns of older adults is "Will I stay sharp?" Although changes in cognitive function vary widely among individuals, actions that would make a difference and promote cognitive health are summarized in Box 8-1 and detailed throughout the discussion and recommendations in this report. Cognitive aging is not just an individual or family or health care system challenge—it is an issue that affects the fabric of society and requires actions by many and varied stakeholders. How society responds to these challenges will reflect the value it places on older adults and how it views their continued involvement and contribution to their families, social networks, and communities.

The committee heard throughout its work on this study that cognitive aging is a concern to many people across all cultural groups and income levels. In recent years a vigorous public health, research, and community response has focused on Alzheimer's disease and other neurodegenerative dementias. These efforts should continue to be strengthened. At the same time, similar efforts should be made in the field of cognitive aging. Attention needs to be paid to the cognitive vulnerabilities of the vast majority of older adults who may experience cognitive decline that is not caused by a neurodegenerative disease. They, too, want to maintain their cognitive health to the fullest extent possible. The committee hopes that a commitment to addressing cognitive aging by many sectors of society will bring about further effective interventions, greater understanding of risk and protective factors, and a society that values and sustains cognitive health.

> **BOX 8-1**
> **Opportunities for Action**
>
> Many of the following actions require multiple efforts involving a number of agencies, organizations, and sectors, as well as individuals and families. These efforts will be greatly strengthened by joint and collaborative efforts.
>
> **Individuals and families:**
> - Be physically active and intellectually and socially engaged, monitor medications, and engage in healthy lifestyles and behavior;
> - Talk with health care professionals about cognitive aging concerns;
> - Be aware of the potential for financial fraud and abuse, impaired driving skills, and poor consumer decision making;
> - Make health, finance, and consumer decisions based on reliable evidence from trusted sources.
>
> **Communities, community organizations, senior centers, residential facilities, housing and transportation planners, local governments:**
> - Provide opportunities for physical activity, social and intellectual engagement, lifelong learning, and education on cognitive aging; expand relevant programs and facilities;
> - Improve walkability and public transportation options in neighborhoods, communities, and cities.
>
> **Health care professionals and professional associations and health care systems:**
> - Learn about cognitive aging and engage patients and families in discussions;
> - Pay attention to cognition during wellness visits, prescribing and reviews of medications, and during hospital stays and post-surgery;
> - Identify useful and evidence-based community and patient resources and make sure patients and families know about them;
> - Develop core professional competencies in cognitive aging as distinct from dementia and other neurodegenerative diseases in treatment and in counseling patients and families;
> - Address factors that lead to delirium in hospitalized patients.

Public health agencies at the federal, state, and local levels; aging organizations; media; professional associations; and consumer groups:
- Strengthen efforts to collect and disseminate population-based data on cognitive aging as separate from dementia and other neurodegenerative diseases;
- Develop and widely disseminate independent authoritative information resources on cognitive aging and criteria for consumer evaluation of products and medications that make claims to enhance cognition;
- Develop, test, and disseminate key messages regarding cognitive aging through social marketing campaigns, media awareness efforts, and other approaches to increase public understanding about cognitive aging; and promote activities that help maintain cognitive health.

Research funders and researchers:
- Explore cognitive aging as separate from dementia and other neurodegenerative diseases in basic, applied, and clinical research;
- Expand research on the trajectories of cognitive aging and improve assessments of cognitive changes and impacts on daily function;
- Focus research on risk and protective factors for cognitive aging and on developing and improving implementation of interventions aimed at preventing or reducing cognitive decline and maintaining cognitive health.

Policy makers, regulators, and consumer advocacy and support organizations:
- Support the resources needed to understand and address cognitive aging;
- Determine (or provide input into the appropriate regulatory review) policies and guidelines for products, medications, and other interventions that claim to enhance cognitive function or that have a negative impact on cognition;
- Develop, validate, and disseminate policies, products, services, and informational materials focused on cognitive aging and addressing potential financial, health, and safety impacts, harms, and vulnerabilities.

Private-sector businesses, including the financial, transportation, and technology industries:
- Develop, validate, and disseminate policies, products, services, and informational materials focused on cognitive aging and addressing potential financial, health, and safety impacts, harms, and vulnerabilities.

A

Meeting Agendas

INSTITUTE OF MEDICINE
National Academy of Sciences
Committee on the Public Health Dimensions of Cognitive Aging
First Committee Meeting
February 3, 2014

National Academy of Sciences Building
Room 125
2101 Constitution Ave., NW
Washington, DC 20001

Monday, February 3, 2014

OPEN SESSION: NAS Building Room 125

10:00 – 10:15 a.m.	Welcome and Introductions *Dan Blazer,* Committee Chair
10:15 a.m. – 12:00 p.m.	Discussion of the Charge to the Committee

10:15 – 11:00 a.m.	Perspectives from Study Sponsors
	McKnight Brain Research Foundation
	  Robert Wah
	  Lee Dockery (via phone)
	National Institute on Aging
	  Molly Wagster
	  Jonathan King

	National Institute of Neurological Disorders and Stroke *Deb Babcock (via phone)* AARP *Sarah Lock* *Susan Reinhard*
11:00 a.m. – 12:00 p.m.	**Committee Discussion with Study Sponsors**
12:00 – 1:00 p.m.	**Lunch**
1:00 – 2:30 p.m.	**Context for the Study** *Francine Grodstein,* Harvard School of Public Health *Lynda Anderson,* Centers for Disease Control and Prevention **Discussion**
2:30 p.m.	**Open Session Adjourns**

APPENDIX A

INSTITUTE OF MEDICINE
National Academy of Sciences

Committee on the Public Health Dimensions of Cognitive Aging

Second Committee Meeting
April 10–11, 2014

National Academy of Sciences Building
Room 120
2101 Constitution Ave., NW
Washington, DC 20001

Thursday, April 10, 2014

OPEN SESSION: NAS 120

9:00 – 9:15 a.m.	Welcome and Opening Remarks *Dan Blazer*, Chair *Kristine Yaffe*, Vice Chair
9:15 – 10:00 a.m.	Opening Speaker *Guy McKhann*, Johns Hopkins University Discussion with the committee
10:00 – 11:30 a.m.	Panel 1: Defining Cognitive Aging Facilitator: *Tia Powell*
10:00 – 10:05 a.m.	Panel introductions
10:05 – 10:20 a.m.	Definitions along the spectrum of cognition—normal to disease *Reisa Sperling*, Harvard Medical School
10:20 – 10:35 a.m.	Cognitive reserve *Yaakov Stern*, Columbia University
10:35 – 10:50 a.m.	Individual assessments of cognitive change *Rich Jones*, Brown University
10:50 – 11:05 a.m.	Cultural and educational impacts *Peggye Dilworth-Anderson*, University of North Carolina
11:05 – 11:30 a.m.	Discussion with the committee
11:30 a.m. – 12:15 p.m.	Lunch
12:15 – 1:45 p.m.	Panel 2: Cognitive Trajectory with Age Facilitator: *Marilyn Albert*
12:15 – 12:20 p.m.	Panel introductions

12:20 – 12:50 p.m.	Animal research *Michela Gallagher,* Johns Hopkins University *Peter Rapp,* National Institute on Aging
12:50 – 1:20 p.m.	Human research *Tim Salthouse,* University of Virginia *David Bennett,* Rush University
1:20 – 1:45 p.m.	Discussion with the committee
1:45 – 2:00 p.m.	**Break**
2:00 – 3:30 p.m.	**Panel 3: Epidemiology and Surveillance** Facilitator: *Bob Wallace*
2:00 – 2:05 p.m.	Panel introductions
2:05 – 2:20 p.m.	Behavioral Risk Factor Surveillance System (BRFSS) *Patricia Lillquist,* New York State Chronic Disease Epidemiology and Surveillance
2:20 – 2:35 p.m.	Health and Retirement Survey (HRS) and ADAMS Study *Jack McArdle,* University of Southern California *(via Webex)*
2:35 – 2:50 p.m.	Midlife in the United States Study (MIDUS) *Margie Lachman,* Brandeis University
2:50 – 3:05 p.m.	National Health and Aging Trends Study (NHATS) *Judith Kasper,* Johns Hopkins University
3:05 – 3:30 p.m.	Discussion with the committee
3:30 – 4:30 p.m.	**Public Testimony—Registered Speakers** Moderator: *Dan Blazer* (3 minutes per speaker)
4:30 p.m.	**Public Session Adjourns**

APPENDIX A

Friday, April 11, 2014
OPEN SESSION: NAS 120

8:45 – 9:00 a.m.	Welcome and Opening Remarks *Dan Blazer*, Chair *Kristine Yaffe*, Vice Chair
9:00 – 10:30 a.m.	Panel 4: Risk Factors for Cognitive Decline (further risk factors and intervention opportunities to be discussed at the June workshop) Facilitator: *Sharon Inouye*
9:00 – 9:05 a.m.	Panel introductions
9:05 – 9:20 a.m.	Medication use *Malaz Boustani*, Indiana University
9:20 – 9:35 a.m.	Cardiovascular risk factors *Jose Luchsinger*, Columbia University
9:35 – 9:50 a.m.	Depression and mental illness *Sarah Tighe*, University of Iowa
9:50 – 10:05 a.m.	Acute illness, delirium, and hospitalization *Edward Marcantonio*, Harvard University
10:05 – 10:30 a.m.	Discussion with the committee
10:30 a.m.	**Public Session Adjourns**

INSTITUTE OF MEDICINE
National Academy of Sciences
Committee on the Public Health Dimensions of Cognitive Aging
Public Workshop
Arnold and Mabel Beckman Center of the National Academies
100 Academy Drive
Irvine, CA

Monday, June 9, 2014

OPEN SESSION: Huntington Room

8:00 – 8:15 a.m.	Welcome and Opening Remarks *Dan Blazer*, Chair, *Kristine Yaffe*, Vice Chair
8:15 – 9:30 a.m.	**Panel 1: Cognitive Stimulation** Facilitators: *Andrea LaCroix* and *Felicia Hill-Briggs*
8:15 – 8:20 a.m.	Panel introductions
8:20 – 8:35 a.m.	Cognitive training *Adam Gazzaley*, University of California, San Francisco
8:35 – 8:50 a.m.	ACTIVE trial *Sherry Willis*, University of Washington
8:50 – 9:05 a.m.	Educational interventions *Fred Wolinsky*, University of Iowa
9:05 – 9:30 a.m.	Discussion with the committee
9:30 – 11:00 a.m.	**Panel 2: Physical Activity and Nutrition** Facilitator: *Art Kramer*
9:30 – 9:35 a.m.	Panel introductions

9:35 – 10:05 a.m.	Physical activity versus sedentary time
	   Kirk Erickson, University of Pittsburgh
	   Deborah Barnes, University of California, San Francisco

10:05 – 10:35 a.m.	Nutrition and supplements
	Diet
	   Martha Clare Morris, Rush University Medical Center
	Supplements and caffeine
	   Steven DeKosky, University of Virginia

10:35 – 11:00 a.m.	Discussion with the committee

11:00 – 11:15 a.m.	Break
11:15 a.m. – 12:30 p.m.	**Panel 3: Social Engagement, Arts, and Sleep** Facilitator: *David Reuben*
11:15 – 11:20 a.m.	Panel introductions
11:20 – 11:35 a.m.	Social engagement *Michelle Carlson*, Johns Hopkins University
11:35 – 11:50 a.m.	Arts *Tony Noice and Helga Noice*, Elmhurst College *(via Webex)*
11:50 a.m. – 12:05 p.m.	Sleep and mindfulness *Sonia Ancoli-Israel*, University of California, San Diego
12:05 – 12:30 p.m.	Discussion with the committee
12:30 – 1:15 p.m.	**Lunch**
1:15 – 1:45 p.m.	**Public Testimony and Questions to Speakers** Facilitator: *Dan Blazer*
1:45 – 3:00 p.m.	**Panel 4: Multi-Domain Trials and Sustaining Behavioral Change** Facilitator: *Sara Czaja*
1:45 – 1:50 p.m.	Panel introductions

1:50 – 2:20 p.m.	Multi-domain trials
	   James Blumenthal, Duke University
	   Miia Kivipelto, Karolinska Institutet *(via Webex)*

2:20 – 2:35 p.m.	Behavioral change *Bonnie Spring*, Northwestern University
2:35 – 3:00 p.m.	Discussion with the committee
3:00 – 4:15 p.m.	**Panel 5: Education of Health Professionals** Facilitators: *Donna Fick and Lisa Gwyther*
3:00 – 3:05 p.m.	Panel introductions

3:05 – 3:35 p.m.	Professional schools
	   Catherine Lucey, University of California, San Francisco
	   Terry Fulmer, Northeastern University

3:35 – 3:50 p.m.	Primary care *Christopher Callahan*, Indiana University
3:50 – 4:15 p.m.	Discussion with the committee

4:15 – 5:30 p.m.	**Panel 6: Public Action**
	Facilitator: *Jason Karlawish*
4:15 – 4:20 p.m.	Panel introductions
4:20 – 5:05 p.m.	Public outreach
	Jennie Chin Hansen, American Geriatrics Society
	Financial issues
	Naomi Karp, Consumer Financial Protection Bureau
	Media/Outreach
	Heidi Keller, Keller Consulting
5:05 – 5:30 p.m.	Discussion with the committee
5:30 p.m.	**Public Session Adjourns**

B

U.S. Surveys and Studies That Include One or More Items to Measure Cognition

Box B-1 provides examples of ongoing and completed surveys and studies relevant to cognitive aging conducted with representative samples of the U.S. population, representative samples of regional or local populations, and samples of community volunteers and other cohorts. All of the surveys and studies include community-living people, and some also include nursing home residents. The list does not include surveys and studies that only include nursing home residents.

Each survey and study includes one or more items to measure cognition. Some surveys and studies include items to measure cognition directly; some include items to measure the survey respondent's awareness and perceptions about his or her cognition; and some include both types of items.

> **BOX B-1**
> **U.S. Surveys and Studies That Include One
> or More Items to Measure Cognition**
>
> A. Surveys and Studies Conducted in Representative Samples of the National Population
>
>   - American Community Survey (ACS)
>   - Asset and Health Dynamics Among the Oldest Old (AHEAD)
>   - Behavioral Risk Factors Surveillance Survey (BRFSS)
>   - Health and Retirement Study (HRS)
>   - Medicare Current Beneficiary Survey (MCBS)
>   - Medicare Expenditure Panel Survey (MEPS)
>   - National Health and Aging Trends Survey (NHATS)
>   - National Health and Nutrition Examination Survey (NHANES)
>   - National Health Interview Survey (NHIS)
>
> B. Surveys and Studies Conducted in Representative Samples of Regional or Local Populations, Community Volunteers, or Other Cohorts
>
>   - Adult Changes in Thought Study (ACT)
>   - Atherosclerosis Risk in Communities Study (ARIC)
>   - Baltimore Longitudinal Study of Aging
>   - Baltimore Memory Study
>   - Cache County Study on Memory Health and Aging
>   - Cardiovascular Health Study (CHS)–Cognition Study
>   - Chicago Health and Aging Project (CHAP)
>   - Established Populations for Epidemiological Studies of the Elderly (EPESE)
>   - Framingham Heart Study
>   - Ginkgo Evaluation of Memory (GEM)
>   - Health Aging and Body Composition (Health ABC)
>   - Hispanic Established Populations for the Epidemiologic Study of the Elderly (HEPESE)
>   - Honolulu-Asia Aging Study (HAAS)

APPENDIX B

- Indianapolis Ibadan Dementia Research Project
- The KAME Study
- MacArthur Studies of Successful Aging
- Mayo Clinic Study of Aging
- Monongahela Valley Independent Elders Survey (MoVIES)
- Multi-Ethnic Study of Atherosclerosis (MESA)
- The National Alzheimer's Coordinating Center/Alzheimer's Disease Centers Study (NACC/ADC)
- National Social Life, Health, and Aging Project
- NCI Surveillance, Epidemiology, and End Results Program (SEER)
- Northern Manhattan Study
- Nun Study
- Nurses' Health Study
- Physicians Health Study
- Precipitating Events Project
- Rancho Bernardo Study
- Religious Orders Study
- Rochester Epidemiology Project
- Rush Memory and Aging Study
- Sacramento Area Latino Study of Aging (SALSA)
- San Antonio Longitudinal Study of Aging
- St. Louis OASIS Study
- Study of Osteoporotic Fractures
- Washington Heights-Inwood Columbia Aging Project (The Epidemiology of Dementia in an Urban Community)
- Wisconsin Longitudinal Study
- Women's Antioxidant Cardiovascular Study
- Women's Health Initiative Memory Study (WHIMS)
- Yale Health and Aging Project

SOURCE: Adapted from Bell, J. F., A. L. Fitzpatrick, C. Copeland, G. Chi, L. Steinman, R. L. Whitney, D. C. Atkins, L. L. Bryant, F. Grodstein, E. Larson, R. Logsdon, and M. Snowden. 2014. Existing data sets to support studies of dementia or significant cognitive impairment and comorbid chronic conditions. *Alzheimer's & Dementia* (September 4).

C

Committee Biographies

Dan G. Blazer, M.D., M.P.H., Ph.D. (*Chair*), is the J.P. Gibbons Professor of Psychiatry Emeritus at Duke. He served nine years as chair of the Department of Psychiatry and Dean of Medical Education at Duke School of Medicine. Dr. Blazer's research interests include the epidemiology of late life substance use disorders and depression, psychosocial predictors of adverse health outcomes, and trajectories of health outcomes. He has worked on the Established Populations for Epidemiologic Study of the Elderly (EPESE) and the National Comorbidity Study. He is the author or editor of 36 books, including *The Age of Melancholy: Depression and Its Social Origins* and a research methods textbook for clinical psychiatry research. He has produced a second edition of *Emotional Problems in Later Life* and authored or co-authored more than 200 published abstracts and more than 450 peer-reviewed articles. Dr. Blazer was president of the American Association of Geriatric Psychiatry and is a current member of the editorial board of *JAMA Psychiatry*. He has been a member of the Institute of Medicine (IOM) since 1995. Currently he is the chair of the IOM Board on the Health of Select Populations. He has served as a member or the chair of many past IOM committees. In 2014, he received the Walsh McDermott Award from the IOM for Lifetime Distinguished Service.

Kristine Yaffe, M.D. (*Vice Chair*), is the Scola Endowed chair and a professor of psychiatry, neurology, and epidemiology and biostatistics at the University of California, San Francisco (UCSF) and vice chair of clinical and translational research in the Department of Psychiatry. Dr. Yaffe was named the first holder of the Roy and Marie Scola Endowed Chair in Psychiatry.

Dr. Yaffe is dually trained in neurology and psychiatry and completed postdoctoral training in epidemiology and geriatric psychiatry, all at UCSF. Dr. Yaffe serves as the director of the UCSF Dementia Epidemiology Research Group, which conducts research relating to cognitive function and dementia in aging populations throughout the United States. A primary focus of the group is determining predictors and outcomes of cognitive decline and dementia in older adults. Dr. Yaffe is also the principal investigator of the data core for the Alzheimer's Disease Research Center at UCSF. In addition to her positions at UCSF, Dr. Yaffe is the chief of geriatric psychiatry and the director of the Memory Disorders Clinic at the San Francisco Veterans Affairs Medical Center. In addition to her research and clinical work, Dr. Yaffe has greatly contributed to training fellows and faculty in clinical research and in career development and mentorship.

Marilyn Albert, Ph.D., is professor of neurology at the Johns Hopkins University School of Medicine, with joint appointments in the Department of Psychiatry and Behavioral Sciences and the Department of Neuroscience at the School of Medicine, the Department of Psychological and Brain Sciences at the School of Arts and Sciences, and the Department of Mental Health in the School of Public Health. She is director of the Division of Cognitive Neuroscience in the Department of Neurology and director of the Johns Hopkins Alzheimer's Disease Research Center. Dr. Albert's major research interests are in the area of cognitive change with age, disease-related changes of cognition (with a particular focus on Alzheimer's disease) and the relationship of cognitive change to brain structure and function, as assessed through imaging. She was a member of the Planning Committee to Organize a Workshop on Alzheimer's Diagnostic Criteria Validation: Exploration of Next Steps.

Sara J. Czaja, Ph.D., is the Leonard M. Miller Professor of Psychiatry and Behavioral Sciences at the University of Miami Miller School of Medicine. She is also the scientific director of the Center on Aging at the University of Miami Miller School of Medicine and the director of the Center for Research and Education for Aging and Technology Enhancement (CREATE), a National Institutes of Health–funded center that focuses on older adults and technology systems. Dr. Czaja's research interests include aging and cognition, e-health, caregiving, human–computer interaction, and functional assessment. She has published extensively in the field of aging, with several books, book chapters, and scientific articles. She is a fellow of the American Psychological Association, the Gerontological Society of America, and the Human Factors and Ergonomics Society. In addition, she is the president of Division 20 (Adult Development and Aging) of the American Psychological Association. She is a member of the Board on Human-Systems Integration and served as a member of the National Research Council Committee on the Role of Human Factors in Home Health Care and was co-chair of the Panel on Human Factors Research Needs for an Aging Population. She is a member of the editorial boards for *The Gerontologist, Human Factors,* and *The Journal of Applied Gerontology.*

Donna Fick, R.N., Ph.D., FGSA, FAAN, is a distinguished professor in the College of Nursing and College of Medicine at Penn State and co-director of the Hartford Center of Geriatric Nursing Excellence at Penn State. Her research focuses on improving detection and management of delirium superimposed on dementia in older adults and inappropriate medication use. She is principal investigator of two large National Institutes of Health–funded multisite randomized clinical trials to decrease the severity and duration of delirium and to improve nurse detection and management of delirium superimposed on dementia. She is board certified as a geriatric clinical nurse specialist by the American Nurses Credentialing Center, Editor of the *Journal of Gerontological Nursing,* and a Fellow of the American Academy of Nursing.

Lisa P. Gwyther, M.S.W., L.C.S.W., is an associate professor in the Duke University Department of Psychiatry and Behavioral Sciences and directs the Duke University Center for Aging's Family Support Program, a state-funded first responder, clearinghouse, training, and technical assistance center for North Carolina families and professionals caring for people with Alzheimer's disease. She also directed education for the National Institute on Aging–funded Bryan Alzheimer's Disease Research Center at Duke Medicine for 26 years. Ms. Gwyther is a past president of the Gerontological Society of America, and she was the first John Heinz Senate Fellow in Aging and Health. Ms. Gwyther has published more than 144 articles, book chapters, and books on Alzheimer's care and family caregiving research. Ms. Gwyther was honored as 1 of 30 founders of the national Alzheimer's Association. Ms. Gwyther received awards for leadership in aging services and won national and state awards for documentaries on Alzheimer's disease, depression in late life, and creativity in Alzheimer's programming.

Felicia Hill-Briggs, Ph.D., A.B.P.P., is professor of medicine at Johns Hopkins University School of Medicine, with joint appointments in the Department of Physical Medicine and Rehabilitation in the School of Medicine, the Department of Health, Behavior and Society in the School of Public Health, the Department of Acute and Chronic Care in the School of Nursing, and the Welch Center for Prevention, Epidemiology, and Clinical Research. She is director of Cognition and Behavior for the Johns Hopkins–University of Maryland Diabetes Research Center and senior director of Population

Health Research and Development for Johns Hopkins Healthcare. Dr. Hill-Briggs's research focuses on assessment and intervention strategies for chronic disease management in high-risk groups, populations of health disparity, and persons with functional impairment and disability. She has been a principal investigator on clinical trials of behavioral and educational interventions, with a focus on decision-making and problem-solving approaches to behavior change and self-management. She collaborates on multicenter epidemiologic and intervention studies examining cognitive and neuropsychological processes in chronic disease. Her research includes translation of research to clinical practice and community-based settings. She has won the Nelson Butters Award for Research Contributions to Clinical Neuropsychology from the National Academy of Neuropsychology.

Sharon K. Inouye, M.D., M.P.H., is a professor of medicine at Harvard Medical School (Beth Israel Deaconess Medical Center), holder of the Milton and Shirley F. Levy Family Chair, and director of the Aging Brain Center at the Institute for Aging Research, Hebrew SeniorLife. Dr. Inouye is board certified in general internal medicine and geriatric medicine and trained in clinical epidemiology and biostatistics. Dr. Inouye's research interests include the epidemiology and outcomes of delirium and functional decline in older persons, reversible contributors to cognitive decline with aging, the interrelationship of delirium and dementia, and improving measurement methods for cognition. Dr. Inouye developed the Confusion Assessment Method, a widely used method for delirium screening, translated into more than 14 languages, and the Hospital Elder Life Program for delirium prevention, which has been implemented in more than 200 hospitals worldwide. She currently directs the Successful AGing after Elective Surgery study, a large program project from the National Institute on Aging exploring innovative risk factors and long-term outcomes of delirium. Dr. Inouye has authored more than 220 scientific articles and was elected to the Institute of Medicine in 2011. Her clinical practice includes dementia and functional assessment for geriatric and homeless populations. In addition to her ongoing clinical and research work, Dr. Inouye has mentored more than 90 students, fellows, and faculty in clinical research and aging.

Jason Karlawish, M.D., is a professor of medicine, medical ethics and health policy, a senior fellow of the Leonard Davis Institute of Health Economics, and a fellow of the Institute on Aging at the University of Pennsylvania. He is the associate director of and a practicing clinician in the Penn Memory Center. He is also director of the Penn Neurodegenerative Disease Ethics and Policy Program and the Alzheimer's Disease Center's Education, Recruitment and Retention Core. Dr. Karlawish's research focuses on ethical and policy issues in human subjects research and on the care of persons with cognitive impairment. He has investigated issues in Alzheimer's disease drug development, informed consent, quality of life, research and treatment decision making, decisional capacity, and voting by persons with dementia.

Arthur F. Kramer, Ph.D., is the director of the Beckman Institute for Advanced Science & Technology and the Swanlund Chair and Professor of Psychology and Neuroscience at the University of Illinois at Urbana-Champaign. He received his Ph.D. in cognitive/experimental psychology from the University of Illinois in 1984. He holds appointments in the Department of Psychology, Neuroscience program, and the Beckman Institute. Dr. Kramer's research projects include topics in cognitive psychology, cognitive neuroscience, aging, and human factors. A major focus of his labs recent research is the understanding and enhancement of cognitive and neural plasticity across the life span. He is a former associate editor of *Perception and Psychophysics* and is currently a member of six editorial boards. Dr. Kramer is also a fellow of the American Psychological Association, American Psychological Society, a former member of the executive committee of the International Society of Attention and Performance, and a recipient of a National Institutes of Health Ten Year MERIT Award. Dr. Kramer's research has been featured in a long list of print, radio, and electronic media, including the *New York Times, Wall Street Journal, Washington Post, Chicago Tribune, CBS Evening News, Today Show, NPR,* and *Saturday Night Live.* He has been a member of multiple National Academies committees.

Andrea Z. LaCroix, Ph.D., is professor of epidemiology and director of the Women's Health Center of Excellence in the Department of Family and Preventive Medicine at the University of California, San Diego (UCSD). She has an extensive research program devoted to studies on factors associated with healthy aging in postmenopausal women. She has conducted numerous randomized clinical trials and observational studies on the prevention of cancer, fracture, heart disease, and frailty in postmenopausal women, as well as large prospective studies of exceptional aging and maintaining function into later life. Prior to joining the faculty of UCSD in October 2013, Dr. LaCroix was co–principal investigator of the Women's Health Initiative Clinical Coordinating Center at the Fred Hutchinson Cancer Research Center in Seattle, Washington. Dr. LaCroix received her doctoral degree in epidemiology from the University of North Carolina at Chapel Hill in 1984, and she completed a postdoctoral fellowship in cardiovascular disease at Johns Hopkins University in Baltimore, Maryland, in 1985. Before going to Seattle, Washington, in 1989, Dr. LaCroix was a federal government epidemiologist at the National Center for Health Statistics and then the National Institute on Aging. She served on the National Advisory Council on Aging for the National Institutes of Health, National Institute on Aging, from 2009 to 2012. In 2010, she received the McDougall Mentoring Award which recognizes and honors faculty members who demonstrate an outstanding investment in their mentees' professional development and success as independent researchers or clinical scientists. She has authored more than 260 scientific publications.

John H. Morrison, Ph.D., is dean of basic sciences and of the Graduate School of Biomedical Sciences, professor of neuroscience, and the Willard T.C. Johnson Professor of Geriatrics and Palliative Medicine (Neurobiology of Aging) at the Icahn School of Medicine at Mount Sinai. He served as chair of the Department of Neuroscience until 2006, when he was appointed as dean. Dr. Morrison earned his bachelor's degree and Ph.D. from Johns Hopkins University and completed postdoctoral studies at the Salk Institute for Biological Studies. He then served as a faculty member at The Scripps Research Institute until he joined the faculty at Mount Sinai in 1989 to develop and lead a new Center for Neurobiology. Dr. Morrison's research program focuses primarily on the neurobiology of aging and neurodegenerative disorders, particularly as they relate to cellular and synaptic organization of cerebral cortex. Dr. Morrison has published more than 300 articles on cortical organization, the cellular pathology of neurodegenerative disorders, the neurobiology of cognitive aging, and more recently the effects of stress on cortical circuitry. He has also edited five books on related topics. He is ranked among the most highly cited investigators in neuroscience (i.e., Institute for Scientific Information Highly Cited/Neuroscience) and has served on numerous editorial boards, advisory boards, National Institutes of Health committees, and the board of directors of the American Federation for Aging Research. Dr. Morrison has served as president of both The Harvey Society and The Cajal Club, and was elected to the Council of the Society for Neuroscience in 2010 and served in that capacity until 2013.

Tia Powell, M.D., founded and directs the bioethics master's program and directs the Center for Bioethics at Montefiore Health System and Albert Einstein College of Medicine, where she is also professor of clinical epidemiology and clinical psychiatry. She has bioethics expertise related to public policy; dementia; decision-making capacity; lesbian, gay, bisexual, and transgender issues; mediation and consultation; and public health disasters. She served 4 years as executive director of the New York State Task Force on Life and the Law, New York State's bioethics commission. She has served the Institute of Medicine on multiple workgroups. Dr. Powell was a 2013–2014 Health and Aging Policy Fellow; based on her work during that fellowship she continues as a senior advisor for the Department of Health and Human Services to assess and develop federal health initiatives related to dementia and ethics. She is a board certified psychiatrist and a Fellow of the New York Academy of Medicine, the American Psychiatric Association, and the Hastings Center.

David Reuben, M.D., is the director of the University of California, Los Angeles (UCLA), Multicampus Program in Geriatric Medicine and Gerontology and director of the UCLA Claude Pepper Older Americans Independence Center. He is a geriatrician-researcher with expertise in studies linking common geriatric syndromes (e.g., functional impairment, sensory impairment, malnutrition) to health outcomes such as mortality. He also has extensive experience with interventional research (e.g., comprehensive geriatric assessment, practice redesign) that has focused on health care delivery to older persons. His most recent work focuses on developing a program of comprehensive, coordinated patient-centered care for patients with dementia and their families. He has served as a member of multiple committees at the Institute of Medicine.

Leslie Snyder, Ph.D., is professor of communication sciences and principal investigator at the Center for Health Intervention and Prevention at the University of Connecticut (UConn). She has master's and Ph.D. degrees in communications from Stanford University, and was director of the Center for Health Communication and Marketing, a Centers for Disease Control and Prevention (CDC) Center of Excellence, at UConn from 2006–2013. She conducts research on media effects, communication campaigns, health, and international communication. Dr. Snyder is particularly interested in the intended and unintended effects of public communication and how individuals interpret messages. Under the CDC Center grant, Dr. Snyder directs a team testing a video game aimed at adults ages 18–26 in urban environments. She has funding from the National Cancer Institute to examine the effects of food ads on child and teen obesity. In the past, she was funded by the National Institute of Alcoholism and Alcohol Abuse to study the effect of advertising exposure on youth alcohol consumption. In addition, Dr. Snyder directs an ongoing meta-analysis project examining the effectiveness of U.S. and international media campaigns on a variety of health topics. She is currently examining the effectiveness of AIDS campaigns under a National Institute of Mental Health Grant and the effectiveness of nutrition campaigns. Dr. Snyder has also served as a consultant on a number of national campaigns, including the National Institute on Drug Abuse (NIDA) media campaign against youth drug abuse, the CDC's Verb campaign promoting youth activity, the March of Dimes and the CDC's folic acid promotion campaign, and NIDA's fetal alcohol syndrome campaign. She has also consulted for the National Academy of Sciences on diversity and campaigns.

Robert B. Wallace, M.D., is the Irene Ensminger Stecher Professor of Epidemiology and Internal Medicine at the University of Iowa College of Public Health and College of Medicine. He is an elected member of the Institute of Medicine, where he has previously chaired two boards and participated in many consensus committees. He has been a member of the U.S. Preventive Services Task Force and the National Advisory Council on Aging of the National Institutes of Health. He is a former chair of the Epidemiology Section of the American Public Health Association. He is the author or co-author of more than 400 peer-reviewed publications and 25 book chapters, and has been the editor of 4 books, including the current edition of Maxcy-Rosenau-Last's *Public Health and Preventive Medicine*. Dr. Wallace received the Walsh McDermott Award from the Institute of Medicine for Lifetime Distinguished Service. Dr. Wallace's research interests concern the causes and prevention of disabling conditions of older persons. He is a co–principal investigator of the Health and Retirement Study, a long-term prospective sample of older Americans exploring health, social, family, and economic policy issues, and is a co–principal investigator of the Women's Health Initiative, a national study exploring the prevention of important chronic diseases of older women. He has been a collaborator in several international studies of the prevention of chronic illness in older persons. Dr. Wallace is currently a member of the Advisory Board for the National Research Council's Division of Behavioral and Social Sciences and Education.